# Anorectal Disease

*Guest Editor*

SCOTT R. STEELE, MD

# SURGICAL CLINICS OF NORTH AMERICA

www.surgical.theclinics.com

*Consulting Editor*
RONALD F. MARTIN, MD

February 2010 • Volume 90 • Number 1

SAUNDERS an imprint of ELSEVIER, Inc.

**W.B. SAUNDERS COMPANY**

*A Division of Elsevier Inc.*

1600 John F. Kennedy Blvd., Suite 1800, Philadelphia, PA 19103-2899

http://www.theclinics.com

**SURGICAL CLINICS OF NORTH AMERICA Volume 90, Number 1**

**February 2010 ISSN 0039–6109, ISBN-13: 978-1-4377-1875-1**

Editor: Catherine Bewick

Developmental Editor: Theresa Collier

*Surgical Clinics of North America* (ISSN 0039–6109) is published bimonthly by Elsevier Inc., 360 Park Avenue South, New York, NY 10010-1710. Months of publication are February, April, June, August, October, and December. Business and Editorial Offices: 1600 John F. Kennedy Blvd., Suite 1800, Philadelphia, PA 19103-2899. Periodicals postage paid at New York, NY and additional mailing offices. Subscription prices are $291.00 per year for US individuals, $475.00 per year for US institutions, $145.00 per year for US students and residents, $356.00 per year for Canadian individuals, $590.00 per year for Canadian institutions, $401.00 for international individuals, $590.00 per year for international institutions and $200.00 per year for Canadian and foreign students/residents. To receive student/resident rate, orders must be accompanied by name of affiliated institution, date of term, and the *signature* of program/residency coordinator on institution letterhead. Orders will be billed at individual rate until proof of status is received. Foreign air speed delivery is included in all *Clinics* subscription prices. All prices are subject to change without notice. POSTMASTER: Send address changes to *Surgical Clinics*, Elsevier Health Sciences Division, Subscription Customer Service, 3251 Riverport Lane, Maryland Heights, MO 63043. **Customer Service (orders, claims, online, change of address): Telephone: 1-800-654-2452 (U.S. and Canada); 314-447-8871 (outside U.S. and Canada). Fax: 314-447-8029. E-mail: journalscustomerservice-usa@elsevier.com (for print support); journalsonlinesupport-usa@elsevier.com (for online support).**

*Reprints.* For copies of 100 or more, of articles in this publication, please contact the Commercial Reprints Department, Elsevier Inc., 360 Park Avenue South, New York, New York 10010-1710. Tel. (212) 633-3812, Fax: (212) 462-1935, e-mail: reprints@elsevier.com.

*The Surgical Clinics of North America* is also published in Spanish by McGraw-Hill Interamericana Editores S.A., P.O. Box 5-237 06500 Mexico D.F. Mexico; and in Portuguese by Interlivros Edicoes Ltda., Rua Comandante Coelho 1085, CEP 21250, Rio de Janeiro, Brazil; and in Greek by Paschalidis Medical Publications, Athens Greece.

*The Surgical Clinics of North America* is covered in *MEDLINE/PubMed (Index Medicus), EMBASE/Excerpta Medica, Current Contents/Clinical Medicine, Current Contents/Life Sciences, Science Citation Index,* and *ISI/BIOMED.*

Printed and bound by CPI Group (UK) Ltd, Croydon, CR0 4YY

Transferred to Digital Print 2011

# Contributors

## CONSULTING EDITOR

**RONALD F. MARTIN, MD**
Staff Surgeon, Department of Surgery, Marshfield Clinic, Marshfield, Wisconsin;
Clinical Associate Professor, University of Wisconsin School of Medicine and Public
Health, Madison, Wisconsin; Colonel, Medical Corps, United States Army Reserve

## GUEST EDITOR

**SCOTT R. STEELE, MD, FACS, FASCRS**
Chief, Department of General Surgery, Colon and Rectal Surgery, Madigan Army Medical
Center, Fort Lewis, Washington; Clinical Assistant Professor of Surgery, University of
Washington, Seattle, Washington

## AUTHORS

**ANDREW BARLEBEN, MD, MPH**
Surgical Resident, Division of Colon and Rectal Surgery, Department of Surgery,
University of California, Irvine, Orange, California

**RICHARD P. BILLINGHAM, MD**
Swedish Colon and Rectal Clinic; Clinical Professor, Department of Surgery, University of
Washington, Seattle, Washington

**BRADLEY J. CHAMPAGNE, MD**
Assistant Professor, Division of Colorectal Surgery, University Hospitals Case Medical
Center, Case Western Reserve University, Cleveland, Ohio; Program Director, American
Society of Colon and Rectal Surgeons Fellowship, University Hospitals Case Medical
Center, Case Western Reserve University, Cleveland, Ohio

**JAMES E. DUNCAN, MD, FACS, FASCRS**
Assistant Professor, Department of Surgery, National Naval Medical Center, Bethesda,
Maryland; Uniformed Services University of the Health Sciences, Bethesda, Maryland

**KELLI BULLARD DUNN, MD**
Associate Professor of Surgery, Department of Surgical Oncology, Roswell Park Cancer
Institute and the University at Buffalo/State University of New York, Buffalo, New York

**KELLY GARRETT, MD**
Clinical Associate, Department of Colorectal Surgery, Digestive Disease Institute,
Cleveland Clinic, Cleveland, Ohio

**JOEL E. GOLDBERG, MD, FACS**
Associate Surgeon, Division of General and Gastrointestinal Surgery, Section of Colon and
Rectal Surgery, Brigham and Women's Hospital, Harvard Medical School, Boston,
Massachusetts

**DANIEL O. HERZIG, MD**
Assistant Professor, Department of Surgery, Oregon Health and Science University, Portland, Oregon

**ASHLEY E. HUMPHRIES, MD**
Department of Surgery, National Naval Medical Center, Bethesda, Maryland

**ERIC K. JOHNSON, MD, FACS, FASCRS**
Chief, Colorectal Surgery and Surgical Endoscopy, Dwight David Eisenhower Army Medical Center, Fort Gordon, Georgia; Assistant Professor of Surgery, Uniformed Services University of the Health Sciences, F. Edward Hebert School of Medicine, Bethesda, Maryland

**MATTHEW F. KALADY, MD, FASCRS**
Staff Surgeon, Department of Colorectal Surgery, Digestive Disease Institute; Department of Cancer Biology, Cleveland Clinic, Cleveland, Ohio

**MUKTA V. KATDARE, MD**
Department of Colon and Rectal Surgery, Lahey Clinic, Burlington, Massachusetts

**PETER K. LEE, MD**
Colon and Rectal Surgery Resident, UMDNJ-Robert Wood Johnson University Hospital, New Brunswick, New Jersey

**ROBERT T. LEWIS, MD**
Resident, Department of Surgery, University of Pennsylvania Health System, Philadelphia, Pennsylvania

**KIM C. LU, MD**
Assistant Professor, Department of Surgery, Oregon Health and Science University, Portland, Oregon

**DAVID J. MARON, MD**
Assistant Professor of Surgery, Division of Colon and Rectal Surgery, University of Pennsylvania Health System, Philadelphia, Pennsylvania

**KATHARINE W. MARKELL, MD**
Major, US Army Medical Corps; Chief, Division of Colon and Rectal Surgery, Brooke Army Medical Center, San Antonio, Texas

**JUSTIN A. MAYKEL, MD**
Assistant Professor, Department of Surgery, Division of Colon and Rectal Surgery, University of Massachusetts Medical School, Worcester, Massachusetts

**ANDERS MELLGREN, MD, PhD, FACS, FASCRS**
Clinical Professor of Surgery, Division of Colon and Rectal Surgery, University of Minnesota, Minneapolis, Minnesota

**MICHAEL F. McGEE, MD**
Administrative Chief Resident and Allen Scholar, Department of Surgery, University Hospitals Case Medical Center, Case Western Reserve University, Cleveland, Ohio; Metrohealth Medical Center, Case Western Reserve University; Louis Stokes Wade Park VA Medical Center, Cleveland, Ohio

**M. SHANE McNEVIN, MD, FASCRS**
Director, Providence Continence Center, Spokane, Washington; Surgical Specialists of Spokane, Spokane, Washington

**STEVEN MILLS, MD, FACS, FASCRS**
Assistant Clinical Professor, Division of Colon and Rectal Surgery, Department of Surgery, University of California, Irvine, Orange, California

**ANNA L. NAIG, MD**
General Surgery Resident, Department of Surgery, Dwight David Eisenhower Army Medical Center, Fort Gordon, Georgia

**JULIE A. RIZZO, MD**
General Surgery Resident, Department of Surgery, Dwight David Eisenhower Army Medical Center, Fort Gordon, Georgia

**ROCCO RICCIARDI, MD, MPH**
Department of Colon and Rectal Surgery, Lahey Clinic, Burlington, Massachusetts

**ERICA B. SNEIDER, MD**
General Surgery Resident, Department of Surgery, University of Massachusetts Medical School, Worcester, Massachusetts

**SCOTT R. STEELE, MD, FACS, FASCRS**
Chief, Department of General Surgery, Colon and Rectal Surgery, Madigan Army Medical Center, Fort Lewis, Washington; Clinical Assistant Professor of Surgery, University of Washington, Seattle, Washington

**KIRSTEN BASS WILKINS, MD, FACS, FASCRS**
Clinical Assistant Professor of Surgery, UMDNJ-Robert Wood Johnson University Hospital, New Brunswick, New Jersey

# Contents

**Foreword**     xiii

Ronald F. Martin

**Preface**     xv

Scott R. Steele

**Anorectal Anatomy and Physiology**     1

Andrew Barleben and Steven Mills

> The rectum and anal canal form the last portion of the gastrointestinal tract. The rectum serves as a reservoir for fecal contents, and the anal canal regulates continence and defecation via synchronization of events regulated by complex interactions between sympathetic and parasympathetic nerves, striated and smooth muscle, and environmental factors. Normal function can be compromised by various pathologies. Investigation into these pathologies includes a detailed history and thorough physical exam and can be augmented by a number of different studies, including manometry, electromyelography, defecography, nerve stimulation, and compliance. Some of these techniques have incorporated the use of ultrasound and magnetic resonance imaging.

**Diagnosis and Management of Symptomatic Hemorrhoids**     17

Erica B. Sneider and Justin A. Maykel

> Hemorrhoidal disease is a common problem that is managed by various physicians, ranging from primary care providers to surgeons. This article reviews the pathophysiology, clinical presentation, and updated treatment of hemorrhoids, including nonoperative options, office-based procedures, and surgical interventions from standard excision to stapled hemorrhoidopexy and Doppler-guided ligation. The article also covers complications and provides guidance for special circumstances, such as pregnancy, hemorrhoidal crisis, and inflammatory bowel disease.

**Anal Fissure**     33

Daniel O. Herzig and Kim C. Lu

> Anal fissure is a common disorder that is effectively treated and prevented with conservative measures in its acute form, whereas chronic fissures may require medical or surgical therapy. This article discusses the nonoperative and operative management strategies, reviews the current literature on expected outcomes, and provides guidance on dealing with fissures in special situations, such as patients with inflammatory bowel disease or hypotonic sphincters.

**Anorectal Abscess and Fistula-in-Ano: Evidence-Based Management**    45

Julie A. Rizzo, Anna L. Naig, and Eric K. Johnson

The management of anorectal abscess and anal fistula has changed markedly with time. Invasive methods with high resulting rates of incontinence have given way to sphincter-sparing methods that have a much lower associated morbidity. There has been an increase in reports in the medical literature describing the success rates of the varying methods of dealing with this condition. This article reviews the various methods of treatment and evidence supporting their use and explores advances that may lead to new therapies.

**Rectovaginal Fistula**    69

Bradley J. Champagne and Michael F. McGee

Despite the prevalence and severe implications of rectovaginal fistula, there is no universally accepted evidence-based approach to surgical management. This article offers a disease-based review of traditional management strategies and highlights the variety of technical approaches that are currently effective for the eradication of this socially disabling condition.

**Anorectal Crohn's Disease**    83

Robert T. Lewis and David J. Maron

Crohn's disease manifests with perianal or rectal symptoms in approximately one-third of patients, and is associated with a more aggressive natural history. Due to the chronic relapsing nature of the disease, surgery has been traditionally avoided. However, combined medical and surgical intervention when treating perianal fistulae has been shown to offer the best chance for success. Endoanal ultrasound examination or pelvic magnetic resonance imaging should be done in conjunction with an examination under anesthesia to characterize the disease. Any abscess should be drained and setons placed if there is active rectal inflammation or complex fistulae. Antibiotics and immunosuppressive therapy (especially with infliximab) should also be initiated. Simple fistulae can be treated surgically by fistulotomy or anal fistula plug. Complex fistulae can be closed with either an anal fistula plug or covered with flaps. Up to 20% of patients anorectal Crohn's disease require proctectomy for persistent and disabling disease.

**Condyloma and Other Infections Including Human Immunodeficiency Virus**    99

Peter K. Lee and Kirsten Bass Wilkins

Sexually transmitted diseases (STDs) are a common public health problem and as such may be more common in a surgical practice than is believed. The recognition that a virus can be responsible for a cancer has profound significant public health implications. This article reviews the presentation and management of the more common perianal STDs including human immunodeficiency virus, as well as the pathogenesis and management of anal intraepithelial neoplasia.

**Evaluation and Management of Pilonidal Disease**     113

Ashley E. Humphries and James E. Duncan

Pilonidal disease is a common condition, ranging from the routine cyst with abscess to extensive chronic infection and sinus formation. It can be associated with significant morbidity and prolonged wound healing after definitive surgery. This article reviews the history and pathogenesis of this often challenging surgical problem and the numerous nonoperative and operative treatment options currently available for it.

**Pruritus Ani: Etiology and Management**     125

Katharine W. Markell and Richard P. Billingham

Pruritus ani is a dermatologic condition characterized by an unpleasant itching or burning sensation in the perianal region. This article briefly discusses the incidence and classification of pruritus ani followed by a more lengthy discussion of primary and secondary pruritus ani. The important points are summarized and a simple algorithm is provided for the clinical management of pruritus ani.

**Anal Stenosis**     137

Mukta V. Katdare and Rocco Ricciardi

Anal stenosis occurs most commonly following a surgical procedure, such as hemorrhoidectomy, excision and fulguration of anorectal warts, endo-rectal flaps, or following proctectomy, particularly in the setting of mucosectomy. Patients who experience anal stenosis describe constipation, bleeding, pain, and incomplete evacuation. Although often described as a debilitating and difficult problem, several good treatment options are available. In addition to simple dietary and medication changes, surgical procedures, such as lateral internal sphincterotomy or transfers of healthy tissue are other potentially good options. Flap procedures are excellent choices, depending on the location of the stenosis and the amount of viable tissue needed. This article presents the definition, pathophysiology, diagnosis, and treatment of anal stenosis, and methods to prevent it.

**Anal Neoplasms**     147

Kelly Garrett and Matthew F. Kalady

A variety of lesions comprise tumors of the anal canal, with carcinoma in situ and epidermoid cancers being the most common. Less common anal neoplasms include adenocarcinoma, melanoma, gastrointestinal stromal cell tumors, neuroendocrine tumors, and Buschke-Lowenstein tumors. Treatment strategies are based on anatomic location and histopathology. In this article different tumors and management of each, including a brief review of local excision for rectal cancer, are discussed in turn.

**Retrorectal Tumors**                                                           163

Kelli Bullard Dunn

> Retrorectal or presacral tumors are rare and can be challenging to diagnose and treat. Because the retrorectal space contains multiple embryologic remnants derived from various tissues, the tumors that develop in this space are heterogeneous. Most lesions are benign, but malignant neoplasms are not uncommon. Lesions are classified as congenital, neurogenic, osseous, inflammatory, or miscellaneous. Although treatment depends on diagnosis and anatomic location, most retrorectal lesions will require surgical resection.

**Rectal Foreign Bodies**                                                        173

Joel E. Goldberg and Scott R. Steele

> Rectal foreign bodies present a difficult diagnostic and management dilemma because of delayed presentation, a variety of objects, and a wide spectrum of injuries. An orderly approach to the diagnosis, management, and post-extraction evaluation of the patient with a rectal foreign body is essential. This article outlines and describes the stepwise evaluation and management of the patient with a rectal foreign body. The authors also describe the varied techniques needed to successfully remove the different foreign bodies that may be encountered.

**Fecal Incontinence**                                                           185

Anders Mellgren

> Fecal incontinence is a debilitating and socially embarrassing condition. Significant advances in the evaluation and treatment of this condition have been made in recent years, and several new treatment modalities are in the pipeline to be made available to affected patients. This article reviews the workup and operative and nonoperative management of fecal incontinence, and it discusses the emerging role of methods, such as bioinjectable agents and sacral nerve stimulation.

**Overview of Pelvic Floor Disorders**                                           195

M. Shane McNevin

> Disorders of the pelvic floor are common sources of morbidity, decreased quality of life, and are unfortunately increasing in incidence. Owing to their complex and often coexistent nature, a comprehensive, multidisciplinary strategy of testing and care is required. Many nonoperative and operative approaches for management of the symptoms of pelvic floor disorders are available. This article reviews the evaluation and management for these difficult disorders.

**Index**                                                                        207

## FORTHCOMING ISSUES

*April 2010*
**Evidence-Based Management of Pancreatic Cancer**
Richard K. Orr, MD, MPH, *Guest Editor*

*June 2010*
**Simulators in Surgery and Assessment of Competency**
Neil E. Seymour, MD and
Daniel J. Scott, MD, *Guest Editors*

*August 2010*
**Liver Surgery**
David Geller, MD, *Guest Editor*

*October 2010*
**General Thoracic Surgery**
Steve DeMeester, MD, *Guest Editor*

*December 2010*
**Wound Healing**
M. Caldwell, *Guest Editor*

## RECENT ISSUES

*December 2009*
**Surgical Practice in Rural Areas**
Randall Zuckerman, MD and
David Borgstrom, MD, *Guest Editors*

*October 2009*
**Endocrine Surgery**
Maratha A. Zeiger, MD, FACS, FACE,
*Guest Editor*

*August 2009*
**Advances in Cardiac and Aortic Surgery**
Irving L. Kron, MD and
John A. Kern, MD, *Guest Editors*

*June 2009*
**Skin Surgery and Minor Procedures**
Frederick Radke, MD, *Guest Editor*

**ISSUE OF RELATED INTEREST**

*Gastroenterology Clinics of North America,* September 2008, Vol 37, Issue 3
**Disorders of the Pelvic Floor and Anorectum**
Satish S.C. Rao, MD, PhD, FRCP (Lon), *Guest Editor*

## THE CLINICS ARE NOW AVAILABLE ONLINE!

Access your subscription at:
**www.theclinics.com**

# Foreword

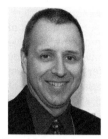

Ronald F. Martin, MD
*Consulting Editor*

I look forward to the day when news broadcasters will say Uranus properly on television without wincing or to when someone of public notoriety goes on one of the influential talk shows and wants to raise public awareness of options for managing stress fecal incontinence. Until then we must provide the best care that we can for these patients as they arrive and present themselves.

Not that many people die from fecal incontinence. Not that many people die from inflamed hemorrhoids. In fact, many of the common problems involving the perianal anatomy are not all that lethal. Moreover, the disorders of the anal canal are not often brought up at cocktail parties or in polite conversation. In short, problems involving the anus and rectum get very little public attention. I would submit, however, that if a person has a malady affecting their anorectal anatomy or function then that problem looms large in their mind. It might even be downright distracting from going about one's business. Distraction though, or even misery, is a difficult thing to quantify.

Lord Kelvin is attributed with the quote, "To measure is to know." He is also attributed with the corollary quote, "If you cannot measure something, you cannot improve it." Perhaps for these reasons, outcomes analyzers are fond of variables such as alive or dead; it is easy to agree on their meaning. Consequently many outcomes studies use mortality, or lack thereof, as an indicator for superiority of a treatment; not because it is a good indicator, necessarily, but because it is easy to measure.

At the time of this writing, we in the United States are perineum deep in a national debate, or at least an argument, about health care reform. Congress is considering multiple bills that will theoretically change the framework for who may be covered by insurance and how the "cost curve will be bent" over time. One of the hot-button topics in the debate is "comparative effectiveness research" although it remains unclear what exactly will be compared; whether it will be clinical effectiveness, cost effectiveness, a combination of the two, or yet some other comparison is not all that well spelled out. It is also not well described how or who will determine which trade-offs for patients are well considered and which are not. One thing that we may be assured of is whoever is going to be responsible for making these decisions are likely to be challenged by nuanced metrics such as discomfort, distraction, or misery.

Surg Clin N Am 90 (2010) xiii–xiv
doi:10.1016/j.suc.2009.11.001
0039-6109/09/$ – see front matter © 2010 Elsevier Inc. All rights reserved.

surgical.theclinics.com

As national figures debate health care for the populace at the stratospheric level, we earth-bound general surgeons must still provide care and comfort to patients one at a time. Some general surgical skills are easily transferred from one set of clinical concerns to another but other skills are not. When it comes to anorectal disorders, much of the knowledge is specific to the clinical problem at hand. A careful study of the best-known ways to understand and manage these issues can often help solve a truly difficult problem for a subsequently most grateful patient. Conversely, a poorly performed initial procedure can generate a challenging problem for even the most expert clinician to repair. To that end, we owe Dr Steele and his associates a debt of thanks for compiling a collection of articles that succinctly and well educate us on the potentially life-threatening and life-altering forms of diseases of the rectum and anus.

Ronald F. Martin, MD
Department of Surgery
Marshfield Clinic
1000 North Oak Avenue
Marshfield, WI 54449, USA

E-mail address:
martin.ronald@marshfieldclinic.org

# Preface: Anorectal Disease

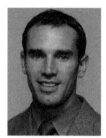

Scott R. Steele, MD, FACS, FASCRS
*Guest Editor*

The American Board of Proctology (now the American Board of Colon and Rectal Surgery) was founded in 1934, and achieved formal approval as an independent specialty board in 1949. Despite this relatively recent acceptance, the wide range of anorectal pathology confronting surgeons has been described since historical times. Over the years, colon and rectal surgery as a specialty, which grew in many instances out of community-based programs, has evolved and transformed through a variety of technological advances and a better understanding of the complex physiology and pathology that occurs in this small region. As such, even the more common anorectal conditions are now often treated by specialists or those with a dedicated interest in the field. Unfortunately, in some cases this has left a void in confidence and proficiency in graduating residents and in experienced general surgeons.

This issue of the *Surgical Clinics of North America* covers a broad spectrum of specifics on anorectal disease such as basic anatomy, physiology, and testing of the anorectal region; and the most current diagnostic and management strategies for many of the common anorectal conditions encountered by surgeons, including hemorrhoids, anal fissures, abscess, and fistula. Also presented are new techniques in the management of pilonidal disease, perianal infections including HIV and condyloma, pruritis ani, and anal stenosis. These difficult conditions often are frustrating for patient and surgeon alike. Two articles are dedicated to the current management of anorectal Crohn's disease and rectovaginal fistulas, including the evolving multidisciplinary approach. In addition, advances in the evaluation and current management of retrorectal tumors and anal neoplasms, including the role of local excision and transanal endoscopic microsurgery for selected rectal tumors, are covered. Rounding out this issue are approaches to the difficult situation of anorectal trauma, including foreign body management, and two articles dedicated to the evaluation of pelvic floor disorders and fecal incontinence.

The authors of each of these articles are experts in their respective fields, and it is my sincere pleasure to thank them for taking time out of their busy schedules to provide the most up-to-date management in these topics. It is my wish that this issue

Surg Clin N Am 90 (2010) xv–xvi
doi:10.1016/j.suc.2009.10.007
0039-6109/09/$ – see front matter

serve as an reference for not only those surgeons well versed in the care of colorectal disease, but also as a guide for surgeons who find themselves confronted with ano-rectal pathology and wish to improve their knowledge, confidence, and care for these patients. Although many of the techniques and practices presented may become outdated, the personal reward and pleasure that comes with caring for patients who are not only ailing, but also often frightened and embarrassed, never will.

Scott R. Steele, MD, FACS, FASCRS
Department of Surgery
Madigan Army Medical Center
9040A Fitzsimmons Drive
Fort Lewis, WA 98431, USA

E-mail address:
scott.steele1@us.army.mil

# Anorectal Anatomy and Physiology

Andrew Barleben, MD, MPH, Steven Mills, MD, FACS, FASCRS*

**KEYWORDS**

- Anus • Anal canal • Anorectal • Rectal
- Anatomy • Physiology

## ANATOMY
### The Rectum

The rectum and anal canal comprise the last portion of the large intestine. The rectum is located in the pelvis, begins at the level of the sacral promontory, and extends 12 to 18 cm distally. This portion of the enteric tract differs from the colon, and its beginning can be marked by noting where the adventitial taeniae bands have coalesced to form outer longitudinal muscle. The rectum has 2 or 3 curves within its lumen, created by submucosal folds called the valves of Houston. The peritoneum covers the upper two-thirds of the rectum anteriorly, but only the upper third laterally. The reflection of the peritoneum is variable but occurs approximately 6 to 8 cm above the anal verge. The lower one-third of the rectum is without peritoneal covering. The endopelvic fascia, also referred to as Denonvilliers fascia, envelops this portion of the rectum. The lateral portion of this fascia is also known as the lateral rectal stalk. The rectum is attached to a strong endopelvic fascia extending from the anterior surface of the sacral bone at about the level of S4. This area of attachment is known as Waldeyer ring (**Fig. 1**).

### The Anal Canal

The anal canal is approximately 2.5 to 5 cm in length. It begins at the level of the levator ani muscle and opens to the anal verge. The anal canal is surrounded by the internal and external anal sphincter muscles. The internal anal sphincter is an extension of the inner circular smooth muscle layer of the rectum. The puborectalis muscle can be palpated digitally, as it helps to form the superior external anal sphincter forming the top of the anorectal ring. The internal anal sphincter is wrapped superiorly by the levator ani muscle, then more distally by the superficial external sphincter muscle (an extension of the anococcygeal ligament), and subsequently by the subcutaneous external striated anal sphincter muscle (**Fig. 2**).

Division of Colon and Rectal Surgery, Department of Surgery, University of California, Irvine, 333 City Boulevard West, Suite 850, Orange, CA 92868, USA
* Corresponding author.
E-mail address: sdmills@uci.edu (S. Mills).

Surg Clin N Am 90 (2010) 1–15
doi:10.1016/j.suc.2009.09.001
0039-6109/09/$ – see front matter. Published by Elsevier Inc.
surgical.theclinics.com

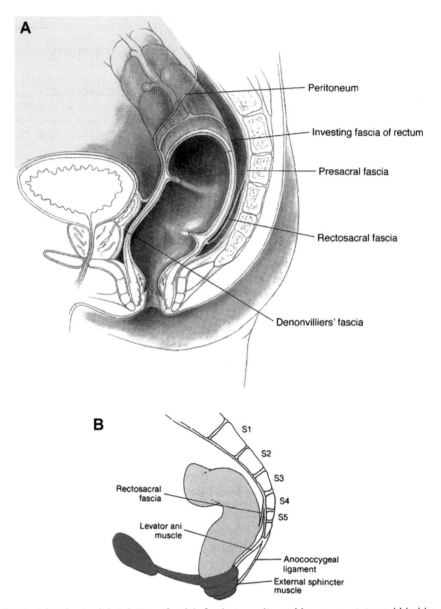

**Fig. 1.** Pelvic fascia. (*A*) Relation of pelvic fascia to peritoneal layers, prostate and bladder. (*B*) Pelvic fascia and Waldeyer ring. *Adapted from* Gordon PH, Nivatvongs S. Principles and practice of surgery for the colon, rectum, and anus. 3rd edition. Informa Healthcare; 2007; with permission.

Histologically, the anal canal has a variable lining. The top of the anal canal contains columnar epithelium. There is a transitional or cloacogenic zone where the mucosa is composed of columnar, transitional, or stratified squamous epithelium. The distal border of this anal transitional zone is called the dentate or pectinate line, which forms an abrupt junction between the anal transitional zone and the squamous epithelium of the external anoderm. Folds in the mucosa parallel to the length of the anal canal

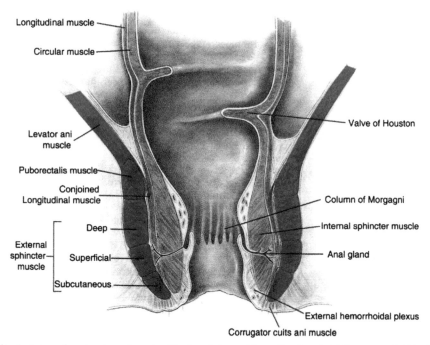

Longitudinal muscle

Circular muscle

Valve of Houston

Levator ani
muscle

Puborectalis muscle

Conjoined
Longitudinal muscle

Column of Morgagni

Internal sphincter muscle

Deep

External
sphincter
muscle    Superficial

Anal gland

Subcutaneous

External hemorrhoidal plexus

Corrugator cuits ani muscle

**Fig. 2.** Internal and external anal sphincter. *Adapted from* Gordon PH, Nivatvongs S. Principles and practice of surgery for the colon, rectum, and anus. 3rd edition. Informa Healthcare; 2007; with permission.

extend above the dentate line called the columns of Morgagni. Between the columns of Morgagni are the anal crypts into which drain several anal glands (**Fig. 3**).

## Pelvic Floor Muscles

The levator ani muscle forms much of the floor of the pelvis. Traditionally the levator ani muscle has been thought to consist of 3 muscles: (1) the iliococcygeal muscle, (2) the pubococcygeal muscle, and (3) the puborectalis muscle. It supports the viscera of the pelvic cavity and aids in defecation with a coordinated action. The levator ani muscle, which is broad and thin, attaches to the inner surface of the lower pelvis. It originates from the posterior surface of the superior pubic rami bilaterally and attaches to the inner surface of the ischium. It is innervated by branches of the pudendal, inferior rectal, perineal, and sacral (S3 and S4) nerves.[1] The iliococcygeal muscle originates from the ischial spine, travels laterally to the rectum, and attaches to the coccyx and anococcygeal raphe, the medial portion of the pubococcygeal muscle. The puborectalis muscle is palpated as forming the top of the anorectal ring. The muscles of the levator ani work in concert in coordinated function during defecation, which is described later.

## Perianal and Perirectal Spaces

There are several spaces around the rectum and anal canal that are clinically significant. These spaces normally contain loose areolar tissue or fat. The intersphincteric space exists between internal and external sphincter muscles and is contiguous with the supralevator space superiorly, which is covered by peritoneum. Lateral to

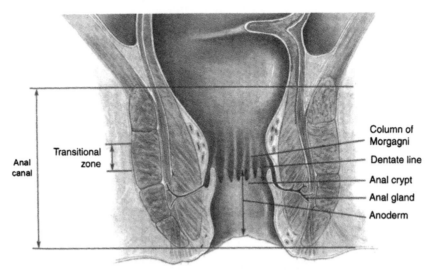

Fig. 3. Rectal and anal mucosas. *Adapted from* Gordon PH, Nivatvongs S. Principles and practice of surgery for the colon, rectum, and anus. 3rd edition. Informa Healthcare; 2007; with permission.

the external sphincter lies the ischioanal space. The triangular ischioanal space is bordered superiorly by the levator ani muscle. Posteriorly, the most caudal space is the superficial postanal space that terminates at the coccyx. Above the superficial postanal space is the anococcygeal ligament, and deep to this ligament, but below the levator ani muscle is the deep postanal space (space of Courtney). This space is continuous laterally with each ischioanal space and when infected can create a large "horseshoe" abscess. Above the levator ani, below and posterior to the rectum, and anterior and superior to the sacrum is the supralevator space that can extend into the retroperitoneum (**Fig. 4**).

### Arterial Supply

The inferior mesenteric artery, the final branch of the aorta before its bifurcation, terminates inferiorly as the superior rectal (hemorrhoidal) artery. This supplies the rectum and the upper third of the anal canal. The middle rectal (hemorrhoidal) arteries, originating from the internal iliac arteries, supply to distal rectum and proximal anal canal. The presence of these arteries is variable.[2] The inferior rectal (hemorrhoidal) arteries arise from the internal pudendal artery, which is a branch of the internal iliac artery. These arteries traverse the ischioanal fossa on both sides of the anal canal feeding the sphincter muscles. Intramural collaterals exist between the superior and inferior rectal arteries at the level of the dentate line in the submucosa. This accounts for the low incidence of rectal ischemia (**Fig. 5**).[3]

### Venous Drainage

Blood returns from the rectum and anal canal into either the portal or systemic systems. Most of the blood from the rectum drains into the superior hemorrhoidal vein that ultimately drains into the portal system via the inferior mesenteric vein. The lowermost portion of the rectum and the anal canal drain into the internal iliac veins directly through the middle rectal veins and the inferior rectal veins (via the pudendal vein) (**Fig. 6**).

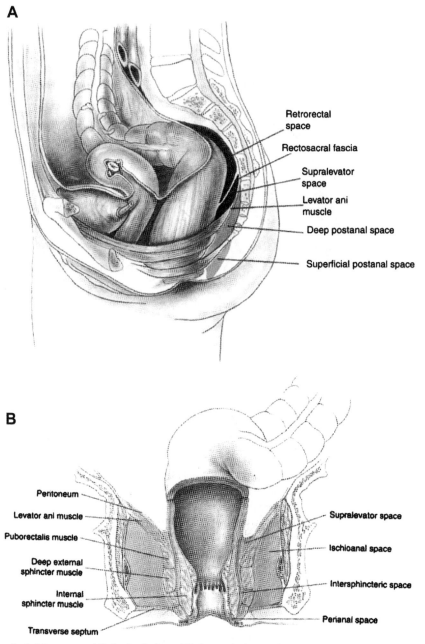

**Fig. 4.** Pelvic spaces. (*A*) Sagittal view. (*B*) Coronal view. *Adapted from* Gordon PH, Nivatvongs S. Principles and practice of surgery for the colon, rectum, and anus. 3rd edition. Informa Healthcare; 2007; with permission.

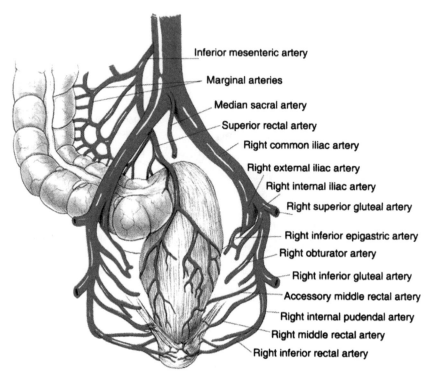

Inferior mesenteric artery

Marginal arteries

Median sacral artery

Superior rectal artery

Right common iliac artery

Right external iliac artery

Right internal iliac artery

Right superior gluteal artery

Right inferior epigastric artery

Right obturator artery

Right inferior gluteal artery

Accessory middle rectal artery

Right internal pudendal artery

Right middle rectal artery

Right inferior rectal artery

**Fig. 5.** Anorectal arterial blood supply. *Adapted from* Gordon PH, Nivatvongs S. Principles and practice of surgery for the colon, rectum, and anus. 3rd edition. Informa Healthcare; 2007; with permission.

### Lymphatic Drainage

Much of the lymphatic drainage of the anal canal and rectum follows the arterial supply. The rectum drains via the superior rectal lymphatics to the inferior mesenteric lymph nodes in the retroperitoneum and laterally to the internal iliac nodes along the middle and inferior rectal vessels through the ischioanal fossa. Lymph drainage from below the dentate line drains to the inguinal nodes. The study of lymphatic drainage in normal anatomy of the rectum revealed the rectal drainage via the superior rectal and inferior mesenteric vessels to the lumboaortic nodes that have no communication with to the internal iliac nodes.[4] However, if distal obstruction occurs, drainage can occur from the anal canal to the superior rectal nodes or laterally to the ischioanal fossa.

### Innervation

Sympathetic nerves arising from the first 3 lumbar segments of the spinal cord are responsible for innervation of the rectum. After leaving the lumbar region, they join at the preaortic plexus and extend caudally from the aortic bifurcation toward the mesenteric plexus before reaching the level of the upper rectum. It then bifurcates into the left and right branches, traveling down both sides of the pelvis before joining the parasympathetic nerve branches. The parasympathetic nerve supply originates from the caudal 3 sacral nerve roots, which form the nervi erigentes. The fibers then rapidly progress anteriorly, joining the sympathetic fibers to create the pelvic plexus. The pelvic plexus is located laterally and superior to the levator ani muscle in the mid

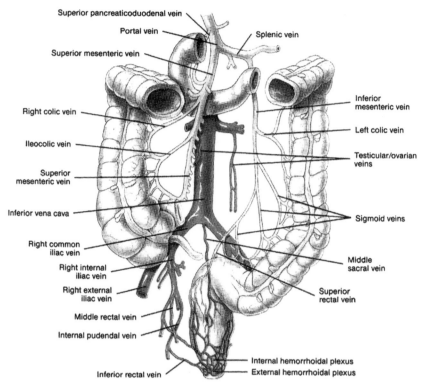

Superior pancreaticoduodenal vein

Portal vein

Splenic vein

Superior mesenteric vein

Inferior mesenteric vein

Right colic vein

Left colic vein

Ileocolic vein

Testicular/ovarian veins

Superior mesenteric vein

Inferior vena cava

Sigmoid veins

Right common iliac vein

Middle sacral vein

Right internal iliac vein

Right external iliac vein

Superior rectal vein

Middle rectal vein

Internal pudendal vein

Internal hemorrhoidal plexus

External hemorrhoidal plexus

Inferior rectal vein

**Fig. 6.** Anorectal venous drainage. *Adapted from* Gordon PH, Nivatvongs S. Principles and practice of surgery for the colon, rectum, and anus. 3rd edition. Informa Healthcare; 2007; with permission.

portion of the lateral stalk. The pelvic plexus then feeds the urinary and genital organs and the rectum with both parasympathetic and sympathetic fibers.

The pelvic plexus also supplies the periprostatic plexus that is important for sexual function in men. This plexus supplies the prostate, prostatic and membranous urethra, seminal vesicles, ejaculatory ducts, and bulbourethral glands. Parasympathetic nerves are involved in erection by increasing blood flow through vasodilation, whereas sympathetic nerves also aid with engorgement and a sustained erection. Sympathetic nerves are substantially more involved in ejaculation, including contraction of the ejaculatory ducts, seminal vesicles, and prostate. Damage to these nerves can result in incomplete erection, lack of ejaculation, retrograde ejaculation or complete impotence.[5]

In women, the hypogastric plexus composed of sympathetic nerve fibers pass through the uterosacral ligament near the rectum. In men, these fibers pass adjacent to the anterolateral wall of the rectum in the retroperitoneal tissue. The pudendal nerves arise from the caudal 3 sacral nerve roots. The nerves cross the ischial tuberosity in the lateral wall of the ischioanal fossa bilaterally. It branches into the inferior rectal, perineal, and dorsal nerves of the penis or clitoris. The branches involved in sensation from the penis or clitoris are anatomically protected during mobilization of the rectum.[5,6]

The anal canal also receives innervation from both sympathetic and parasympathetic fibers. Both inhibit the internal anal sphincter. The external sphincter relies on innervation from the perineal branch of the fourth sacral nerve and the inferior rectal branch of the internal pudendal nerve. As previously mentioned, the levator ani muscle is innervated by branches of the pudendal, inferior rectal, perineal, and sacral (S3 and S4) nerves.[1] Sensation of the anal canal comes from the inferior rectal nerve, also a branch of the pudendal nerve. The epithelium of the anal canal is extensively innervated up to 2 cm proximal to the dentate line (**Fig. 7**).

## PHYSIOLOGY
### Anal Continence

Anal continence is very complex, and investigation continues to further elucidate its mechanism. Several types of studies can be used to evaluate anorectal function, including anorectal manometry, electromyography, defecography, nerve stimulation testing, and radiographic studies, including endorectal ultrasound and magnetic resonance imaging (MRI).

Anal continence relies upon the ability of the anorectum to discriminate between the states of fecal matter, solid, liquid, or gas. Its presence also depends on both voluntary and involuntary control and a multitude of other factors, adding to its complexity.

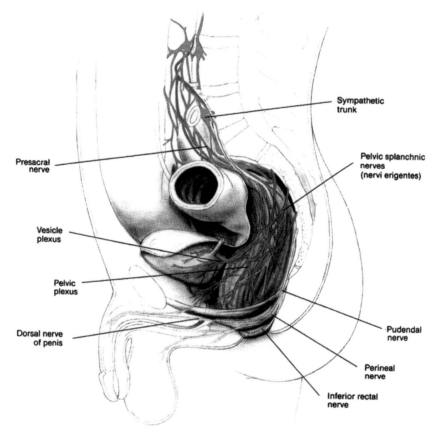

**Fig. 7.** Anorectal parasympathetic, sympathetic, and somatic nerve supply. *Adapted from* Gordon PH, Nivatvongs S. Principles and practice of surgery for the colon, rectum, and anus. 3rd edition. Informa Healthcare; 2007; with permission.

Patients' symptoms of incontinence may vary depending on the state of fecal matter. It is thought that this is the most common factor affecting continence.[7] If patients are continent of solid stool but not liquid or gas, maneuvers to change the consistency may be enough to ameliorate symptoms and regain fecal control. The rectum acts as a reservoir where stool accumulates (reservoir continence). Other possible contributing factors to reservoir function include the adaptive compliance of the rectum, differences in pressure patterns, and angulations between the rectum and anal canal, which is due to continuous tonic activity of the puborectalis muscle.

The internal anal sphincter is the major contributor to the high-pressure zone. When the external sphincter is paralyzed, resting anal pressure changes minimally, suggesting that the internal sphincter is primarily responsible for resting anal continence.[8] Control of the internal anal sphincter is thought to be a complex interaction between the intrinsic and extrinsic neuronal systems and myogenic neurons.[9,10] The external anal sphincter also has continuous tonic activity at rest and even during sleep.[11] Thus, the external sphincter is unique because other striated muscles are electrically silent at rest. Postural changes and other increases in intra-abdominal pressure such as sneezing, coughing, and the Valsalva maneuver increase the resting tone of the external sphincter by an anal reflex. The second sacral spinal segment modulates the external sphincter, which can be contracted voluntarily for 40- to 60-second periods.[12]

It was traditionally thought that nerve endings responsible for the determination of the fecal state exist in the levator ani muscle outside the anal wall; however, Ruhl and colleagues[13] demonstrated that sacral dorsal roots contain some afferents from low-threshold mechanoreceptors located in the rectal wall and that these afferents monitor the filling state and the contraction level of the rectum.[14] Sensation within the anal canal is carried out by several types of sensory receptors, including free intraepithelial nerve endings (pain), Meissner corpuscles (touch), bulbs of Krause (cold), Pacini corpuscles and Golgi-Mazzoni corpuscles (pressure and tension), and genital corpuscles (friction).[15] Despite an extensive network of nerves within the anal mucosa, anal continence does not rely heavily on input from these nerve endings. They are thought to play only a minor role in discrimination between the states of fecal matter. Thus, when this area is anesthetized, discrimination between solid and gas is impaired; however, continence is maintained.[16]

### Defecation

At rest, the aforementioned factors keep stool within the rectum. Once this reservoir is distended, the stimulus for initiating defecation is sent. The resultant process of the left colon initiating peristaltic waves that result in propulsion of the fecal mass downward into the rectum occurs once or several times a day.[17] Once the rectum is distended, the internal sphincter relaxes (rectoanal inhibitory reflex) and the external sphincter contracts maintaining continence. Squatting straightens the angle between the rectum and the anal canal. Adding the pressure of a Valsalva maneuver overcomes the resistance of the external sphincter and the pelvic floor descends. If the external anal sphincter receives inhibiting signals causing relaxation, the fecal bolus passes. Timing results from the balance of environmental factors acting through cortical inhibition and basic reflexes of the anorectum.

## PHYSIOLOGIC TESTING

Multiple techniques have been developed to assess the physiologic function of the pelvic floor, rectum, and sphincters. In conjunction with a detailed history and physical exam, these techniques should be used to assess and detail function, identify and locate a lesion, or solidify a diagnosis.

## Manometry

Manometry measures pressure, and when performed in the rectum, the function of the internal and external anal sphincters can be quantified. There is no one standardized method when performing anorectal manometry, and each method has advantages and disadvantages.

The oldest method incorporates a balloon that is placed in the rectum filled with noncompressible material, and pressure of the material is measured when attached to a sensor in an open system. Open-tip catheters are smaller than balloons (an advantage to the patient in terms of comfort); however, they require perfusion, which can leak and stimulate perianal skin, causing reflex activity. Microtransducers overcome the errors with the previous 2 methods by using a closed but small system, yet they have higher equipment costs. Anal pressure profiles are obtained from the rectum to the anal canal in either stepwise fashion or the pull-through technique. This is often performed 3 times to obtain the maximal resting anal pressure (MRAP) (**Fig. 8**).

In general, normal values of resting and maximal resting and squeeze pressures have shown to vary among sex and decade of age and should be interpreted as such.[18] Studies have shown that normal MRAP ranges between 65 to 85 mm Hg above the rectal intraluminal pressure and is located 1 to 1.5 cm from the distal end of the sphincter where the bulk of the internal anal sphincter is located. To determine function of all segments of the external anal sphincter, the probe must be removed in stepwise fashion, demonstrating the maximal squeeze anal pressure (MSAP). Although the normal values have again been shown to vary, basal pressures usually do not differ among men and women and are in the range of 60 mm Hg, whereas MSAP varies significantly from men to women (183 vs 102 mm Hg).[19,20] These values decrease with age. Finally, although the range of length of the sphincter is 2.5 to 5.0 cm, normal sphincter length in men is on average statistically longer than women (4.1 vs 3.5 cm).[20]

## Electromyography

Although endoanal ultrasound and MRI have shown superiority over electromyography (EMG) for localization of sphincter defects and elimination of the need for painful probe placement and the need for ionizing radiation, EMG can be used as an alternative technique. EMG characterizes muscle function by recording the electrical activity or action potential of a contracting muscle. As previously mentioned, the external anal

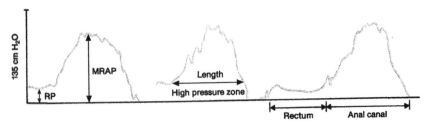

**Fig. 8.** Anorectal manometry. *Adapted from* Gordon PH, Nivatvongs S. Principles and practice of surgery for the colon, rectum, and anus. 3rd edition. Informa Healthcare; 2007; with permission.

sphincter and puborectalis striated and voluntary muscles are unique in that they exhibit electrical activity at rest and even during sleep. It ceases only during defecation. Traditional concentric EMG uses a probe that is inserted manually either into the puborectalis or external anal sphincter (**Fig. 9**). Maneuvers, such as rectal balloon distention, saline infusion or perianal pinprick, are then performed to elicit reflex contraction of the sphincter. For a more specific definition of electronic function of the sphincter, single-fiber EMG can be used. This technique can analyze both innervation and reinnervation after injury to determine the number of fibers supplying 1 motor unit (fiber density). The latter has shown to be associated with primary "idiopathic" anal incontinence or secondary incontinence from neurologic disorders.[21]

### Defecography/MR Defecography

This technique uses a contrast agent, usually liquid barium suspension or paste, which is placed within the rectum, and a series of radiographs or fluoroscopy are obtained. Defecography can be used to investigate several anorectal abnormalities. It can measure the anorectal angle, the position of the pelvic floor at rest or during Valsalva (perineal descent), the presence of a rectocele, rectal intussusception, and function, including the ability to expel rectal contents.[22,23] Balloon proctography can simplify the procedure of examining the ability to evacuate by providing a quick and clean test with minimal radiation.[24] In the largest series to date, when defecography was performed for defecation disorders, 67% of patients had one abnormal finding (eg, rectal intussusception, prolapse, rectocele) and 21% of patients had multiple disorders.[25] MRI technology has been added to the armamentarium of defecographic techniques.[26] It has shown excellent capabilities in diagnosing structural and

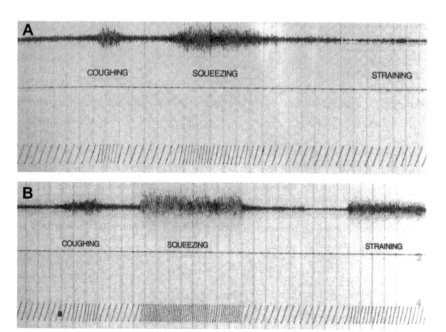

**Fig. 9.** Anorectal electromyelography. (*A*) Normal. (*B*) Puborectalis dysfunction. *Adapted from* Gordon PH, Nivatvongs S. Principles and practice of surgery for the colon, rectum, and anus. 3rd edition. Informa Healthcare; 2007; with permission.

functional disturbances, including those diagnosed with traditional defecography, and the improved characterization of the perirectal soft tissues and surrounding structures. This provides assessment of other abnormalities, including pelvic floor abnormalities and descending perineum syndrome. All of this is completed without exposure to harmful ionizing radiation. Unfortunately, there is extensive morphologic variability among normal healthy individuals and interobserver variability.

Defecography can be used with other technologies to obtain more information on anatomy and function. Simultaneous dynamic proctography and peritoneography identifies rectal and pelvic floor pathologic conditions, such as hernia sacs, and pelvic floor dynamics during defecation.[27,28] When combined together, they provide a large amount of information in the patient with obstructed defecation to determine which patients may benefit from surgical intervention and those that are likely to need nonoperative measures such as biofeedback.

### Nerve Stimulation Techniques

Nerve stimulation can further characterize neuromuscular function, providing even more precise identification of the anatomic site of the nerve (either proximal or distal) or muscle lesions. Spinal nerves are evaluated when a stimulus electrode is placed vertically across the lumbar spine. The induced response of the puborectalis or external sphincter can be detected. The latency of the response can be measured, and longer times are associated with anal incontinence. A similar technique can be performed on the pudendal nerve to evaluate the external sphincter and periurethral striated sphincter muscles (pudendal nerve motor latency). This device consists of 2 electrodes at the tip of a rubber glove and 2 recording electrodes at the base of the glove (**Fig. 10**). The latency is again measured, and an increase can be associated with multiple different disorders; it has been associated with worse outcomes after overlapping sphincteroplasty in some series.

### Ultrasound

Ultrasonography can evaluate anal sphincter integrity and augment manometry and assess anorectal angles and puborectalis function. Ultrasonography evaluates discontinuity in anal sphincters, indicating a prior injury that may be seen in up to 30% of postvaginal deliveries. The internal and external sphincters can be evaluated separately. Various angles are measured with the patient at rest and during maximal voluntary contraction of the puborectalis. Significant differences have been noted between incontinent and normal patients. Ultrasonography does have the advantage of avoiding exposure to radiation and allows for longer viewing time. Anal ultrasonography relies on the operator for accuracy, but in experienced hands, it can be the mainstay for anal anatomic investigations. In addition, it can provide information regarding the presence and location of anorectal abscess and fistula and staging of tumors.

### Compliance

Rectal compliance refers to the amount of force required to distend the rectal wall. Rectal compliance is measured by inserting an ultrathin polyethylene bag into the rectum.[29] Once in place, the bag is inflated to different volumes, and the pressures from the rectal wall are measured. Multiple measurements are taken and are plotted on a pressure-volume curve. The slope of this curve reflects the compliance of the rectum. There are 3 phases of the compliance curve. The first phase corresponds to the initial resistance and compliance of the rectal wall. The second phase is more compliant as evidenced by the increased volume with pressure changes and

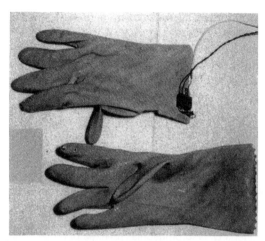

**Fig. 10.** Gloves used in nerve stimulation. *Adapted from* Gordon PH, Nivatvongs S. Principles and practice of surgery for the colon, rectum, and anus. 3rd edition. Informa Healthcare; 2007; with permission.

represents "adaptive relaxation" of the rectal wall. The last phase represents the terminal compliance of the rectal wall and is generally less compliant than the other phases. Urge of defecation occurs during the second phase of compliance. Multiple studies have analyzed the association between anorectal pathologies and rectal compliance findings, and there is still controversy regarding its utility.[30–32] This technique is also highly variable because of variations in readings of the equipment, variations in patient's physiology, and interobserver variations in readings.[33]

## SUMMARY

The anorectal area consists of a relatively small but complex region where multiple anatomic and physiologic interactions occur to help aid continence and defecation. A thorough understanding of the anatomy and the available testing modalities is imperative to diagnose and treat the wide range of pathologic conditions that may occur.

## REFERENCES

1. Grigorescu BA, Lazarou G, Olson TR, et al. Innervation of the levator ani muscles: description of the nerve branches to the pubococcygeus, iliococcygeus, and puborectalis muscles. Int Urogynecol J Pelvic Floor Dysfunct 2008;19:107–16.
2. DiDio LJ, Diaz-Franco C, Schemainda R, et al. Morphology of the middle rectal arteries. A study of 30 cadaveric dissections. Surg Radiol Anat 1986;8:229–36.
3. Kirschner MH. [Vascular anatomy of the anorectal transition]. Langenbecks Arch Chir 1989;374:245–50 [in German].
4. Miscusi G, Masoni L, Dell'Anna A, et al. Normal lymphatic drainage of the rectum and the anal canal revealed by lymphoscintigraphy. Coloproctology 1987;9: 171–4.
5. Bauer JJ, Gelernt IM, Salky B, et al. Sexual dysfunction following proctocolectomy for benign disease of the colon and rectum. Ann Surg 1983;197:363–7.

6. Schlegel PN, Walsh PC. Neuroanatomical approach to radical cystoprostatectomy with preservation of sexual function. J Urol 1987;138:1402–6.

7. Devroede G, Arhan P, Schang JC, et al. Orderly and disorderly fecal continence. In: Kodner IJ, Fry RD, Roe JP, editors. Colon, rectal and anal surgery: current techniques and controversies. St Louis (MO): CV Mosby Co; 1985. p. 40–62.

8. Duthie HL, Watts JM. Contribution of the external anal sphincter to the pressure zone in the anal canal. Gut 1965;6:64–8.

9. Gunterberg B, Kewenter J, Petersen I, et al. Anorectal function after major resections of the sacrum with bilateral or unilateral sacrifice of sacral nerves. Br J Surg 1976;63:546–54.

10. Meunier P, Mollard P. Control of the internal anal sphincter (manometric study with human subjects). Pflugers Arch 1977;370:233–9.

11. Kumar D, Waldron D, Williams NS, et al. Prolonged anorectal manometry and external anal sphincter electromyography in ambulant human subjects. Dig Dis Sci 1990;35:641–8.

12. Varma KK, Stephens D. Neuromuscular reflexes of rectal continence. Aust N Z J Surg 1972;41:263–72.

13. Ruhl A, Thewissen M, Ross HG, et al. Discharge patterns of intramural mechanoreceptive afferents during selective distension of the cat's rectum. Neurogastroenterol Motil 1998;10:219–25.

14. Sun WM, Read NW, Prior A, et al. Sensory and motor responses to rectal distention vary according to rate and pattern of balloon inflation. Gastroenterology 1990;99:1008–15.

15. Duthie HL, Gairns FW. Sensory nerve-endings and sensation in the anal region of man. Br J Surg 1960;47:585–95.

16. Cherry DA, Rothenberger DA. Pelvic floor physiology. Surg Clin North Am 1988; 68:1217–30.

17. Lubowski DZ, Meagher AP, Smart RC, et al. Scintigraphic assessment of colonic function during defaecation. Int J Colorectal Dis 1995;10:91–3.

18. Jameson JS, Chia YW, Kamm MA, et al. Effect of age, sex and parity on anorectal function. Br J Surg 1994;81:1689–92.

19. Cali RL, Blatchford GJ, Perry RE, et al. Normal variation in anorectal manometry. Dis Colon Rectum 1992;35:1161–4.

20. Felt-Bersma RJ, Gort G, Meuwissen SG. Normal values in anal manometry and rectal sensation: a problem of range. Hepatogastroenterology 1991;38:444–9.

21. Gooszen HG. Disordered defaecation: current opinion on diagnosis and treatment. Boston: Kluwer Academic Pub; 1987.

22. Halligan S, Thomas J, Bartram C. Intrarectal pressures and balloon expulsion related to evacuation proctography. Gut 1995;37:100–4.

23. Jorge JM, Habr-Gama A, Wexner SD. Clinical applications and techniques of cinedefecography. Am J Surg 2001;182:93–101.

24. Preston DM, Lennard-Jones JE, Thomas BM. The balloon proctogram. Br J Surg 1984;71:29–32.

25. Mellgren A, Bremmer S, Johansson C, et al. Defecography. Results of investigations in 2,816 patients. Dis Colon Rectum 1994;37:1133–41.

26. Kruyt RH, Delemarre JB, Doornbos J, et al. Normal anorectum: dynamic MR imaging anatomy. Radiology 1991;179:159–63.

27. Bremmer S, Ahlback SO, Uden R, et al. Simultaneous defecography and peritoneography in defecation disorders. Dis Colon Rectum 1995;38:969–73.

28. Sentovich SM, Rivela LJ, Thorson AG, et al. Simultaneous dynamic proctography and peritoneography for pelvic floor disorders. Dis Colon Rectum 1995;38:912–5.

29. Toma TP, Zighelboim J, Phillips SF, et al. Methods for studying intestinal sensitivity and compliance: in vitro studies of balloons and a barostat. Neurogastroenterol Motil 1996;8:19–28.

30. Gosselink MJ, Hop WC, Schouten WR. Rectal compliance in females with obstructed defecation. Dis Colon Rectum 2001;44:971–7.

31. Rasmussen OO, Sorensen M, Tetzschner T, et al. Dynamic anal manometry in the assessment of patients with obstructed defecation. Dis Colon Rectum 1993;36: 901–7.

32. Varma JS. Autonomic influences on colorectal motility and pelvic surgery. World J Surg 1992;16:811–9.

33. Kendall GP, Thompson DG, Day SJ, et al. Inter- and intraindividual variation in pressure-volume relations of the rectum in normal subjects and patients with the irritable bowel syndrome. Gut 1990;31:1062–8.

# Diagnosis and Management of Symptomatic Hemorrhoids

Erica B. Sneider, MD[a], Justin A. Maykel, MD[b],*

**KEYWORDS**

• Hemorrhoid • Treatment • Complication

Hemorrhoidal disease is a common problem in the United States, affecting approximately 1 million Americans each year.[1] It has been estimated that 5% of the general population is affected by symptoms from hemorrhoids, with 50% of people over the age of 50 having experienced symptoms related to hemorrhoids at some point in time.[2] Studies have shown that symptomatic hemorrhoids are more common in Caucasians and those of higher socioeconomic status—speculated to be a result of a low fiber diet—although equally affecting men and women.[1,3,4]

Despite hemorrhoid disease being a benign condition, it has been studied extensively. Numerous surgical treatment options have been outlined, including office-based procedures that allow for treatment without anesthesia. The goals of this article are to review the pathophysiology and presentation of hemorrhoids, to outline the treatment options, and to highlight the current literature.

## PATHOPHYSIOLOGY

Hemorrhoids are cushions of highly vascular tissue found within the submucosal space and are considered part of the normal anatomy of the anal canal. The anal canal contains 3 main cushions that are found in the left lateral, right anterior, and right posterior positions. Within these hemorrhoidal cushions, blood vessels, elastic tissue, connective tissue, and smooth muscle are found.[3,5,6] Together, these tissues contribute to 15% to 20% of the resting pressure within the anal canal.[3] Each cushion surrounds arteriovenous communications between the terminal branches of the superior and middle rectal arteries and the superior, middle, and inferior rectal veins.[4]

[a] Department of Surgery, University of Massachusetts Medical School, 55 Lake Avenue North Worcester, MA 01655, USA
[b] Division of Colon and Rectal Surgery, Department of Surgery, University of Massachusetts Medical School, 67 Belmont Street, Worcester, MA 01605, USA
* Corresponding author.
*E-mail address:* maykelj@ummhc.org (J.A. Maykel).

Surg Clin N Am 90 (2010) 17–32
doi:10.1016/j.suc.2009.10.005
0039-6109/09/$ – see front matter © 2010 Elsevier Inc. All rights reserved.

surgical.theclinics.com

Hemorrhoidal cushions have several important functions within the anal canal. By engorging with blood and causing closure of the anal canal, they contribute to the maintenance of anal continence and prevention of stool leakage during coughing, straining, or sneezing.[7] When engorged with blood, these cushions also serve as protection for the underlying anal sphincters during the act of defecation.[1,3] This tissue also plays a key role in sensory function, which is central to the differentiation between liquid, solid, and gas and the subsequent decision to evacuate.[3,4]

Many factors contribute to the development of pathologic changes within the hemorrhoidal cushions, including constipation, prolonged straining, exercise, gravity, nutrition (low-fiber diet), pregnancy, increased intra-abdominal pressure, irregular bowel habits (constipation/diarrhea), genetics, absence of valves within the hemorrhoidal veins, and aging.[1,3–9] These factors lead to increased pressure within the submucosal arteriovenous plexus and ultimately contribute to swelling of the cushions, laxity of the supporting connective tissue, and protrusion into and through the anal canal.[4,10]

## CLASSIFICATION

There are 2 types of hemorrhoids, external and internal, which are classified anatomically based on their location relative to the dentate line (**Fig. 1**). External hemorrhoids are located distal to the dentate line and are covered by modified squamous epithelium (anoderm), which is richly innervated tissue, making external hemorrhoids extremely painful on thrombosis.[8] Internal hemorrhoids are located proximal to the

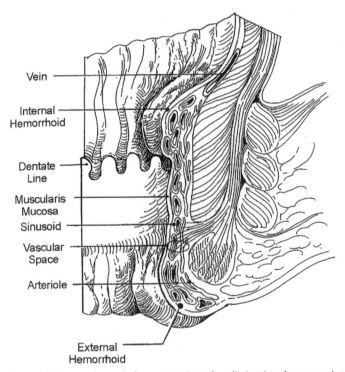

**Fig. 1.** Anatomy of the anal canal demonstrating the distinction between internal and external hemorrhoids relative to the dentate line. (*From* Cintron J, Abcarian H. Benign anorectal: hemorrhoids. In: The ASCRS textbook of colon and rectal surgery. New York: Springer-Verlag, Inc; 2007. p. 156–77; with kind permission of Springer Science+Business Media.)

dentate line and are covered by columnar epithelium. The overlying columnar epithelium is viscerally innervated; therefore these hemorrhoids are not sensitive to pain, touch or temperature.[1,3]

Internal hemorrhoids are further classified by a grading system. First-degree hemorrhoids do not prolapse and are merely protrusions into the lumen of the anal canal. These hemorrhoids have the potential to bleed at the time of defecation and they cannot be visualized on examination without the aid of an anoscope. Second-degree hemorrhoids prolapse outside of the anal canal during defecation, but reduce spontaneously to their original location. Third-degree hemorrhoids prolapse but require manual reduction, whereas fourth-degree hemorrhoids are prolapsed but irreducible.[1,11–13]

## DIFFERENTIAL DIAGNOSIS

Often, patients are referred to a surgeon already diagnosed with hemorrhoids or "piles", but it is still important to rule out other causes of similar symptoms. The differential diagnosis of hemorrhoids includes anal fissure, perirectal abscess, anal fistula, anal stenosis, malignancy, inflammatory bowel disease (IBD, Crohn's disease and ulcerative colitis), anal condyloma, pruritus ani, rectal prolapse, hypertrophied anal papilla, and skin tags.[3] Although not all-inclusive, this list does emphasize that many other conditions may be concomitantly present or cause similar symptoms. Consequently, problems in the anorectal region cannot be simply attributed to hemorrhoids without a proper examination.

## CLINICAL PRESENTATION

Like all medical problems, it is important to take a thorough history and to complete a physical examination to confirm a diagnosis of hemorrhoids. Internal hemorrhoids typically cause painless bleeding, tissue protrusion, mucous discharge, or the feeling of incomplete evacuation.[3,4,11] Symptoms of external hemorrhoids tend to be different, including anal discomfort with engorgement, pain with thrombosis, and itching caused by difficult perianal hygiene due to the presence of skin tags.[3,4] At times, it can be difficult to establish whether symptoms are due to internal or external hemorrhoids, particularly when patients present with mixed disease. Despite years of advanced symptoms, many patients defer evaluation because of fear and embarrassment.

### Thrombosed External Hemorrhoids

When a patient presents with an exquisitely painful lump in the perianal area, the diagnosis can often be made by history alone. The pain tends to be acute at onset, typically following straining, at the time of bowel movement or physical exertion. Most patients who present early benefit from complete excision of the thrombosed external hemorrhoid (**Fig. 2**).[1,7] Obviously, not all patients follow this timeframe, and there are some who have persisting symptoms beyond 72 hours who would benefit from excision. Partial removal or incision of the hemorrhoid is generally ineffective, because the remaining loculated clot causes persisting pain, tissue edema, and bleeding, and the redundant skin tags persist. For those patients whose symptoms are resolving or who decline intervention, a more conservative approach can be successfully followed. Therapy consists of stool texture modification with fiber supplementation, oral hydration, analgesia (typically with nonsteroidal anti-inflammatory drugs [NSAIDs] rather than narcotics to avoid the constipating side effects of narcotics), sitz baths, and rest. It is important to warn patients that the body will either absorb or extrude

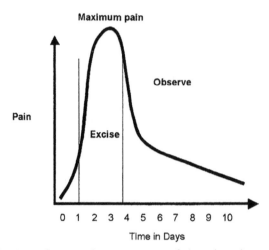

**Fig. 2.** Timing of pain and appropriate treatment of thrombosed external hemorrhoids. (*From* Cintron J, Abcarian H. Benign anorectal: hemorrhoids. In: The ASCRS textbook of colon and rectal surgery. New York: Springer-Verlag, Inc; 2007. p. 156–77; with kind permission of Springer Science+Business Media.)

the clot with time, so patients should be advised to wear a protective pad to avoid social embarrassment.

## TREATMENT

The treatment of symptomatic hemorrhoids varies and ranges from conservative therapy involving dietary and lifestyle changes to use of various pharmacological agents and creams, office-based nonoperative procedures, and operative hemorrhoidectomy.

## MEDICAL MANAGEMENT
### Dietary/Lifestyle Changes

Whether treating symptomatic hemorrhoids with medical or operative management, several dietary and lifestyle changes should be encouraged, to help prevent the recurrence of symptoms. The ultimate treatment goal should be the maintenance of soft, bulked stools that pass easily without straining at the time of defecation. A diet high in fiber, approximately 20 to 35 g/d, or intake of fiber supplements, such as psyllium (Konsyl), methylcellulose (Citrucel), or calcium polycarbophil (FiberCon), is recommended as the best means to consistently modify stool texture.[3] In addition to a high-fiber diet, it is also important to increase fluid intake, which adds moisture to stool, thus decreasing constipation. Changes in bathroom habits that exacerbate hemorrhoid symptoms, such as spending less time on the commode and avoiding reading while on it, will ultimately lead to a decrease in straining and downward pressure.[8]

### Medical Agents/Creams

There is little information in the literature supporting the use of pharmacological agents for the treatment of hemorrhoids or the symptoms related to hemorrhoid disease. Despite the lack of evidence supporting their use, there are a plethora of agents available to the general population, including topical anesthetics, topical corticosteroids, phlebotonics, suppositories, and physical therapies, such as ice and sitz baths. The most effective of the therapies listed earlier is the sitz bath, which is a warm-water (40°C) bath that relieves tissue edema and sphincter spasm.[3] Suppositories are awkward and painful to insert, and they are generally ineffective in the treatment of hemorrhoids because they usually end up in the rectum rather than the anal canal. Topical creams usually have a soothing effect but do not actually cure the underlying condition. Patients are advised not to use these agents for long periods because of local reactions and sensitization of the skin.[3]

Most patients associate the use of Preparation H (Wyeth Consumer Healthcare, Inc, Madison, New Jersey, USA) with treatment of symptoms associated with hemorrhoids. Preparation H is available in many different forms, including ointment, cream, cooling gel, cream with pain reliever, cream with 1% Hydrocortisone, suppositories, and medicated portable wipes. The active ingredients are light mineral oil (14%), petrolatum (71.9%), phenylephrine hydrochloride (HCl; 0.25%) and shark liver oil (3%).[14] Three of these ingredients are considered protectants (light mineral oil, petrolatum and shark liver oil), whereas phenylephrine HCl is a vasoconstrictor. Preparation H is used for relief of local itching and discomfort associated with hemorrhoids, temporary shrinkage of hemorrhoids, relief from burning, and temporary protection of the inflamed and irritated anorectal surface to make defecation less painful.[14] This agent is commonly purchased by patients with symptomatic hemorrhoids but is rarely recommended by surgeons, because it only provides temporary relief of localized symptoms and does not treat the underlying disorder.

## OFFICE-BASED PROCEDURES FOR TREATMENT OF INTERNAL HEMORRHOIDS
### Rubber Band Ligation

Rubber band ligation (RBL) is a common procedure for treatment of first-, second-, or third-degree hemorrhoids, performed in the office without administration of local anesthesia and without preparation of the bowel with an enema. Barron[15] initially described this technique in 1963 with successful results in the 50 patients enrolled in the original study. This procedure is performed by placing a rubber band on the mucosa of the hemorrhoid approximately 1 cm or more above the dentate line (**Fig. 3**). Placement of the rubber band causes strangulation of the blood supply to the banded redundant mucosa (**Fig. 4**A, B). The resulting tissue necrosis sloughs off

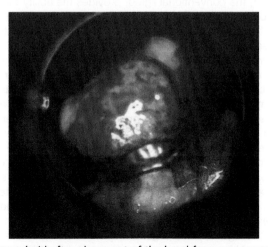

**Fig. 3.** View of hemorrhoid after placement of the band from an anoscope.

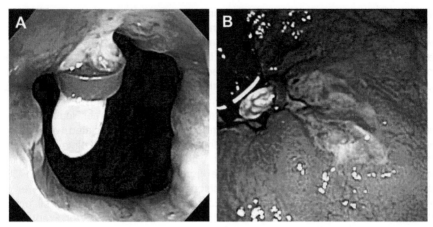

**Fig. 4.** (A) and (B). Ischemic hemorrhoid after placement of the rubber band, viewed during a colonoscopy.

5 to 7 days after band application, leaving behind a small ulcer that heals and fixes the surrounding tissue to the underlying sphincter.[3,4] It is recommended that only one hemorrhoid complex, usually the largest, be banded during the first visit to determine the patient's tolerance to the procedure. During subsequent visits, 2 or more complexes can safely be banded at the same time, although multiple applications may increase the potential for complications.[1,4]

There are several different commercially available hemorrhoid ligators that use either manual graspers or suction to pull rectal mucosa tissue into the instrument. The McGown ligator (George Percy McGown, NY, USA) is an instrument that uses suction to bring the redundant mucosa into the ligating barrel. Closure of the handle deploys a band around the neck of the hemorrhoid, making it easy for the surgeon to perform this procedure without an assistant. The main disadvantage of this ligator is that the ligating barrel is fairly small, therefore decreasing the amount of tissue banded.[3] Conventional ligators require the surgeon to grasp the hemorrhoid tissue and apply the band with a second hand; therefore, an assistant is needed.[1,3] Unlike the McGown ligator, the conventional ligator provides the ability to check the sensation of the tissue before band application; bands applied too close to the dentate line can cause instantaneous and exquisite pain mandating immediate band removal, which can be a real challenge.

Complications from RBL occur in 0.5 to 0.8% of patients and are typically benign.[4] The complication rate has been found to correlate with the number of bands placed during one session.[4] Potential complications include pressure/discomfort, severe pain, abscess formation, urinary retention, bleeding, band slippage, and sepsis.[1,3,4,16] Postprocedure pain is experienced in approximately 30% of patients but is usually minor and can be controlled with mild analgesics.[3,16]

RBL has a success rate varying from 50% to 100%, depending on the length of time between procedure and follow-up and the degree of hemorrhoids ligated (first- and second-degree hemorrhoids have higher success rates).[4,11] Several studies have suggested that approximately 68% of patients experience recurrence of symptoms at 4 to 5 years follow-up, although these symptoms often resolve with repeat RBL; only 10% of patients progress to needing surgical hemorrhoidectomy.[4,17,18]

El Nakeeb and colleagues,[19] in a large retrospective study, evaluated the effectiveness, safety, quality of life, and early and long-term results of RBL in 750 patients. One session ligation was performed in 63% of the patients, multiple hemorrhoid ligations were performed in 2 sessions in 34%; and 3 sessions, in 2%. Successful results were seen in 92.8% of patients who had undergone RBL, and 86.6% of patients were cured at the end of their treatment. This study did not detect a significant difference in outcome of RBL between second- and third-degree hemorrhoids. Seven percent of patients experienced complications after RBL, including pain, mild rectal bleeding, postbanding vasovagal symptoms, and perineal abscess. On follow-up, 11% of patients experienced recurrence of symptoms 2 years after their initial treatment. There was no significant difference in manometric studies before or after banding.

Discussing anticoagulant usage with the patient before performing any procedure for the treatment of hemorrhoids is important. An absolute contraindication to RBL is the use of sodium warfarin (Coumadin) or heparin (Heparin) because of the risk of hematoma formation and bleeding, particularly when the tissue sloughs off 5 to 7 days after the procedure.[4] Patients taking aspirin or platelet-altering drugs, such as clopidogrel bisulfate (Plavix), should be advised to avoid these drugs for a period of 5 to 7 days before and after the banding procedure, to minimize the risk of bleeding.[4] If patients are unable to stop taking sodium warfarin, heparin, or platelet-altering drugs, they may be better candidates for a procedure, such as sclerotherapy, which has a theoretically lower risk of postprocedure bleeding.

### Sclerotherapy

First described by Morgan in 1869, sclerotherapy is a procedure commonly used in the treatment of first and second-degree hemorrhoids. Injection of approximately 5 mL of a sclerosing agent (5% phenol in oil or hypertonic saline) into the submucosa at the base of the hemorrhoid causes vessel thrombosis and sclerosis of the surrounding connective tissue.[4,20] During each office visit, only 2 sites should be sclerosed to decrease the risk of complications, such as postprocedure pain, urinary retention, and sepsis. Approximately 70% of patients experience a dull pain after this procedure. No anesthetic is required and the injection of a sclerosing agent can be performed in the office through an anoscope, using a small gauge spinal needle. Recurrence of symptoms occurs in approximately 30% of patients 4 years after the initial injection of a sclerosing agent.[4]

### Bipolar Diathermy and Infrared Photocoagulation

Bipolar diathermy and infrared photocoagulation (IPC) cause coagulation and ultimately lead to sclerosis of the hemorrhoidal vascular pedicle and fixation of the tissue to the underlying structures at the treated site.[3,4] IPC has been shown to successfully treat first- and second-degree hemorrhoids, and bipolar diathermy can adequately treat first-, second-, and third-degree hemorrhoids in 88% to 100% of patients.[3]

Bipolar diathermy is a method of electrocautery that is applied in 1-second pulses of 20 watts at the base of the hemorrhoid until the underlying tissue coagulates. The depth of penetration is 2.2 mm, which is slightly more superficial then IPC.[1] IPC uses infrared radiation generated by a tungsten-halogen lamp that is applied onto the hemorrhoid tissue via a polymer probe tip. The infrared light is converted to heat, coagulates tissue proteins, and leads to an inflammatory response, eschar formation, and scarring.[3] The tip of the probe must be applied to the base of the hemorrhoid to successfully deliver pulses of energy lasting 0.5 to 2 seconds. The depth of penetration from each application is 2.5 mm. Three or 4 applications of energy are needed for each hemorrhoidal complex and several hemorrhoids can be treated during each session. Complications are infrequent but pain can be experienced after the procedure and fissures may develop, particularly if the tip of the probe is too close to the dentate line during application.[3]

### Phlebotonics

Micronized purified flavonoid fraction (MPFF), a flavonoid venotonic agent, is an alternative treatment for first- and second-degree hemorrhoids, which is commonly used in Europe and Asia. MPFF improves venous tone, inhibits the release of prostaglandins, and has been shown to reduce the acute symptoms associated with first- and second-degree hemorrhoids.[20] Injection of MPFF can be accomplished in the office setting and no bowel preparation is necessary. When compared with sclerotherapy, Yuksel and colleagues[20] found MPFF to have lower long-term success rates, most likely because MPFF does not lead to scar formation at the site of injection.

## SURGICAL MANAGEMENT
### Open/Closed Excision

Historically, numerous procedures have been described for the surgical treatment of symptomatic hemorrhoids, including those by Buie, Fansler, Ferguson, Milligan-Morgan, Parks, Salmon, and Whitehead.[1] Operative hemorrhoidectomy is indicated in the treatment of combined internal and external hemorrhoids or third- and fourth-degree hemorrhoids, especially in patients who are unresponsive to other methods of treatment or those with extensive disease.[2,3] The need for operative intervention is rare, with only 5% to 10% of patients with symptomatic hemorrhoid disease requiring an invasive procedure, such as surgical hemorrhoidectomy.[3] In counseling patients regarding hemorrhoid surgery, it remains essential to set expectations at the time of consultation, detailing expected postoperative recovery, potential complications, and functional result.

The open hemorrhoidectomy, otherwise known as the Milligan-Morgan hemorrhoidectomy (MMH), is most commonly performed in the United Kingdom.[3] This technique involves excision of the internal and external components of the hemorrhoid, with suture ligation of the hemorrhoidal pedicles. The internal defect of the mucosa is closed and the skin incision is left open to heal by secondary intention over a 4- to 8-week period of time.[1,3,4] The closed hemorrhoidectomy, or Ferguson hemorrhoidectomy (FH), more commonly used in the United States, is a similar technique to the MMH except that the skin is closed primarily with a running suture.[1,3]

Although open and closed hemorrhoidectomy result in extremely high success rates, significant postoperative pain remains a major obstacle. Unlike the office-based procedures where patients are able to return to their normal activities fairly quickly, patients who undergo operative hemorrhoidectomy are not able to return to their normal routine for approximately 2 to 4 weeks.[3] Severe pain can be successfully managed using a combination of narcotic analgesics, NSAIDs, muscle relaxants, and local treatments, such as sitz baths and ice packs.

Gencosmanoglu and colleagues[2] performed a study evaluating the open and closed technique to determine any difference, comparing operating time, analgesic requirement, hospital stay, morbidity rate, duration of inability to work, and healing time. The investigators found operative time to be significantly shorter when the open technique was performed (35 ± 7 minutes) compared with the closed technique (45 ± 8 minutes). There was also no significant difference observed in the duration of hospital stay or the duration of inability to work. The average healing time was significantly shorter in the closed hemorrhoidectomy group, 2.8 ± 0.6 weeks, compared with 3.5 ± 0.5 weeks for open hemorrhoidectomy. The patients who had undergone hemorrhoidectomy with the Ferguson technique were more likely to require pain medication initially, and they were also more likely to develop complications, such as urinary retention and anal stenosis.

## Harmonic Scalpel

The Harmonic Scalpel (Ethicon EndoSurgery, Inc, Cincinnati, OH, USA) can also be used to perform an open or closed hemorrhoidectomy.[21] Some benefits have been associated with the use of the Harmonic Scalpel, such as less eschar formation, less desiccation of tissue, decreased postoperative pain, and improved wound healing.[21]

Sohn and colleagues[21] compared the open versus closed technique for performing hemorrhoidectomy with the use of the Harmonic Scalpel. Of the 42 patients enrolled in the study, 13 underwent closed hemorrhoidectomy, whereas 29 underwent open hemorrhoidectomy. The open group experienced higher complication rates of 13.8% (compared with 7.7% in the closed group) and were more likely to experience postoperative pain and bleeding. The most common postoperative complication in both groups was urinary retention, experienced by patients who had spinal anesthesia for the procedure. This study, although small, found that leaving the mucosal defect open significantly reduces operative time and therefore operative cost, despite the additional cost of using the Harmonic Scalpel.

## LigaSure

Another alternative to the Milligan-Morgan (open) hemorrhoidectomy is the LigaSure Vessel Sealing System (Valleylab, Boulder, CO, USA), which can be used for treatment of third- and fourth-degree hemorrhoids.[22] This device, through a combination of pressure and electrical energy, allows coagulation of blood vessels up to 7 mm in diameter and limits the thermal spread within 0.5 to 2 mm of the adjacent tissue.[22–24]

In a randomized clinical trial, Tan and colleagues (in 2008)[22] compared outcomes of hemorrhoidectomy with the LigaSure tissue-sealing device with open diathermy. Although there was no statistically significant difference in postoperative pain, there was a significantly shorter operative time, less intraoperative bleeding, and superior wound healing in the LigaSure group. Sixty percent of patients treated by LigaSure hemorrhoidectomy had wounds that were completely epithelialized after 3 postoperative weeks compared with 19% in the diathermy group.

Bessa[23] also evaluated the use of the LigaSure device compared with diathermy and found that the daily median pain score for the first 7 postoperative days was significantly lower in the LigaSure group than in the diathermy group. Postoperative complications occurred in 3.6% of patients who had undergone hemorrhoidectomy with the LigaSure device, compared with 12.7% in the diathermy group, but the difference did not reach statistical significance. There were no cases of hemorrhage in the LigaSure group, whereas 3.6% of patients in the diathermy group experienced hemorrhage on the night of the operation, requiring packing under anesthesia. Although re-examination at the end of the first postoperative week demonstrated that all the wounds in the LigaSure group were open rather than closed, all wounds were completely healed by the sixth postoperative week in the LigaSure group and only 80% in the diathermy group.

## Doppler-guided Transanal Hemorrhoidal Ligation

In 1995, a new treatment for hemorrhoid disease was introduced, called Doppler-guided transanal hemorrhoidal ligation or de-arterialization. A Doppler transducer can be inserted into the anal canal and rotated to identify the terminal branches of the superior hemorrhoidal arteries for ligation. The arterial sound emitted from the transducer demarcates the location of the hemorrhoidal artery, which can then be suture ligated.[1] Complications include bleeding, thrombosis, pain, and fissure. Post-procedure pain has been shown to be less than that experienced with other procedures.[25,26] A recent case series of 100 patients followed for 3 years resulted in a 12% recurrence rate and low complication rate (6%).[25] This technique has gone through several iterations of instrumentation since its release, and although not widely used, has consistent literature demonstrating less pain at the cost of slightly higher recurrence when compared with operative excision.

### Procedure for Prolapsed Hemorrhoids

In 1998, Longo[27] proposed a technique of circular stapled hemorrhoidopexy (SH), or procedure for prolapsed hemorrhoids (PPH), as an alternative to the more traditional Milligan-Morgan (open) hemorrhoidectomy for the surgical treatment of symptomatic internal hemorrhoids. This technique removes a cylindrical "donut" of mucosa and submucosa (including hemorrhoid tissue) proximal to the dentate line. The stapling device creates a circumferential anastomosis between the proximal and distal mucosa and the submucosa, using 33 mm titanium staples placed approximately 2 to 3 cm above the dentate line (**Fig. 5**). The stapler divides the terminal branches of the superior hemorrhoidal arteries and decreases the blood supply to the distal hemorrhoidal venous plexus.[10,13,27,28]

Although the stapled hemorrhoidopexy or PPH has been shown to be associated with significantly less postoperative pain than the more traditional open hemorrhoidectomy, several studies, including a Cochrane meta-analysis, have demonstrated that the recurrence after this procedure is higher than that seen after hemorrhoidectomy (5.7% versus 1% at 1 year, and 8.5% versus 1.5% in the long term at all time points).[29–31,32,33]

Stolfi and colleagues[10] compared the SH to the MMH procedure in a randomized, prospective study. A total of 200 patients with either grade 3 or 4 hemorrhoids were

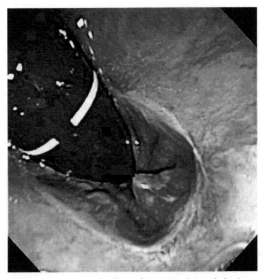

**Fig. 5.** Appearance of the circular staple line after PPH viewed during a colonoscopy.

enrolled into the study and were equally randomized into 2 treatment groups: SH and MMH. Surgical time was not significantly different for SH and MMH. Following the first 2 postoperative days, patients who had undergone the SH procedure had significantly less pain when compared with the MMH group. Prolonged hospital stay due to postoperative pain or urinary retention and postoperative anal fissure and skin tags were significantly higher in the SH group.[10]

Sgourakis and colleagues[34] performed a meta-analysis of 5 randomized controlled trials that compared the circular SH with the FH between 1998 and 2007. SH had comparable results to FH in terms of hospital stay, postoperative hemorrhage requiring an intervention, and early and late postoperative bleeding, but was superior when it came to operative time, postoperative pain, urinary retention, and wound healing.[34]

## POSTOPERATIVE COMPLICATIONS

Surgeons learn over time when it is appropriate to recommend an operation. This is particularly true in the management of hemorrhoidal disease. Rarely are hemorrhoids life-threatening; more commonly, symptoms represent an excessive nuisance. Yet, there are definitely certain patients who benefit from a surgical excision. By understanding the potential operative risks, one can weigh the risks of surgery and guide the patient towards an appropriate treatment option. The following potential complications must be considered for every case.

### Bleeding

The submucosal vessels that are cut, cauterized, or ligated at the time of surgery can be the source of significant postoperative hemorrhage. This may be a result of suture ligature failure, energy sealant or staple device failure, or local trauma during stool passage. The risk of postoperative hemorrhage (immediate, early, or delayed) is approximately 2%.[35] Occasionally, the bleeding will cease without intervention or manual pressure or anal canal packing may be enough to promote clotting. With adequate exposure and patient cooperation, suture ligation may be performed at the bedside but more frequently requires a return trip to the operating room. The risk of bleeding does increase with the use of blood thinning agents such as aspirin, Plavix, or warfarin. In general, these agents should be avoided during the perioperative period.

### Urinary Retention

Urinary retention is considered the most frequent complication of hemorrhoid surgery, up to 34% being reported in some series. The pelvic nerves that innervate the bladder are in close proximity to the rectum and tend to be irritated at the time of hemorrhoidectomy. Additionally, the sacral nerve roots can be affected by the choice of anesthesia, particularly under spinal or caudal block. Severe pain leads to sphincter spasm, and perioperative fluid overload may exacerbate the situation. One approach to avoiding this complication is to run patients dry in the operating room—to avoid overdistention of the bladder—allowing time for bladder function to recover after surgery. More frequently, surgeons maintain a policy that requires the patient to urinate before hospital discharge. If unable to void, a Foley catheter can be placed and left in place for high bladder residuals. Removal is typically successful after 24 to 48 hours.

### Wound Infections

The excellent blood supply and the routine bacterial exposure and subsequent impact on local immunity probably contributes to the low incidence of postoperative wound infections. This may seem counterintuitive because this area of the body is considered "dirty". The use of sitz or warm tub baths after bowel movements helps to keep the wounds clean. Pelvic or perineal sepsis is an extremely rare consequence of hemorrhoidectomy. One must always be cautious in high-risk patients, whether immunosuppressed by medications (ie, transplant patients) or comorbidities (ie, diabetic patients). The key to management is early detection and subsequent broad spectrum antibacterial coverage, local debridement, and rarely, fecal diversion.

### Continence

Traditionally, there has been excessive concern about the loss of continence after anorectal surgery. As outlined earlier, hemorrhoids serve multiple roles, including functioning as a "cushion" that assists continence. In addition, particularly with long-standing disease, the internal sphincter can be intimately scarred to the hemorrhoids. Using proper technique and avoiding radical tissue excision, any continence changes in the postoperative period should be unlikely. Because this tends to be affected by patient selection, operative intervention for patients with marginal baseline continence should be avoided.

### Anal Stricture and Ectropion

Complications, including anal stricture formation and ectropion, are rarely seen today (**Fig. 6**). This is probably a result of an evolution in operative technique, because one learns from the long-term results of predecessors. Strictures can still result from excessive tissue excision or infection, but they can be minimized by preserving at least 1cm of anoderm between the specimens in a 3-column hemorrhoidectomy. Ectropion formation can be avoided by preserving the tissue at the anal verge and keeping the rectal mucosa within the anal canal. Treatment includes local dilation and tissue flap advancement procedures.

### SPECIAL CIRCUMSTANCES
### Hemorrhoid Strangulation/Crisis

When a patient presents with a severe hemorrhoid attack, it is perceived unquestionably as a crisis (**Fig. 7**). When considering treatment options, determining whether there is loss of tissue viability is a key step. At times, this can be difficult based on a limited examination secondary to severe pain and tissue edema. Considering other clues, such as fever, tachycardia, foul odor, and leukocytosis is important. If necrotic

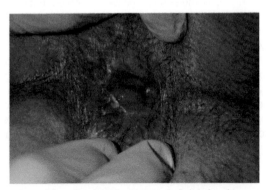

**Fig. 6.** Ectropion occurs when the rectal mucosa is brought down and sutured to the perianal skin, causing mucous drainage and irritation of the surrounding skin.

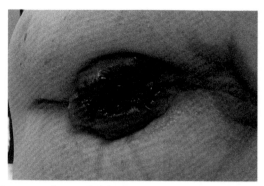

**Fig. 7.** Patient with a severe hemorrhoid crisis.

tissue is encountered, urgent excision and debridement must be undertaken in the operating room. Otherwise, the patient can be offered several treatment options. Medical management consists of stool softeners, analgesics, rest, and local care, such as warm soaks and ice packs. At 1-week follow-up, most patients are well on their way to recovery. Recurrence can often be prevented through regular fiber supplementation or subsequent in-office RBL. Patients may also be offered surgical intervention in the form of an excisional hemorrhoidectomy. In the emergent setting, it can be difficult to preserve perianal skin and mucosa, and the rate of stricture formation rises. The local injection of hyaluronic acid (Wydase) has been described, but experience is limited, typically due to overall low incidence and medication availability.

### Rectal Varices

Although to the untrained eye, it can be difficult to distinguish rectal varices from hemorrhoids (**Fig. 8**), these 2 entities deserve distinction because their management is very different. Typically the physician learns of potential liver disease from the history (eg, alcohol use, hepatitis) and explosive, recurrent episodes of rectal bleeding. On examination, the varices are noted below the surface of the anorectum, and the overlying tissue friability/abrasions that are seen with chronically traumatized hemorrhoids are absent. The treatment should be directed to the portal hypertension in the form of a transjugular intrahepatic portosystemic shunt procedure, portacaval shunt, or liver transplantation. Although direct suture ligation may be possible, any manipulation may result in life-threatening hemorrhage. Even when successful, ligation is not a reliable long-term solution.

### IBD

The management of hemorrhoids in IBD continues to be an area of debate. The frequent loose stools associated with active disease often lead to hemorrhoid exacerbation. Particular concern arises regarding local wound healing, especially in the setting of Crohn's disease and when patients are on immunosuppressive medications. Although traditional surgical teaching opposes hemorrhoid surgery in patients with IBD, Wolkomir and Luchtefeld[36] suggest that it may be safe to perform hemorrhoidectomy on patients with quiescent anorectal disease (proctitis). Of 17 patients undergoing surgery for symptomatic hemorrhoids, 15 wounds healed without complication at a median follow-up of 11.5 years.

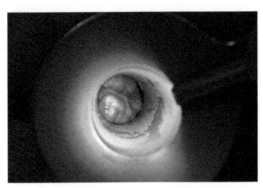

**Fig. 8.** Appearance of rectal varices through an anoscope.

## Pregnancy

Because of increased intra-abdominal pressure, dehydration, and constipation, hemorrhoids commonly develop during pregnancy. Rarely do hemorrhoids have to be addressed surgically during the pregnancy, because symptoms tend to resolve after delivery. In fact, one should be cautioned against surgical intervention until the pregnancy is completed, because of the potential impact on the induction of labor, perineal infection, and post-procedure urinary retention. When severe symptoms arise toward the end of the pregnancy, the epidural may be left in place after delivery and used as the anesthetic for the subsequent hemorrhoidectomy. When making management recommendations, it is essential to determine whether hemorrhoid symptoms preceded the pregnancy. If the symptoms resolve, then a conservative approach makes most sense. Long-standing symptoms that have been aggravated by pregnancy should be addressed. One of the more common conditions that physicians may encounter is thrombosis of external hemorrhoid disease. The authors recommend proceeding similarly to the approach for nonpregnant patients, with liberal use of local anesthesia for cases requiring operative management.

## SUMMARY

Symptomatic hemorrhoidal disease is extremely common, and a complete understanding of the normal anatomy and physiology of the anorectum facilitates management recommendations. With a firm diagnosis in hand, treatment options include topical applications, office-based procedures, and operative interventions. Postprocedure complication rates tend to be low, and durable long-term results are offered. With all available options on hand, the surgeon can confidently select the proper treatment for each individual patient's distressing, and often long-standing, symptoms.

## REFERENCES

1. Corman ML. Hemorrhoids. In: Brown B, McMillan E, LaPlante MM, editors. Colon and rectal surgery. 5th edition. New York: Lippincott Williams and Wilkins, Inc; 2002. p. 177–248.
2. Gencosmanoglu R, Orhan S, Demet K, et al. Hemorrhoidectomy: open or closed technique? Dis Colon Rectum 2002;45(1):70–5.

3. Cintron J, Abcarian H. Benign anorectal: hemorrhoids. In: Wolff BG, Fleshman JW, Beck DE, et al, editors. The ASCRS textbook of colon and rectal surgery. New York: Springer-Verlag, Inc; 2007. p. 156–77.
4. Fleshman J, Madoff R. Hemorrhoids. In: Cameron J, editor. Current surgical therapy. 8th edition. Philadelphia: Elsevier; 2004. p. 245–52.
5. Thomson WH. The nature of haemorrhoids. Br J Surg 1975;62(7):542–52.
6. Haas P, Fox T, Haas G. The pathogenesis of hemorrhoids. Dis Colon Rectum 1984;27:442–50.
7. Aigner F, Gruber H, Conrad F, et al. Revised morphology and hemodynamics of the anorectal vascular plexus: impact on the course of hemorrhoidal disease. Int J Colorectal Dis 2009;24:105–13.
8. Welton ML, Chang GJ, Shelton AA. Hemorrhoids. In: Doherty GM, editor. Current surgical diagnosis and treatment. 12th edition. New York: Lange; 2006. p. 738–64.
9. What to do about hemorrhoids. Harvard women's health watch 2008;4–5. Available at: http://www.health.harvard.edu/newsweek/Hemorrhoids_and_what_to_do_about_them.htm.
10. Stolfi VM, Sileri P, Micossi C, et al. Treatment of hemorrhoids in day surgery: stapled hemorrhoidopexy vs Milligan-Morgan hemorrhoidectomy. J Gastrointest Surg 2008;12:795–801.
11. Beck DE. Benign rectal, anal, and perineal problems. In: Barie PS, Cance WG, Jerkovich JG, et al, editors. ACS surgery: principles and practice. New York: WebMD; 2005. p. 739–51.
12. Gerjy R, Lindhoff-Larson A, Nystrom PO. Grade of prolapse and symptoms of haemorrhoids are poorly correlated: result of a classification algorithm in 270 patients. Colorectal Disease 2007;10:694–700.
13. Ceci F, Picchio M, Palimento D, et al. Long-term outcome of stapled hemorrhoidopexy for grade III and grade IV hemorrhoids. Dis Colon Rectum 2008;51:1107–12.
14. Preparation H. Available at: http://www.preparationh.com. Accessed May 24, 2009.
15. Barron J. Office ligation treatment of hemorrhoids. Dis Colon Rectum 1963;6: 109–13.
16. Bernal JC, Enguix M, Garcia L, et al. Rubber-band ligation for hemorrhoids in a colorectal unit: a prospective study. Rev Esp Enferm Dig 2003;96:38–45.
17. Savioz D, Roche B, Glauser T, et al. Rubber band ligation of hemorrhoids: relapse as a function of time. Int J Colorectal Dis 1998;13:154–6.
18. Walker AJ, Leicester RJ, Nicholls RJ, et al. A prospective study of infrared coagulation, injection and rubber band ligation in the treatment of haemorrhoids. Int J Colorectal Dis 1990;5:113–6.
19. El Nakeeb AM, Fikry AA, Omar WH, et al. Rubber band ligation for 750 cases of symptomatic hemorrhoids out of 2200 cases. World J Gastroenterol 2008;14(42):6525–30.
20. Yuksel BC, Armagan H, Berkem H, et al. Conservative management of hemorrhoids: a comparison of venotonic flavonoid micronized purified flavonoid fraction (MPFF) and sclerotherapy. Surg Today 2008;38:123–9.
21. Sohn VY, Martin MJ, Mullenix PS, et al. A comparison of open versus closed techniques using the harmonic scalpel in outpatient hemorrhoid surgery. Mil Med 2008;173(7):689–92.
22. Tan KY, Zin T, Sim HL, et al. Randomized clinical trial comparing LigaSure haemorrhoidectomy with open diathermy haemorrhoidectomy. Tech Coloproctol 2008;12:93–7.
23. Bessa SS. Ligasure™ vs. conventional diathermy in excisional hemorrhoidectomy: a prospective, randomized study. Dis Colon Rectum 2008;51:940–4.

24. Mastakov MY, Buettner PG, Ho YH. Updated meta-analysis of randomized controlled trials comparing conventional excisional haemorrhoidectomy with LigaSure for haemorrhoids. Tech Coloproctol 2008;12:229–39.

25. Faucheron JL, Gangner Y. Doppler-guided hemorrhoidal artery ligation for the treatment of symptomatic hemorrhoids: early and three year follow-up results in 100 consecutive patients. Dis Colon Rectum 2008;51:945–9.

26. Conaghan P, Farouk R. Doppler-guided hemorrhoid artery ligation reduces the need for conventional hemorrhoid surgery in patients who fail rubber band ligation treatment. Dis Colon Rectum 2009;52:127–30.

27. Longo A. Treatment of hemorrhoids disease by reduction of mucosa and hemorrhoidal prolapsed with a circular suturing device: a new procedure. In: Montori A, Lirici MM, Montori J, editors. Proceedings of the 6th world congress of endoscopic surgery. Bologna (Italy): Monduzzi Editori; 1998. p. 777–84.

28. De Nardi P, Corsetti M, Passaretti S, et al. Evaluation of rectal sensory and motor function by means of the electronic barostat after stapled hemorrhoidopexy. Dis Colon Rectum 2008;51:1255–60.

29. Pescatori M, Gagliardi G. Postoperative complications after procedure for prolapsed hemorrhoids (PPH) and stapled transanal rectal resection (STARR) procedures. Tech Coloproctol 2008;12:7–19.

30. Nisar PJ, Acheson AG, Neal K, et al. Stapled haemorrhoidopexy compared with conventional haemorrhoidectomy: systematic review of randomized controlled trials. Dis Colon Rectum 2004;47:1837–45.

31. Jayaraman S, Colquhoun PH, Malthaner RA. Stapled haemorrhoidopexy is associated with a higher long-term recurrence rate of internal hemorrhoids compared with conventional excisional hemorrhoidal surgery. Dis Colon Rectum 2007;50: 1297–305.

32. Mehigan BJ, Monson JR, Hartley JE. Stapling procedure for haemorrhoids versus Milligan-Morgan haemorrhoidectomy: randomized controlled trial. The Lancet 2000;355:782–5.

33. Ganio E, Altomare DF, Gabrielli F, et al. Prospective randomized multicentre trial comparing stapled with open haemorrhoidectomy. Br J Surg 2001;88(5): 669–74.

34. Sgourakis G, Sotiropoulos GC, Dedemadi G, et al. Stapled versus Ferguson hemorrhoidectomy: is there any evidence-based information? Int J Colorectal Dis 2008;23:825–32.

35. Bleday R, Pena JP, Rothenberger DA, et al. Symptomatic hemorrhoids: current incidence and complications of operative therapy. Dis Colon Rectum 1992; 35(5):477–81.

36. Wolkomir AF, Luchtefeld MA. Surgery for symptomatic hemorrhoids and anal fissures in Crohn's disease. Dis Colon Rectum 1993;36(6):545–7.

# Anal Fissure

Daniel O. Herzig, MD*, Kim C. Lu, MD

**KEYWORDS**

- Anal fissure • Anorectal disease • Nonoperative treatment
- Sphincterotomy

An anal fissure is a tear in the epithelial lining of the anal canal. Although this is an extremely common condition, it is surprisingly difficult to know exactly how widespread it is. Many people avoid seeking treatment, and many fissures will resolve without intervention. Nevertheless, the combination of anal pain and bleeding is sufficiently worrisome that patients often seek medical attention. As such, anal fissure represents one of the most common, if not the single most common, anorectal problems encountered in practice. It has been cited as the cause of over 1200 office visits to a single colon and rectal surgery clinic over a 5-year period.[1]

Fissures may be delineated as acute versus chronic and typical versus atypical. Acute fissures cause bright red bleeding with bowel movements and anal pain or spasm that can last for hours after the bowel movement. Physical findings include a linear separation of the anoderm, at times visible with just separation of the buttocks (**Fig. 1**). Often, elevated anal resting pressures are revealed on digital rectal examination. If tolerated by the patient, the suspected diagnosis can be confirmed by visualizing the break in the anoderm with office anoscopy after using an anesthetic lubricant. If only one area can be examined, the posterior midline should be evaluated first, as it is the site of up to 90% of typical anal fissures. The remaining minority of typical fissures are found in the anterior midline.[2] Acute fissures generally resolve within 4 to 6 weeks of appropriate management; therefore, chronic fissures are defined as those producing symptoms beyond 6 to 8 weeks. Chronic fissures have additional physical findings of a sentinel tag at the external apex, exposed internal sphincter muscle, and a hypertrophied anal papilla at the internal apex (**Fig. 2**). Typical fissures are usually in the posterior or anterior midline, have the characteristic findings described earlier, and are not associated with other diseases. In contrast, atypical fissures can occur anywhere in the anal canal, can have a wide variety of findings, and tend to be associated with other diseases, including Crohn's Disease, human immunodeficiency virus (HIV) infection, cancer, syphilis, and tuberculosis.

Department of Surgery, Oregon Health and Science University, 3181 SW Sam Jackson Park Road, Mail Code L-223A, Portland, OR 97239, USA
* Corresponding author.
*E-mail address:* herzigd@ohsu.edu (D.O. Herzig).

Surg Clin N Am 90 (2010) 33–44
doi:10.1016/j.suc.2009.09.002
0039-6109/09/$ – see front matter © 2010 Elsevier Inc. All rights reserved.

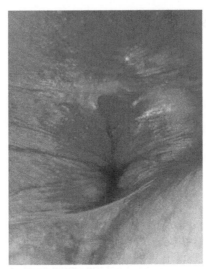

**Fig. 1.** With the patient in prone jackknife position, an posterior acute anal fissure is visible once the buttocks are separated. (*Courtesy of* Richard P. Billingham, MD, Seattle, WA.)

## PATHOGENESIS

Despite the common nature of this longstanding problem, the exact cause remains uncertain. Many patients relate the occurrence of a fissure to the passage of a large stool or anal trauma. There may be mechanical factors in the posterior midline, secondary to the anorectal angle, that creates the greatest stress at that location.[3] The common finding of sphincter hypertonicity has been described in early reports of the disease and documented by manometry in multiple studies, and it is the leading hypothesis behind the pathogenesis.[4,5] However, it remains unclear whether the elevated pressures are a direct cause of the disease or an effect.[6] Another common theory relates to the relative ischemia at the posterior midline anoderm. This area of the anal canal has been shown to be fairly ischemic by arteriographic studies and laser

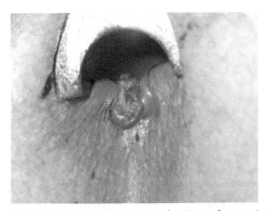

**Fig. 2.** With the patient in lithotomy position at the time of a surgical sphincterotomy, a chronic posterior fissure is seen, with a sentinel tag and rolled edges.

Doppler flow studies.[7,8] The theories of hypertonicity and ischemia may be intertwined to some extent, particularly in that hypertonicity may aggravate the relative ischemia. Nevertheless, tears in the anoderm undoubtedly occur with great frequency, whether from a large stool, anorectal intercourse, or instrumentation from surgical procedures. In fact, the evolution to a chronic fissure is probably only seen in a minority of these instances. Furthermore, fissures can occur in the absence of any trauma or constipation, and may even be present in patients with diarrheal states or sphincter hypotonia.

## NONOPERATIVE TREATMENT

Practice parameters from the American Society of Colon and Rectal Surgeons state that conservative therapy is safe, has few side effects, and should usually be the first step in therapy for all fissure types.[9] The benefits of conservative management have been repeatedly demonstrated in the control groups of trials testing various interventions for fissure treatment. Jensen[10] reported a randomized trial done in patients with acute anal fissures, examining the outcome of topical anesthestics versus steroid cream. The control group in this trial was instructed to take 10 g of unprocessed bran twice daily with a warm sitz bath for 15 minutes twice daily and after bowel movements, if possible. With 91% of patients able to follow the study protocol, this "control" group with fiber alone had fissure healing in 87% of patients.

A more frequent problem for the surgeon is the patient who presents with symptoms for several weeks and has failed an initial approach similar to that described by Jensen. In these patients with more chronic fissures, spontaneous healing is, unfortunately, likely to be seen in only a minority of cases. A recent Cochrane review of the nonoperative treatment of anal fissure addressed this scenario, analyzing over 50 randomized trials of various nonoperative therapies for chronic anal fissures.[11] Unlike the acute fissure population, the healing rate in the combined placebo group is only 34%. Therefore, these patients are felt to benefit from a more aggressive technique that may involve a stepwise approach with initial topical or local therapies. The widely held belief is that internal anal sphincter hypertonicity is a determining factor in the development and continued presence of an anal fissure. Hence, initial nonoperative treatment strategies are targeted at alleviating this internal anal sphincter smooth muscle activity, mainly through 2 topical agents, nitrates and calcium channel blockers, and 1 injectable agent, botulinum toxin A.

### Nitroglycerin

Nitric oxide was reported to be the neurotransmitter mediating relaxation of the internal anal sphincter muscle in the early 1990's.[12] Since then, development and topical application of 0.2% glyceryl trinitrate ointment (GTN) has subsequently been found to result in relaxation of the anal sphincter by manometric studies.[13] A landmark randomized trial was reported in 1997, demonstrating a healing rate of 68% with GTN treatment, compared with only 8% in the placebo group.[14] Despite these initial impressive results, subsequent experience has failed to confirm these findings. In fact, a recent Cochrane analysis of 15 trials, including GTN, showed a healing rate of 48.6% with GTN treatment, compared with 37% in the placebo or control group ($P = .004$).[11] The most common side effect of topical GTN treatment is headache, at a reported rate of 27% in the pooled analysis, and may be as high as 50% depending on the severity.[15] Although often minor and temporary, it may lead to discontinuation of therapy in 10% to 20% of patients.[16–18] A second potential drawback is tachyphylaxis, which eventually does not respond to escalations in dose or frequency. In the United States, this indication is not approved by the Food and Drug

Administration (FDA), and the topical form of nitroglycerin is supplied as a 2% ointment. To achieve a 0.2% concentration, the prescription often needs to be filled at a compounding pharmacy. Jonas and colleagues[15] reported that after application of 0.2% GTN, the reduction in mean anal resting pressure lasted only about 2 hours, which may explain some of the treatment failures seen with GTN. Despite these somewhat disappointing results, there are few major drawbacks to initial attempts with topical GTN, and it is frequently the first medication used in a escalating or stepwise plan of care. Yet, patients should be counseled to have realistic expectations of the outcomes with GTN use.

### Calcium Channel Blockers

Diltiazem and nifedipine, in either oral or topical form, have been described as causing relaxation of the smooth muscle of the internal anal sphincter. Oral and topical nifedipine have also been shown to lower mean resting anal pressure[19] as has diltiazem in which, however, the effect is greater with the topical rather than oral formulations.[20,21] Because studies done with calcium channel blockers have more variability in medication, dosages, and routes, it is difficult to pool data for analysis. Yet, multiple small trials suggest healing rates at least equivalent to GTN, although with fewer side effects.[22,23] As both are also used as blood pressure agents, there is a small chance of postural dizziness or an unanticipated drop in blood pressure, although this happens in less than 5% of patients and is almost unheard of in the topical forms. Again, although diltiazem and nifedipine are not FDA-approved for the treatment of anal fissure, there is a plethora of literature detailing their use and expected outcomes. As with GTN, there is no topical formulation available in the United States, so a compounding pharmacy needs to make a topical gel from an oral formulation (typical doses: diltiazem 2%; nifedipine 0.2%–0.5%). Patients should again be thoroughly counseled on anticipated results and the differences in side effect profile to nitrates.

### Botulinum Toxin Type A

Botulinum toxins are a family of neuroparalytic proteins synthesized by *Clostridium botulinum*. They inhibit the release of acetylcholine at neuromuscular junctions.[24,25] These agents can be used to induce a local paralysis that lasts for several months, depending on the subtype used. The toxins are labeled A through G, according to immunologic specificity, with type A being most commonly used in the United States. Although commonly associated with curing wrinkles, botulinum toxins are FDA-approved for treatment of certain spastic disorders, but not anal fissure. They have been used "off-label" in many other disorders, such as drooling, speech impediments, hair loss, headaches, phantom limb pain, and chronic anal fissures. At present, there is no uniformly recommended dose or method (unilateral vs bilateral, location at the verge) of injection. Botulinum toxin type A is supplied as a powder in 100-unit single-patient–use vials. Because most dosing regimens range from 20 to 50 IU, once reconstituted, any remaining solution must be discarded—providing a potential cost problem outside of multiple scheduled injections. After the initial report of a technique in 1994, various methods of injection, including injection into the internal or external sphincter, at single or multiple sites, and in various doses, have been described.[26] Relaxation of the muscle occurs within days, and lasts for 2 to 4 months. Just as in other forms of treatment, the goal is to allow the fissure to heal, followed by lifestyle changes to avoid its recurrence. Theoretically, the sphincter could become completely relaxed, resulting in alterations in continence, though this is a rarity outside of case reports. A much more common side effect, though minimal and short-lived, is local pain with injection. Even for those who may experience incontinence, this has the theoretical advantage of allowing fissure healing while avoiding permanent fecal incontinence due to the defined half-life of the medication.

Botulinum toxin injections of the internal anal sphincter have been compared with placebo and other treatments with mixed results. In a widely referenced double-blind, placebo-controlled, randomized crossover trial of 30 patients, botulinum toxin A injection was superior to placebo, with a healing rate of 73% after 20 IU of botulinum toxin, compared with 13% with placebo at 2 months follow-up ($P$ = .003).[27] In those placebo failures, 70% had subsequent healing of their fissures with botulinum injection. The same group then went on to compare 20 IU of botulinum toxin with 0.2% GTN over 6 weeks in another randomized controlled trial of 50 patients, demonstrating the superiority of the botulinum toxin (96% vs 60%, $P$ = .005).[17] A meta-analysis by Sajid and associates[28] including 180 patients was more tempered, demonstrating no statistically significant difference between the 2 pharmacotherapies (relative risk [RR] 1.29; 95% confidence interval [CI] 0.98–1.70), with a higher rate of total side effects and headache in the GTN cohort. Additional trials have compared botulinum toxin injection with lateral internal sphincterotomy for fissures refractory to medical management. Arroyo and colleagues[29] reported a randomized controlled trial of 80 patients and showed healing rates of 92.5% for the lateral internal sphincterotomy group compared with 45% in the botulinum toxin group. However, they concluded that botulinum toxin is still their preference in patients older than 50 years or at risk of incontinence due to a higher, but not statistically significant, incidence of incontinence following sphincterotomy. Other small studies support the finding of higher numbers of treatment failures, but fewer complications in the botulinum toxin group.[30,31] Shao and Zhang[32] recently attempted to answer this question in a meta-analysis encompassing 4 studies and 279 patients. They found a significant improvement in healing following sphincterotomy (RR 1.31), and lower recurrence, at the expense of a higher rate of minor anal incontinence. Unfortunately, there still remains little data regarding the long-term effectiveness of botulinum toxin, though initial data have demonstrated a higher rate of overall recurrence that may be amenable to repeat injections or sphincterotomy.[33]

## OPERATIVE TREATMENT

One of the earliest forms of treatment was anal dilation, first described in 1829, and studied in trials for anal fissure as recently as 2007.[34,35] Although extensively studied, there is considerable variability in the technique along with a wide range of reported outcomes, because few well-controlled studies exist. The recent Cochrane review included an analysis of 7 randomized controlled trials meeting their inclusion standards.[36] The investigators demonstrated that dilation was less effective than sphincterotomy, and had a much higher rate of fecal incontinence (odds ratio [OR] = 4.03, 95% CI = 2.04–7.46). A more standardized, controlled, and objective method of anal stretch, pneumatic balloon dilation, has been reported. Renzi and colleagues[37] evaluated the use of balloon dilation compared with lateral internal sphincterotomy in a prospective randomized trial using a 40-mm balloon insufflated to 1.4 atmospheres for 6 minutes. Healing rates were high and no different in both groups (overall 94%). However, after 24 months of follow-up, no patients in the balloon cohort developed incontinence compared with 16% in the lateral internal sphincterotomy group ($P$<.001). Although manual dilation is now rarely indicated for anal fissure, balloon dilation may be a preferable alternative, though formal recommendations await increased experience and longer follow-up.

Although described in various forms since the early 1800s, in the 1950s, Eisenhammer[38] was the first person to advocate and effectively describe the anatomy and physiology behind isolated division of the internal anal sphincter muscle (sphincterotomy) for anal fissure. Although successful at healing the fissure, regrettably, his technique of posterior internal sphincterotomy at the site of the fissure led to a posterior midline "gutter" or "keyhole" deformity with subsequent fecal soiling in 30% to 40% of patients. Notaras[39] then described a simple modification: performing the sphincterotomy laterally, which eliminated this problem and providing similar success rates. Since then, lateral internal anal sphincterotomy has become the primary surgical intervention on failure of medical management. The procedure can be done under local anesthesia, and the authors' preference is to perform this as a same-day surgical procedure. The variations currently include open versus closed technique and conservative versus traditional sphincterotomy. The closed technique is performed by inserting the scalpel blade in the intersphincteric groove or submucosa and then turning it to divide the distal fibers of the internal sphincter. The open technique is done through a radial incision just outside the intersphincteric groove, allowing dissection and visualization of the internal anal sphincter before division (**Fig. 3**). Division is traditionally described to the level of the dentate line, though recent reports describe a more conservative approach, with division of the muscle to either the fissure apex or until the band of hypertrophied muscle is released.

Although there are strong proponents on both sides, a Cochrane Library systematic review on the operative procedures for anal fissures was updated in 2009.[36] The techniques of open and closed sphincterotomy have been compared in multiple reports, including 5 randomized studies meeting inclusion criteria for the Cochrane analysis.[40–44] Combined, these reports show no difference in either persistence of fissure or incontinence using these 2 techniques. A recent prospective cohort study evaluated 140 consecutive patients undergoing open or closed sphincterotomy.[45] Postoperative endoanal ultrasound showed that open sphincterotomy was associated with

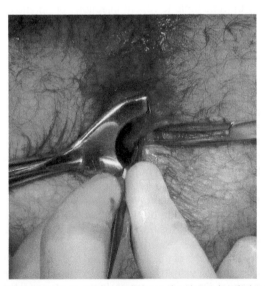

**Fig. 3.** An open sphincterotomy is performed through a lateral radial incision just outside the anal verge. The hypertrophied internal sphincter muscle is isolated between the intersphincteric groove and submucosal plane before being divided under direct vision.

a significantly higher proportion of complete sphincterotomies. The rate of incontinence and treatment failure was not different between the open and closed groups; although an increasing proximal extent of sphincterotomy was associated with a significant increase in incontinence scores ($P<.001$) and decrease in recurrence rates ($P<.001$).

There remains a fine balance between minimizing incontinence and maximizing healing, though the two may be inversely proportional to the degree of division. Thus, the decision regarding the extent of sphincterotomy performed in the operating room is a controversial topic, which may explain some variation in outcomes. Excessive division increases the risk of incontinence, but inadequate division increases the risk of persistence or recurrence. Although many texts have noted division to the dentate line when describing the procedure, recent studies have examined a more conservative sphincterotomy. Mentes and colleagues[46] prospectively randomized 76 patients with chronic anal fissure to lateral internal sphincterotomy to the dentate line or to the apex of the fissure. Treatment failure was nil in the traditional dentate line group compared with 13% in the conservative group after 1 year of follow-up, with most treatment failures occurring after 2 months. There was no difference in the postoperative incontinence scores between the 2 treatment groups. However, there was a statistically significant increase in the postoperative incontinence score in the traditional group, suggesting that the study may have been underpowered to detect a possible difference. In a similar manner, Elsebae[47] prospectively randomized 92 patients to sphincterotomy to the dentate line (traditional) or sphincterotomy to the apex of the fissure (conservative). Similar to the Mentes study, there were no treatment failures in the traditional group versus 4% in the conservative group ($P$ not significant), whereas persistent incontinence was 4% in the traditional group compared with 0% in the conservative group ($P$ not significant). However, the follow-up period was only 18 weeks, leaving some question as to eventual outcome.

Although the techniques of division to the dentate line or to the fissure apex have objective definitions, many surgeons approach the sphincterotomy as a more subjective task. The band of hypertrophied internal anal sphincter muscle may or may not relate to either of these 2 landmarks. As such, the division of the hypertrophied muscle segment becomes more subjective. A subsequent report from Mentes and colleagues[48] attempted to evaluate this method by creating a sphincterotomy that achieves an anal caliber of 30 mm, in a prospective comparison to division to the apex of the fissure. Their findings showed that the average anal caliber was greater in the group that underwent division to the apex, the incontinence rates were higher, and there was no significant difference in treatment failure. With all these various techniques, it is imperative that surgeons thoroughly counsel patients about the different methods and expected outcomes, and that they feel confident and competent in performing the technique chosen.

The hallmark of chronic fissure is the triad of a hypertrophied internal sphincter, a hypertrophied anal papilla, and an external sentinel tag. Excision of the papilla and tag, or complete fissurectomy, are optional but particularly useful if the fissure edges appear rolled and epithelialized, because this may promote faster wound healing. In addition, many chronic fissures are associated with a small subcutaneous tract that extends into the anal canal. Interest has been expressed in the laying open of this tract, the subcutaneous fissurotomy, as primary treatment of the fissure. It is believed that unroofing this tract results in widening of the distal anal canal, thus rendering the sphincterotomy pointless.[49] Although there remains little data at this stage, the initial reports are promising with failure rates of less than 2% and no changes in incontinence. Detractors point out that the simultaneous dilation occurring in the course of the procedure may account for some of its success. Its ultimate role in the operative management of fissures remains to be seen.

In addition to the randomized controlled trials detailing lateral internal sphincterotomy, a myriad of additional nonrandomized reports are available describing a wide range of outcomes with this procedure. Although most reports cite low rates of treatment failure, the incontinence rate is widely variable, with some studies citing rates as high as 30% to 40%.[50,51] Part of this reflects the definition of incontinence and study design (ie, temporary vs permanent, flatus vs liquid or solid stool, prospective vs retrospective data collection), although the exact reasons for such a wide range of results remain unclear. What is clear is that this remains a significant issue. With a multimodal and often stepwise approach designed to minimize the risk of permanent incontinence, the trend seems to be to move away from lateral internal sphincterotomy and toward more medical therapy or botulinum toxin. Unfortunately, it is not clear whether this strategy will be the most effective long-term solution with respect to morbidity, cost, patient satisfaction, and, ultimately, healing. However, the disease is largely measured by the subjective experience of the patient, so they remain the best judge of which treatment is worth pursuing and which risks are worth taking. A recent review by Floyd and colleagues[52] reported that with the increasing trend of multiple options available to patients, the ultimate time to healing is prolonged, although 72% of patients can avoid operative treatment and 97% of patients can eventually be healed. Further support for this approach was recently reported by Lysy and associates,[33] where an escalating regimen from topical agents to botulinum toxin to sphincterotomy led to a 71% cure rate at 47 months without the need for sphincterotomy. Similar to Floyd and colleagues, they also noted that the low rate of sphincterotomy comes at the price of increased recurrence before complete healing, prolonged symptoms, and of a longer time spent in treatment.

## SPECIAL SITUATIONS
### Fissures Without Anal Hypertonicity

The presumption that relief of anal hypertonicity leads to healing is the basis of treatments directed at relaxation of the anal sphincter, either pharmacologically or surgically. However, a subset of patients with fissure will not demonstrate hypertonicity, and hypotonicity may actually be profound. As such, concerns exist regarding the effect of further decreasing sphincter tone, leading to higher rates of incontinence. In this situation, anal advancement flap is a useful option. Giordano and colleagues[53] recently reported results from their prospective study of simple cutaneous advancement flaps in 51 patients over a 6-year period, for all patients regardless of hyper- or hypo- anal tone. They found the procedure to be well tolerated, with an overall 98% treatment success rate. Similarly, Nyam and colleagues[54] evaluated 21 patients with fissures and less than normal anal pressures with the use of an island advancement flap, demonstrating complete healing and no incontinence in all patients. An earlier report from St Marks in 2002 also noted favorable results with advancement flaps for fissures with hypertonicity in a small series, with successful treatment in 7 of 8 patients at a median follow-up of 7 months.[55] Although this technique may be useful for all patients with refractory fissures, it holds particular promise in addressing the fissure in the setting of a hypotonic anus.

### Crohn's Disease

Fissures are commonly seen in people with Crohn's disease, affecting approximately 30% of patients.[56,57] When they occur, they tend to be in more atypical locations, deeper, and associated with other pathology, especially fistula. These fissures also have an atypical appearance, often creating deep ulcerations and potentially creating significant deformity. As with other manifestations of Crohn's, it is reasonable to intervene only as complications dictate. Some investigators have reported acceptable outcomes from operative procedures in these patients,[58,59] though caution should be the rule, and sphincter salvage is prudent. Multidisciplinary care is crucial in addressing anorectal disease in the patient with Crohn's, because appropriate medical management of the disease may lead to resolution of the anorectal disorders in 50% or more of these cases.[60,61] Careful evaluation for more proximal disease should also be done, because often, anal manifestations may herald a generalized flare.

### Human Immunodeficiency Virus

HIV-related anal disease includes typical fissures and anorectal ulcers, which, similar to Crohn's, can appear as deep, broad-based, or cavitating lesions. Poor sphincter tone and diminished function is a more frequent finding than the hypertonicity that generally accompanies typical, non-HIV–related fissures. Small studies have reported successful treatment of typical fissures that may also occur in patients with HIV, though surgeons should be wary in the setting of active proctitis, poorly-controlled or advanced disease, and those with baseline continence impairment.[62,63] Although the medical treatment of HIV continues to improve, concerns about delayed wound healing and increased infectious complications remain, especially in those with advanced disease.

### SUMMARY

Anal fissure is a common disorder that is effectively treated and prevented with conservative measures in its acute form. Chronic fissures usually require medical therapy, which can be effective in a small majority of patients. Initial therapy includes bulking agents, control of constipation, and topical medications to relax the internal anal sphincter. Botulinum toxin and lateral internal sphincterotomy can both be considered for treatment of refractory anal fissures, and the popularity of botulinum toxin is increasing. Sphincterotomy remains an effective operation, with a high rate of resolution of symptoms, but at the price of an increased risk of temporary or permanent incontinence.

### REFERENCES

1. Fleshman JW. Fissure-in-ano and anal stenosis. In: Becker DE, Wexner SD, editors. Fundamentals of Anorectal Surgery. London: W.B. Saunders: 1998. p. 557.
2. Fazio VW, Church JM, Delaney CP, editors. Current therapy in colon and rectal surgery. Philadephia, Penn: Elsevier Mosby, the Curtis Center; 2005.
3. Perry GG. Fissure in ano–a complication of anusitis. South Med J 1962;55:955–7.
4. Nothmann BJ, Schuster MM. Internal anal sphincter derangement with anal fissures. Gastroenterology 1974;67(2):216–20.
5. Farouk R, Duthie GS, MacGregor AB, et al. Sustained internal sphincter hypertonia in patients with chronic anal fissure. Dis Colon Rectum 1994;37(5):424–9.
6. Gibbons CP, Read NW. Anal hypertonia in fissures: cause or effect? Br J Surg 1986;73(6):443–5.
7. Klosterhalfen B, Vogel P, Rixen H, et al. Topography of the inferior rectal artery: a possible cause of chronic, primary anal fissure. Dis Colon Rectum 1989; 32(1):43–52.

8. Schouten WR, Briel JW, Auwerda JJ, et al. Ischaemic nature of anal fissure. Br J Surg 1996;83(1):63–5.
9. Orsay C, Rakinic J, Perry WB, et al. Practice parameters for the management of anal fissures (revised). Dis Colon Rectum 2004;47(12):2003–7.
10. Jensen SL. Treatment of first episodes of acute anal fissure: prospective randomised study of lignocaine ointment versus hydrocortisone ointment or warm sitz baths plus bran. Br Med J (Clin Res Ed) 1986;292(6529):1167–9.
11. Nelson RL. Non surgical therapy for anal fissure. Cochrane Database Syst Rev 2009;(2):CD003431.
12. O'Kelly T, Brading A, Mortensen N. Nerve mediated relaxation of the human internal anal sphincter: the role of nitric oxide. Gut 1993;34(5):689–93.
13. Loder PB, Kamm MA, Nicholls RJ, et al. 'Reversible chemical sphincterotomy' by local application of glyceryl trinitrate. Br J Surg 1994;81(9):1386–9.
14. Lund JN, Scholefield JH. A randomised, prospective, double-blind, placebo-controlled trial of glyceryl trinitrate ointment in treatment of anal fissure. Lancet 1997;349(9044):11–4.
15. Jonas M, Barrett DA, Shaw PN, et al. Systemic levels of glyceryl trinitrate following topical application to the anoderm do not correlate with the measured reduction in anal pressure. Br J Surg 2001;88(12):1613–6.
16. Lund JN, Armitage NC, Scholefield JH. Use of glyceryl trinitrate ointment in the treatment of anal fissure. Br J Surg 1996;83(6):776–7.
17. Brisinda G, Maria G, Bentivoglio AR, et al. A comparison of injections of botulinum toxin and topical nitroglycerin ointment for the treatment of chronic anal fissure. N Engl J Med 1999;341(2):65–9.
18. Watson SJ, Kamm MA, Nicholls RJ, et al. Topical glyceryl trinitrate in the treatment of chronic anal fissure. Br J Surg 1996;83(6):771–5.
19. Chrysos E, Xynos E, Tzovaras G, et al. Effect of nifedipine on rectoanal motility. Dis Colon Rectum 1996;39(2):212–6.
20. Carapeti EA, Kamm MA, Phillips RK. Topical diltiazem and bethanechol decrease anal sphincter pressure and heal anal fissures without side effects. Dis Colon Rectum 2000;43(10):1359–62.
21. Jonas M, Neal KR, Abercrombie JF, et al. A randomized trial of oral vs. topical diltiazem for chronic anal fissures. Dis Colon Rectum 2001;44(8):1074–8.
22. Kocher HM, Steward M, Leather AJ, et al. Randomized clinical trial assessing the side-effects of glyceryl trinitrate and diltiazem hydrochloride in the treatment of chronic anal fissure. Br J Surg 2002;89(4):413–7.
23. Bielecki K, Kolodziejczak M. A prospective randomized trial of diltiazem and glyceryltrinitrate ointment in the treatment of chronic anal fissure. Colorectal Dis 2003;5(3):256–7.
24. Cheng CM, Chen JS, Patel RP. Unlabeled uses of botulinum toxins: a review, part 1. Am J Health Syst Pharm 2006;63(2):145–52.
25. Tjandra JJ. Ambulatory haemorrhoidectomy - has the time come? ANZ J Surg 2005;75(4):183.
26. Gui D, Cassetta E, Anastasio G, et al. Botulinum toxin for chronic anal fissure. Lancet 1994;344(8930):1127–8.
27. Maria G, Cassetta E, Gui D, et al. A comparison of botulinum toxin and saline for the treatment of chronic anal fissure. N Engl J Med 1998;338(4):217–20.
28. Sajid MS, Vijaynagar B, Desai M, et al. Botulinum toxin vs glyceryltrinitrate for the medical management of chronic and fissure: a meta-analysis. Colorectal Dis 2008;10(6):529–30.

29. Arroyo A, Perez F, Serrano P, et al. Surgical versus chemical (botulinum toxin) sphincterotomy for chronic anal fissure: long-term results of a prospective randomized clinical and manometric study. Am J Surg 2005;189(4):429–34.

30. Iswariah H, Stephens J, Rieger N, et al. Randomized prospective controlled trial of lateral internal sphincterotomy versus injection of botulinum toxin for the treatment of idiopathic fissure in ano. ANZ J Surg 2005;75(7):553–5.

31. Mentes BB, Irkorucu O, Akin M, et al. Comparison of botulinum toxin injection and lateral internal sphincterotomy for the treatment of chronic anal fissure. Dis Colon Rectum 2003;46(2):232–7.

32. Shao WJ, Zhang ZK. Systematic review and meta-analysis of randomized controlled trials comparing botulinum toxin injection with lateral internal sphincterotomy for chronic anal fissure. Int J Colorectal Dis 2009;24(9):995–1000.

33. Lysy J, Israeli E, Levy S, et al. Long-term results of "chemical sphincterotomy" for chronic anal fissure: a prospective study. Dis Colon Rectum 2006;49(6):858–64.

34. Steele SR, Madoff RD. Systematic review: the treatment of anal fissure. Aliment Pharmacol Ther 2006;24(2):247–57.

35. Saad AM, Omer A. Surgical treatment of chronic fissure-in-ano: a prospective randomised study. East Afr Med J 1992;69(11):613–5.

36. Nelson RL. Operative procedures for fissure in ano. Cochrane Database Syst Rev 2009;(2):CD002199.

37. Renzi A, Izzo D, Di Sarno G, et al. Clinical, manometric, and ultrasonographic results of pneumatic balloon dilatation vs. lateral internal sphincterotomy for chronic anal fissure: a prospective, randomized, controlled trial. Dis Colon Rectum 2008;51(1):121–7.

38. Eisenhammer S. The evaluation of the internal anal sphincterotomy operation with special reference to anal fissure. Surg Gynecol Obstet 1959;109:583–90.

39. Notaras MJ. Lateral subcutaneous sphincterotomy for anal fissure – a new technique. Proc R Soc Med 1969;62:713.

40. Kortbeek JB, Langevin JM, Khoo RE, et al. Chronic fissure-in-ano: a randomized study comparing open and subcutaneous lateral internal sphincterotomy. Dis Colon Rectum 1992;35(9):835–7.

41. Arroyo A, Perez F, Serrano P, et al. Open versus closed lateral sphincterotomy performed as an outpatient procedure under local anesthesia for chronic anal fissure: prospective randomized study of clinical and manometric longterm results. J Am Coll Surg 2004;199(3):361–7.

42. Wiley M, Day P, Rieger N, et al. Open vs. closed lateral internal sphincterotomy for idiopathic fissure-in-ano: a prospective, randomized, controlled trial. Dis Colon Rectum 2004;47(6):847–52.

43. Filingeri V, Gravante G. A prospective randomized trial betwen subcutaneous lateral internal sphincterotomy with radiofrequency bistoury and conventional parks' operation in the treatment of anal fissures. Eur Rev Med Pharmacol Sci 2005;9(3):175–8.

44. Boulos PB, Araujo JG. Adequate internal sphincterotomy for chronic anal fissure: subcutaneous or open technique? Br J Surg 1984;71(5):360–2.

45. García-Granero E, Sanahuja A, García-Botello SA, et al. The ideal lateral internal sphincterotomy: clinical and endosonographic evaluation following open and closed internal anal sphincterotomy. Colorectal Dis 2009;11(5):502–7.

46. Mentes BB, Ege B, Leventoglu S, et al. Extent of lateral internal sphincterotomy: up to the dentate line or up to the fissure apex? Dis Colon Rectum 2005;48(2):365–70.

47. Elsebae MM. A study of fecal incontinence in patients with chronic anal fissure: prospective, randomized, controlled trial of the extent of internal anal sphincter division during lateral sphincterotomy. World J Surg 2007;31(10):2052–7.

48. Mentes BB, Guner MK, Leventoglu S, et al. Fine-tuning of the extent of lateral internal sphincterotomy: spasm-controlled vs. up to the fissure apex. Dis Colon Rectum 2008;51(1):128–33.

49. Pelta AE, Davis KG, Armstrong DN. Subcutaneous fissurotomy: a novel procedure for chronic fissure-in-ano. A review of 109 cases. Dis Colon Rectum 2007; 50(10):1662–7.

50. Garcia-Aguilar J, Belmonte C, Wong WD, et al. Open vs. closed sphincterotomy for chronic anal fissure: long-term results. Dis Colon Rectum 1996;39(4):440–3.

51. Madoff RD, Fleshman JW. AGA technical review on the diagnosis and care of patients with anal fissure. Gastroenterology 2003;124(1):235–45.

52. Floyd ND, Kondylis L, Kondylis PD, et al. Chronic anal fissure: 1994 and a decade later—are we doing better? Am J Surg 2006;191(3):344–8.

53. Giordano P, Gravante G, Grondona P, et al. Simple cutaneous advancement flap anoplasty for resistant chronic anal fissure: a prospective study. World J Surg 2009;33(5):1058–63.

54. Nyam DCNK, Wilson RG, Stewart KJ, et al. Island advancement flaps in the management of anal fissures. Br J Surg 2005;82(3):326–8.

55. Kenefick NJ, Gee AS, Durdey P. Treatment of resistant anal fissure with advancement anoplasty. Colorectal Dis 2002;4(6):463–6.

56. Sangwan YP, Schoetz DJ Jr, Murray JJ, et al. Perianal Crohn's disease. Results of local surgical treatment. Dis Colon Rectum 1996;39(5):529–35.

57. Platell C, Mackay J, Collopy B, et al. Anal pathology in patients with Crohn's disease. Aust N Z J Surg 1996;66(1):5–9.

58. Wolkomir AF, Luchtefeld MA. Surgery for symptomatic hemorrhoids and anal fissures in Crohn's disease. Dis Colon Rectum 1993;36(6):545–7.

59. Fleshner PR, Schoetz DJ Jr, Roberts PL, et al. Anal fissure in Crohn's disease: a plea for aggressive management. Dis Colon Rectum 1995;38(11):1137–43.

60. Ouraghi A, Nieuviarts S, Mougenel JL, et al. Traitement par anticorps anti-TNF alpha (infliximab, remicade) des lesions anoperineales de la maladic de Crohn [Infliximab therapy for Crohn's disease anoperineal lesions][see comment]. Gastroenterol Clin Biol 2001;25(11):949–56 [in French].

61. Sweeney JL, Ritchie JK, Nicholls RJ. Anal fissure in Crohn's disease. Br J Surg 1988;75(1):56–7.

62. Weiss EG, Wexner SD. Surgery for anal lesions in HIV-infected patients. Ann Med 1995;27(4):467–75.

63. Viamonte M, Dailey TH, Gottesman L. Ulcerative disease of the anorectum in the HIV+ patient. Dis Colon Rectum 1993;36(9):801–5.

# Anorectal Abscess and Fistula-in-Ano: Evidence-Based Management

Julie A. Rizzo, MD[a], Anna L. Naig, MD[a],
Eric K. Johnson, MD, FACS, FASCRS[b,c],*

KEYWORDS

• Anorectal abscess • Anal fistula • Incontinence

Anorectal abscess, and the fistula that may result, are long established processes that were originally described at the beginning of recorded medical history as part of the "Corpus Hippocraticum" in a treatise termed "On Fistulae."[1] The basic principles regarding the treatment of this disease have remained the same: resolution of perianal sepsis, and treatment of the resulting fistula without leading to impairment in continence. This second principle remains a challenge, and there are continued efforts to achieve an optimal form of therapy. A recent surge of interest in this disease process occurred after the release of the collagen anal fistula plug. Hopefully this will lead to an improvement in the care of patients with this inconvenient and embarrassing condition.

## PATHOPHYSIOLOGY

Anorectal abscess occurs commonly in normal, healthy individuals. The most widely recognized cause is described in the cryptoglandular theory, which suggests that an anal crypt gland becomes obstructed with inspissated debris and leads to infection. These glands penetrate the anal sphincter complex to varying degrees, and the suppuration tends to follow the path of least resistance. The abscess collects in whichever anatomic space the gland terminates, or wherever the path of least resistance leads. A basic understanding of anorectal anatomy and the perianal and perirectal spaces is critical for grasping this concept.

[a] Department of Surgery, Dwight David Eisenhower Army Medical Center, 300 Hospital Road, Fort Gordon, GA, USA
[b] Colorectal Surgery and Surgical Endoscopy, Dwight David Eisenhower Army Medical Center, 300 Hospital Road, Fort Gordon, GA, USA
[c] Uniform Services University of Health Sciences, F. Edward Hebert School of Medicine, Bethesda, MD, USA
* Corresponding author. Colorectal Surgery and Surgical Endoscopy, Dwight David Eisenhower Army Medical Center, 300 Hospital Road, Fort Gordon, GA.
*E-mail address:* eric.k.johnson@us.army.mil (E.K. Johnson).

Surg Clin N Am 90 (2010) 45–68
doi:10.1016/j.suc.2009.10.001
0039-6109/09/$ – see front matter. Published by Elsevier Inc.
surgical.theclinics.com

Anal fistulas develop in approximately one-third of patients who undergo drainage of an anorectal abscess. In a series[2] of 170 patients without previous fistulas who were followed for an average of 99 months after abscess drainage, a fistula occurred in 37% and recurrent abscess was reported in an additional 10%. A retrospective cohort study[3] of 148 patients with anorectal abscesses showed a 37% rate of fistula formation. Patients younger than 40 years and nondiabetic patients had a higher likelihood of developing a fistula-in-ano over the mean follow-up of 38 months. Any recurrent abscess that occurs at the same site as a previous abscess can be considered a fistula and treated as such. There are other notable causes of atypical/complicated abscess and fistula, including inflammatory bowel disease, fungal infection, mycobacterial infection, neoplasm, and trauma. Fistulas that are secondary to these processes are classified as complex and require the use of nonstandard methods of management.

## CLASSIFICATION

Anorectal abscesses are classified based on their location. Four types of anorectal abscesses are commonly described: perianal (superficial), ischiorectal (perirectal), intersphincteric, and supralevator. Perianal is the most common type and is the simplest to treat. The collections are located in the superficial perianal tissues and are typically located close to the anal verge. Ischiorectal abscesses are located more deeply in the ischiorectal fossa and may communicate to the contralateral side via the deep postanal space; this would be a classic example of a horseshoe abscess. Intersphincteric abscesses are often difficult to diagnose as they may reside completely within the anal canal. They are located in the intersphincteric space between the internal and external sphincter muscles. Patients affected by this process complain of severe anal pain and often cannot tolerate an examination without anesthesia. The fluctuant collection may be found only by performing a digital rectal examination or anoscopy. Supralevator abscesses are rare and are typically diagnosed through computed tomographic scanning. A patient presenting with this condition might complain of pelvic and rectal pain with tenesmus. The abscess can sometimes be palpated through a digital rectal examination performed by an experienced examiner. These abscesses are often related to perforated diverticular disease, inflammatory bowel disease, or rarely neoplastic disease in the pelvis. Sometimes an abscess occurs in the supralevator location because cryptoglandular suppuration followed the path of least resistance. Simple internal drainage often ameliorates this problem. The management of the processes already mentioned outside drainage is complex and is beyond the scope of this discussion. A study of more than 1000 patients who presented with anorectal abscess revealed that perianal abscess occurred in 42.7%, ischiorectal in 22.7%, intersphincteric in 21.4%, and supralevator in 7.33%.[4]

A question that often arises is whether or not to treat a fistula that is noted during a procedure performed to drain perianal sepsis. A randomized clinical trial comparing simple drainage alone to drainage plus fistula tract treatment was published in 2002.[5] The investigators randomized 200 patients to one of the two treatment arms, excluding any patient who had incontinence or a history of inflammatory bowel disease. Internal openings were found in 83% of the patients and they were treated with simple fistulotomy or seton fistulotomy if they had been randomized to the tract-treatment arm. Recurrence was noted in 29% of the group who received drainage only compared with 5% of the group who received tract treatment. In low fistulas treated by fistulotomy, incontinence was seen in only 2.8%. Patients who had high fistulas that were managed by seton (delayed) fistulotomy developed incontinence 37% of the time. This result illustrates a major concern in the treatment of high fistula tracts. A later meta-analysis addressing this same issue evaluated 5 trials containing 405 patients and found an 83% reduction in recurrence in those who had their fistula tracts addressed at the initial procedure with no significant increase in the rate of postoperative incontinence.[6]

Fistulas are classified based on their relation to the anal sphincter complex. They are typically divided into 5 common classifications: submucosal, intersphincteric (**Fig. 1**), trans-sphincteric (divided into high and low) (**Fig. 2**), suprasphincteric (**Fig. 3**), and extrasphincteric (**Fig. 4**). Trans-sphincteric fistulas cross through the internal and external sphincter muscles to varying degrees. Low fistulas involve only the outer or distal one-third of the external sphincter muscle, whereas high fistulas involve greater degrees of the external sphincter. This characteristic is clinically significant because division of greater amounts of the external sphincter leads to higher rates of fecal incontinence. Intersphincteric fistulas cross through the internal sphincter and exit through the intersphincteric plane. They do not involve the external sphincter muscle and can therefore be opened without high risk of incontinence. Submucosal fistulas typically originate at an offending crypt at the level of the dentate line, but track only just beneath the submucosa and do not involve the sphincter complex. These fistulas may be opened without fear of compromising continence. Suprasphincteric fistulas typically originate at the dentate line internally, cross above the external sphincter but below the puborectalis, and exit onto the perianal skin through the ischiorectal

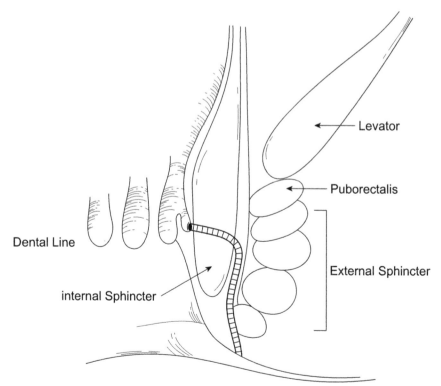

**Fig. 1.** An intersphincteric fistula. (*From* Belliveau P. Anal fistula. In: Fazio VM, Church JM, Delaney CP, editors. Current therapy in colon and rectal surgery. 2nd edition. Philadelphia: Elsevier Mosby; 2005. p. 28; with permission.)

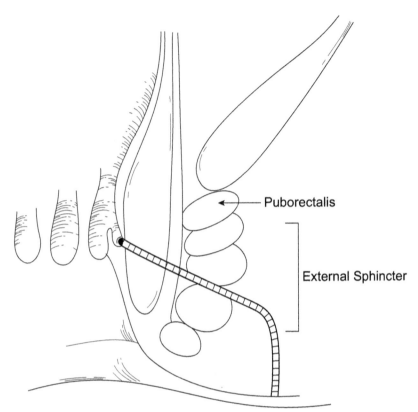

**Fig. 2.** A trans-sphincteric fistula. (*From* Belliveau P. Anal fistula. In: Fazio VM, Church JM, Delaney CP, editors. Current therapy in colon and rectal surgery. 2nd edition. Philadelphia: Elsevier Mosby; 2005. p. 28; with permission.)

fossa. Extrasphincteric fistulas are rare and do not involve the sphincter complex. They typically arise from the pelvis or rectum above the dentate line, cross proximal to the sphincter complex into the ischiorectal fossa, and exit onto the perianal skin. These fistulas do not have a cryptogenic origin and are often associated with inflammatory bowel disease, pelvic inflammatory processes, and neoplasia.

## TREATMENT

The treatment of anal fistula is dictated by the classification and the amount of sphincter complex that is involved with the tract. Simple fistulas, intersphincteric, and low trans-sphincteric of cryptoglandular origin, can be treated easily with a fistulotomy with minimal risk to continence. Complex fistulas, high fistulas, and those related to inflammatory bowel disease must be treated through more intricate methods. The primary surgical approach to successful resolution of an anal fistula is appropriately addressing the internal opening, which requires the internal opening to be located with certainty, and then either closed through various methods or opened widely and allowed to heal by secondary intention. Obliteration of the internal opening is key to the success of treatment.[7]

Simple observation is a viable option in a patient who is minimally symptomatic or presents a prohibitive operative risk. The most significant risk associated with

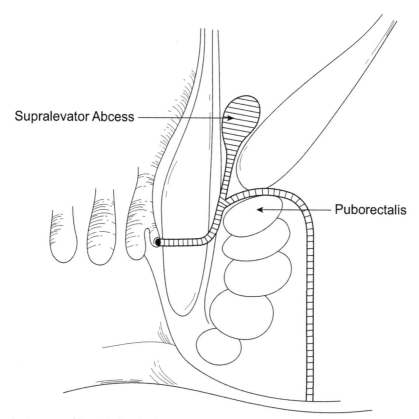

**Fig. 3.** A suprasphincteric fistula. (*From* Belliveau P. Anal fistula. In: Fazio VM, Church JM, Delaney CP, editors. Current therapy in colon and rectal surgery. 2nd edition. Philadelphia: Elsevier Mosby; 2005. p. 29; with permission.)

observation of an anal fistula is recurrent anorectal abscess. This abscess can usually be managed by simple repeat incision and drainage, although this may lead to a more complex fistula if the process is repeated indefinitely. There have been rare case reports of malignancies arising in long-standing anal fistula tracts,[8] but this unusual occurrence should not drive a clinician's treatment plan. Multiple methods can be used to address this problem, and as previously stated, this decision is based on fistula anatomy, cause, prior attempts at treatment, the patient's preoperative fecal continence, and comorbid conditions.

## MEDICAL MANAGEMENT

The major morbidity associated with the surgical treatment of fistula-in-ano is fecal incontinence. Kim and colleagues[9] retrospectively studied 404 male patients with fecal incontinence and found that in patients younger than 70 years, the second most common association was a prior surgical fistulotomy or hemorrhoidectomy. Lindsey and colleagues[10] performed anal manometry and endoanal ultrasonography in 93 patients being evaluated for fecal incontinence after anal surgery. They had universal findings of internal sphincter disruption and reversal of the normal resting pressure gradient seen in the anal canal. They caution clinicians to investigate sphincter-sparing alternatives in the primary management of anorectal maladies.

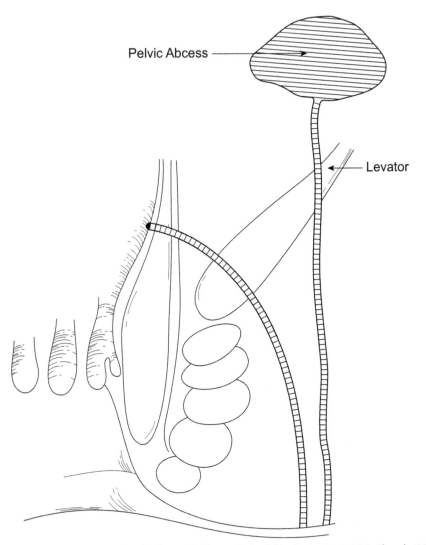

Pelvic Abcess

Levator

**Fig. 4.** An extrasphincteric fistula. (*From* Belliveau P. Anal fistula. In: Fazio VM, Church JM, Delaney CP, editors. Current therapy in colon and rectal surgery. 2nd edition. Philadelphia: Elsevier Mosby; 2005. p. 29; with permission.)

Medical management of fistula-in-ano is most often associated with patients suffering from inflammatory bowel disease. As mentioned previously, there is little harm in observing a fistula that is minimally symptomatic. After first draining the perianal suppuration, simple observation and medical treatment of associated Crohn's disease led to healing in 8 of 15 patients followed for 10 years.[11] Halme and Sainio[12] noted a similar healing rate of 50% in patients with Crohn's disease with anal fistulas who were only observed. Oral metronidazole is a useful agent in the medical management of fistula-in-ano in the population with Crohn's disease. A dosage of 20 mg/kg/d divided into 3 or 4 doses has been shown to eliminate drainage, erythema, and induration in as many as 80% of patients treated within 8 weeks.[13] Compliance with this regimen can be poor secondary to associated nausea, metallic taste, and peripheral neuropathy from the use of the drug. Other investigators have evaluated the use of topical metronidazole preparations to assist with nonoperative management without the side effects associated with oral use of the drug. A prospective, nonrandomized study of 14 patients with anorectal Crohn's disease evaluated the perianal Crohn's disease activity index (PCDAI) in patients treated with 10% topical metronidazole cream for 4 weeks.[14] The investigators showed a significant decrease in the PCDAI after 4 weeks of therapy. The largest improvements noted were diminished perianal pain, discharge, and induration.

Surgery is not contraindicated in patients with Crohn's-associated anal fistulas, but should be undertaken cautiously. A retrospective review of 66 patients with perianal Crohn's disease showed that surgery was performed to treat fistula-in-ano in 71%.[15] Fistulotomies were performed in 35 patients and draining setons were placed in 24. Of this group, 61% retained a functional anus during the 10-year study. The investigators state that fistulotomy involving the lower portion of the sphincter complex is safe. Another study[16] evaluating the use of long-term draining setons in patients with high, Crohn's-associated fistulas showed that simple removal of the seton resulted in a 39% recurrence rate, but that staged fistulotomy resulted in no recurrences with a 12% rate of fecal incontinence. A more recent 10-year retrospective review of Crohn's-associated anal fistula disease showed that 45% of patients with complex fistula-in-ano or rectovaginal fistulas recur in the long term after surgery.[1] The investigators also showed that 20% of patients who demonstrated recurrence went on to require a proctectomy. Observations like these encourage the clinician to exhaust medical therapy before undertaking surgery in this group of patients.

The use of infliximab (Remicade, Centocor Ortho Biotech Inc, Horsham, PA, USA), a monoclonal antibody to tumor necrosis factor, has been shown to be effective in the treatment of luminal Crohn's disease.[17] A short-term trial of infliximab use showed its effectiveness in the closure of anal fistulas, although there was a high recurrence rate and the median duration of response was only 12 weeks.[18] Sands and colleagues[19] showed that in patients who have an initial favorable response to infliximab, maintenance therapy for 54 weeks resulted in sustained fistula closure in 36%, although those treated with placebo healed only 19% of the time ($P = .009$). Although these are compelling data, surgeons cannot free themselves of responsibility to these patients. Gaertner and colleagues[20] reviewed their experience with the operative treatment of Crohn's-related perianal fistulas and found that healing was no better in patients who underwent surgery alone compared with those treated with surgery and concomitant infliximab therapy. Based on these data it seems wise to use medical therapy as primary treatment of anal fistulas associated with Crohn's disease with surgery reserved for those that fail in the long term. It should also be noted that surgical drainage of perianal suppuration and the liberal use of draining setons should be employed in the "medical" management of these patients.

## PREOPERATIVE PLANNING

Simple submucosal, intersphincteric, and low trans-sphincteric fistulas are effectively managed by fistulotomy with minimal risk to fecal continence. In the past, the patient had to undergo an examination under anesthesia to determine the type of fistula and the amount of sphincter mechanism that was involved. If a simple fistula was found, then definitive management was typically undertaken. Complex fistulas would be managed through staged approaches. These decisions hinge on the clinician's intraoperative physical diagnostic skill. Techniques such as palpation of the offending crypt and tract injection with hydrogen peroxide or methylene blue assist the surgeon in identification of the internal opening, with the subsequent procedure being dictated by its location and the path of the tract. A review of 101 patients showed that primary crypt palpation was possible in 93% of patients. Hydrogen peroxide was seen to drain through the internal opening of 83% of those who underwent injection via the external opening of the fistula.[21] Newer technologies are available to the clinician that may assist in preoperative planning in these patients so that definitive management may be undertaken immediately, and appropriate patients may be selected for sphincter-sparing alternatives. A prospective study[22] in which 102 patients with anal fistula were examined preoperatively with a 3-dimensional endoanal ultrasonography system showed that the anatomy of the primary fistula tract was correctly identified in 94% of patients and that internal openings were correctly localized in 91%. The imaging was augmented by the injection of hydrogen peroxide into the external openings of the tracts and the imaging findings were confirmed or refuted during examination under anesthesia. The investigators showed that preoperative imaging with this system assisted in preoperative planning and counseling. Another study of preoperative imaging showed that tract angulation, as imaged by magnetic resonance imaging, correlated with internal opening location.[23] Tracts that showed acute angulation from the internal opening tended to be high transsphincteric tracts, whereas those exhibiting obtuse angulation tended to be lower fistulas. Both studies demonstrate the ability of noninvasive preoperative imaging to assist the surgeon in preoperative planning, counseling, and selection of the appropriate procedure.

## FIBRIN GLUE

Because traditional methods to repair complex fistulas, including fistulectomies, fistulotomies, and advancement flaps, have resulted in high rates of incontinence, investigations into less invasive procedures have been performed. Fibrin glue first made its appearance in surgery during World War I, when it was used for hemostasis, and then later in the 1940s as a sealant for skin-graft procedures.[24] In 1992, Hjortrup and colleagues[25] first used it as a sealant for anal fistulas and since that time there have been several publications regarding its use in this complex disease.

The principle of its sealant properties is based on clot formation and to understand its mode of action, knowledge of the clotting cascade is mandatory. Fibrin glue is a mixture of fibrinogen, thrombin, and calcium ions, which when combined form a soluble clot, because fibrinogen is cleaved into fibrin. This soluble clot is transformed into an insoluble, stable clot as the thrombin and calcium activate factor XIII. This reaction seals the fistula tract within 30 to 60 seconds as the glue sets. The glue also stimulates the migration and proliferation of fibroblasts and pluripotent endothelial cells to heal the fistula. Between days 7 and 14, plasmin that is present in the surrounding tissue lyses the fibrin clot as the tract is replaced by synthesized collagen.[26]

There are 2 forms of fibrin glue preparation: autologous, which is prepared from pooled human blood, and a commercial preparation, which first became widely available in the United States in 1998.[24] The autologous product carries rare but potentially lethal disadvantages, such as the risk of viral transmission (mainly hepatitis B, C and human immunodeficiency virus). Both formulations also carry the rare risk of allergic reaction.[27] Studies have promoted the commercial glue as having a higher fibrinogen concentration, with the result being a stronger and more consistent plug[27,28] and easier and quicker preparation than autologous glue.[29] Other studies, however, have demonstrated no success advantage between the 2 preparations.[30]

The procedure is promoted as simple and repeatable with no significant learning curves, in direct contrast to other procedures, such as the advancement flap. Both openings of the tract are identified and the tract is mechanically curetted and irrigated with normal saline or hydrogen peroxide. The double-barreled syringe, containing the 2 components of the glue, is inserted through the external opening until the tip is seen at the internal opening. The syringe is depressed, which mixes the 2 components as they are injected into the canal. The tract is filled completely until a blob of glue is seen at the external opening. The glue is allowed to set for 30 to 60 seconds to form its stable clot. Different investigators have advocated suturing the internal or external opening around the bead of glue,[31] although others have demonstrated no statistically significant benefit.[27,29] Postoperatively, the use of antibiotics and diet restrictions was variable, but sitz baths, excessive straining, or vigorous exercise were prohibited uniformly to prevent dislodgement of the plug.[32] Preoperative bowel preparations, the use of perioperative antibiotics, and the use of setons is widely variable with none shown to confer a benefit.[27,33]

A variable range of success has been achieved, from 31% to 85%, because of the complexity of the disease and the variation in tactics used to tackle the problem (Table 1). Each investigator has postulated various reasons for success or lack thereof, either in the technical aspects of the procedure or perioperative care. Sentovich[34] dedicated much of his success to using the commercial fibrin glue preparation, which he believes forms a stronger plug than autologous glue. This initial study had a follow-up of 10 months and the data held up over a longer follow-up period of 22 months, with success decreasing to 69%.[35] This result raises an important element of the fibrin glue procedure: the length of follow-up of these patients is crucial as most failures have been shown to occur within 6 months.[33] Some investigators advocate as long as 2 years for follow-up[26] but the optimum time has been almost universally agreed on to be no less than 6 months.[27,34,35]

Reasons for failure of the glue have been postulated by many, with dislodgement being most common. For this reason, patients are instructed not to take sitz baths and to avoid vigorous exercise and excessive straining (some are given stool softeners or put on a liquid diet to aid with this).[27] Recurrence of fistulas is another issue and is

**Table 1**
Fibrin glue studies, cited in order of most to least successful

| Author (Reference Number) | Year | No. of Subjects | Success Rate (%) | Follow-up Interval (Months) |
|---|---|---|---|---|
| Sentovich[34] | 2001 | 20 | 85 | 10 |
| Maralcan[32] | 2005 | 36 | 83 | 12 |
| Patrlj[38] | 2000 | 69 | 74 | 28 |
| Sentovich[35] | 2002 | 48 | 69 | 22 |
| Lindsey[36] | 2001 | 42 | 63 | 4 |
| Adams[33] | 2007 | 36 | 61 | 3 |
| Witte[39] | 2007 | 34 | 55 | 7 |
| Zmora[37] | 2005 | 60 | 53 | 6 |
| Parades[27] | 2008 | 30 | 50 | 12 |
| Gisbertz[31] | 2005 | 27 | 33 | 7 |
| Dietz[29] | 2006 | 39 | 31 | 23 |

believed to be caused by inadequate removal of granulation tissue during tract preparation with mechanical curetting and irrigation[26] and the natural course of fistula disease. Another cause of failure is abscess formation, which has been quoted as high as 5% in some studies.[33] This is believed to be caused by a lack of complete tract filling with glue, representing a technical error,[36] or a lack of proper tract cleansing before glue instillation.[35,36] Some investigators have sought to prevent this by making a glue/antibiotic mixture,[37] whereas others have irrigated the tract before glue instillation with an antibiotic irrigant.[38]

A controversy continues to exist regarding the length of the tract and its impact on glue success. Patrlj and colleagues[38] and Lindsey and colleagues[36] demonstrated greater success with longer tracts, attributing this to the ability of glue to leak from shorter tracts (<3.5 cm) more easily. On the contrary, Sentovich,[34,35] Cintron and colleagues[30] and Maralcan and colleagues[32] had greater success with shorter tracts. To date, there is no consensus on the tract length most amenable to success with glue and therefore no patient should be excluded by tract length.

Two main advantages of glue that should be remembered are that no patient experienced a decrease in level of continence from the procedure,[29] and that treatment with fibrin glue does not preclude the patient from receiving other treatments, such as repeat fibrin glue instillation, or conventional fistula treatments.[39] Despite its varying success to date, fibrin glue offers the patient a less invasive option for first-line fistula treatment.

## FISTULA PLUG

Fibrin glue studies failed to achieve results that were reproducible, but did show promise in muscle-sparing, noninvasive operative techniques for anal fistulas. This result led to the development of additional sphincter-sparing therapies. The concept of a plug was first introduced in 2006 by Robb and colleagues[40] and Johnson and colleagues[41] with the idea that securing the plug into the primary opening of a fistula tract could close the tract more reliably than previous procedures, without compromising continence because the sphincters were not incised or divided. The biologic plug (Surgisis Anal Fistula Plug, Cook Surgical, Bloomington, IN) is made of lyophilized porcine small intestinal submucosa, which has an inherent resistance of infection, generates no foreign body or giant cell reaction, and is repopulated by host cell tissue within 3 months.[42] Its conical shape allows for added mechanical stability as high pressures within the anal canal maintain the plug in its proper position, avoiding dislodgement during straining.

Regarding the procedure, the critical points for correct plug insertion are as follows: the plug must be rehydrated first, usually in a 0.9% normal saline solution for 3 to 5 minutes, before insertion; it must be inserted in the internal (also known as primary) opening and then pulled through the tract until light resistance is met; and it must be sutured securely in the primary opening. Various suture types have been used for securing the plug. Champagne and colleagues[43] noticed plug dislodgement as the primary cause of failure in their study, prompting them to use a 2–0 Vicryl (Ethicon Inc, Sommerville, NJ) to provide a stronger securing suture. This choice resulted in a lower incidence of dislodgement and consequently a lower failure rate. Trimming excess plug from the external (secondary) opening at the skin level and irrigating the tract with hydrogen peroxide before insertion are options during the procedure. The external (secondary) opening must be partially open at the end of the procedure as this is the path that allows drainage and prevents a closed-space infection.[44] The use of a bowel preparation, choice of preoperative antibiotics, patient position (lithotomy verses prone jackknife), and the concurrent use of setons are dictated by surgeon preference. A recent consensus statement of 15 colorectal surgeons certified by the American Board of Medical Specialties stated that a seton should always be temporally employed until there is no evidence of acute inflammation or drainage. There was no consensus on the use of bowel preparation or best patient position.[45]

Since introduction of the plug in early 2006, it has achieved a wide range of success, reported between 14% and 87% (**Table 2**). Several investigations have been undertaken to elucidate variables that are predictors of success and reasons for failure. In one of the pioneer studies, Johnson and colleagues[41] achieved 87% success in a follow-up of nearly 14 weeks in a prospective study of 25 patients. Along with following the critical operative technique as outlined earlier, these patients underwent mechanical bowel preparation, had their tracts irrigated with hydrogen peroxide before plug placement, received topical metronidazole after the procedure, and had strict activity limitations for 2 weeks. This success rate persisted for a longer median follow-up time of 12 months, with 83% success shown in the Champagne and colleagues[43] study, which followed Johnson's patients in the long term. Other studies aimed to reproduce this success rate, and a few investigators came close with a modified technique. O'Connor and colleagues[46] achieved 80% success in Crohn's patients by using a similar technique to Johnson and colleagues,[41] except nearly all their patients had setons placed to "mature" the tract and facilitate plug placement by identifying the primary opening and narrowing the diameter of the tract to make it more amenable to plugging. Garg[48] achieved a slightly lower success rate of 71%, with the only technical difference being not using hydrogen peroxide to clean the tract before plug placement, which may offer a reason for decreased success as all epithelial and granulation tissue was not cleansed from the fistula tract, leading to a barrier to cell migration. This explanation was also theorized as a reason for failure by Schwander and colleagues,[49] who reported an overall success rate of 61%, with fistula persistence being the cause of 40% of their failures.

Regarding reasons for failure of the plug, the first important issue is proper securing of the plug to the primary opening in an effort to create immediate closure. Plug dislodgement continues to be the most common reason for failure in numerous

**Table 2**
**Collagen fistula plug studies, cited in order of most to least successful**

| Author (Reference Number) | Year | No. of Subjects | Success Rate (%) | Follow-up Interval (Months) |
|---|---|---|---|---|
| Johnson[41] | 2006 | 25 | 87 | 3 |
| Champagne[43] | 2006 | 46 | 83 | 12 |
| O'Connor[46] | 2006 | 20 | 80 | 10 |
| Ellis[47] | 2007 | 18 | 78 | 10 |
| Garg[48] | 2008 | 21 | 71 | 10 |
| Schwander[49] | 2007 | 19 | 61 | 9.3 |
| Ky[50] | 2007 | 45 | 55 | 6.5 |
| Thekkinkatti[51] | 2008 | 43 | 44 | 11 |
| Christofordis[54] | 2007 | 47 | 43 | 6.5 |
| Van Koperen[53] | 2007 | 17 | 41 | 7 |
| El-Gazzaz[55] | 2008 | 33 | 25 | 7.4 |
| Lawes[69] | 2008 | 20 | 24 | 7.4 |
| Safar[52] | 2009 | 35 | 14 | 4 |

studies. Steps to prevent dislodgement include adequately securing the plug to the primary opening, ensuring it is not dangling,[44] and instructing the patient to avoid strenuous activity for at least 2 weeks.[43,45,46] Avoidance of securing the plug at the secondary opening has been advocated because it provides countertraction to the suture at the primary opening, leading to dislodgement. Another cause of dislodgement is enlarging the fistula tract, which has been done by curetting or overdebridement of the tract. Multiple fistula tracts are often associated with a higher failure rate caused by the persistence of 1 or more tracts, usually those not treated by the plug at the time of the initial procedure.[46] These tracts are candidates for plug insertion at a later date. The importance of ensuring that the secondary opening remains open as a site for drainage cannot be overemphasized because this prevents the formation of abscesses, which is not only a cause of failure but also a cause of mortality in these patients because of perineal sepsis.[52]

There are a few controversies about the various modifications of the procedure that can be performed and their influence on the success rate. The most published modification is the concurrent use of the seton. The concept of the seton maturing the tract, making the wall more fibrotic, which results in increased healing, has been proposed by several investigators[54,55] and is recommended by a recent consensus.[45] It has also been shown to minimize sepsis and facilitate fistula closure when used in conjunction with other procedures, such as an advancement flap.[56] O'Connor and colleagues[46] and Champagne and colleagues[43] found no correlation between seton placement and increasing healing rates. They stated that the presence of the seton resulted in a technically easier insertion of the plug because it helped define the anatomy of the primary and secondary opening and helped "pull" the plug through the tract.

There is little doubt that the anal fistula plug is a promising new method of treating this complex problem but with the variable success rates, more studies need to be performed to elucidate the best procedure and postoperative care to ensure the highest chance of success.

## ADVANCEMENT FLAP

Before the advent of the collagen anal fistula plug or the use of fibrin glue, surgeons devised the endorectal/endoanal advancement flap as a sphincter-sparing method to treat complex anal fistulas. It was believed that this would preserve continence because there is no surgical division of the anal sphincter complex. There are several methods, but the technical aspects common to all methods are cleaning/debridement of the fistula tract, mobilization of a well-vascularized rectal mucosal or anodermal flap, and coverage of the internal opening of the tract with or without closure of the tract before coverage. Healing rates have been reported to be from 77% to 100% in various studies.[1,2,4,57–64] Length of follow-up is important when evaluating the success of various methods of the surgical treatment of fistula-in-ano. Ortiz and colleagues[4] performed a retrospective study of 91 patients who underwent flap repair of complex fistulas. The median follow-up was 42 months and there was a recurrence rate of 19%. These investigators noted that the median time to relapse was 5 months and that no recurrences were noted beyond 1 year of follow-up. Van Koperen and colleagues[62] evaluated their long-term outcomes from flap repair of high anal fistulas and noted that after 76 months of follow-up, recurrence was seen in 21% of patients and fecal soiling was reported in 40%.[59] This addresses an important issue and dispels the myth that incontinence is not a potential risk of flap repair.

A recent study[2] reported a transient minor incontinence rate of 8% with complete resolution by 2 months of follow-up after advancement flap repair. Additional studies have reported minor incontinence rates of 0% to 23% associated with advancement flap procedures.[57,58,63,65] Uribe and colleagues[58] performed a prospective study of 56 patients with complex fistulas who underwent advancement flap repair. Preoperative and postoperative anal manometry were performed in all patients. A significant reduction was demonstrated in mean resting pressure and maximal squeeze pressure in the study subjects 3 months postoperatively. A 21% rate of incontinence was reported, with 9% of patients reporting major disturbances in fecal continence. Perez and colleagues[60] performed a manometric study of patients who were randomized to undergo either advancement flap repair of complex fistulas or fistulotomy with concomitant sphincter repair. Their data revealed that mean resting pressure was significantly diminished postoperatively in both groups, but that maximal squeeze pressure was reduced only in the group undergoing flap repair. This finding did not equate to any difference in continence between the groups. The study results showed equivalent rates of healing between the 2 methods.

Various methods have been espoused to improve the success rates of flap repairs. Van der Hagen and colleagues[65] evaluated their experience with the treatment of complex anal fistula disease and included patients with Crohn's disease in their study group. They propose that the initial placement of a loose seton allows for resolution of sepsis and improves subsequent outcomes with advancement flap repair. They reported only 1 flap failure in 26 patients who underwent the procedure. Others have suggested that combining the use of fibrin glue obliteration of the fistula tract with endorectal advancement flap repair would potentially improve the rates of healing. Ellis and Clark[61] and van Koperen and colleagues[62] settled this argument with 2 studies that showed higher failure rates in patients who had fibrin glue instilled into their fistula tracts as an adjunct to flap repair. Perhaps the glue instillation prevents adequate drainage of fluid trapped under the flap through the external opening. It is easy to imagine how this might lead to flap failure.

The question of whether to use a partial or full thickness advancement flap was addressed in a study in 2008 by Dubsky and colleagues.[66] These investigators demonstrated a higher flap failure rate in the partial thickness group (35% vs 5%). They also demonstrated a higher incontinence score in the patients treated with partial thickness flaps, although the statistical significance of this result was not reported. There were no differences in continence that correlated to flap failure. It is difficult to draw any definitive conclusion regarding incontinence from this small data set. The likely causes of incontinence after flap repair are partial division of the internal sphincter during flap mobilization, and sphincter trauma from unintentional anal dilation during retraction for operative exposure. At present these technical aspects of the procedure seem to be unavoidable and must be taken into consideration when counseling a patient preoperatively. Tyler and colleagues[63] reported their success in treating anal fistulas using a "sphincter-sparing only" algorithm. They performed fistulotomies only when simple submucosal fistulas were present. All other fistulas were treated with loose setons followed by fibrin glue injection or advancement flaps. Glue failures went on to repeat therapy with fibrin glue or advancement flap repair. These investigators reported a 100% success rate using this algorithm with no resulting fecal incontinence. These data support the recommendation of sphincter-sparing surgery for all anal fistulas.

## SETONS

Setons are a viable treatment option for high trans-sphincteric fistulas, fistulas involving greater than half the bulk of the sphincter complex, and anterior trans-sphincteric fistulas in women. Setons are preferred to surgical fistulotomy because of the high incontinence rate associated with that technique in these patient populations.[67,68] The risk of and concern about incontinence are not eliminated with the use of cutting/tight setons. More conservative sphincter-sparing measures that do not pose a risk of incontinence, such as fistula plugs and fibrin glue, have a higher rate of recurrence than that associated with cutting setons when used to treat these complex fistulas.[35,69–71]

Numerous materials have been used for setons, including nonabsorbable suture, Penrose drains, rubber bands, vessel loops, silastic catheters, and ayurvedic thread (kshara sutra). Kshara sutra is the earliest known seton, and dates to 1000 BC. It is a linen thread soaked in kshara (an alkaline chemical made from plant extracts) that has caustic properties, resulting in slow cutting through tissue.[72]

The 2 types of setons used are cutting setons (**Fig. 5**), which slowly incise through tissue, and noncutting setons, which are primarily for drainage. With cutting setons, the skin and anal mucosa overlying the sphincter are typically divided once the internal

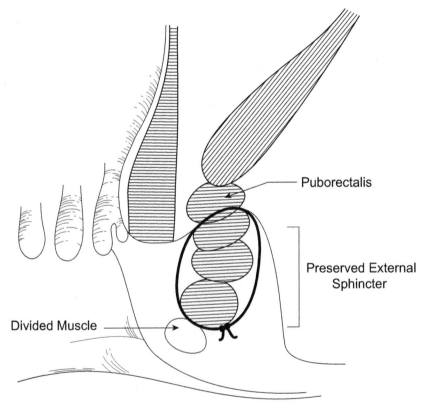

**Fig. 5.** A cutting seton, or seton fistulotomy. (*From* Belliveau P. Anal fistula. In: Fazio VM, Church JM, Delaney CP, editors. Current therapy in colon and rectal surgery. 2nd edition. Philadelphia: Elsevier Mosby; 2005. p. 30; with permission.)

and external openings of the fistula are identified. The seton is then placed through the fistula tract and tightened at varying intervals (from a few days to every 2 weeks). There may be no need for further tightening if elastic materials are used and are secured tightly at the time of surgery.[73] The time it takes to heal can range from 1 month to more than a year.[70,71] These patients require numerous follow-up visits, which require tightening of the seton, examination of the fistula tract, and potentially performance of a second procedure. For this reason Mentes and colleagues[73] used pieces of surgical gloves as cutting setons in 20 patients. These setons were secured tightly at the initial procedure and slowly cut through the sphincter mechanism without additional tightening. The average time for the seton to cut through the sphincter completely was 19 days, and a 20% rate of minor incontinence was reported. This seton has the advantages of avoiding numerous postoperative visits for adjustment, the pain associated with tightening, and the need for secondary procedures.

Noncutting (or draining) setons are typically used for patients with chronic sepsis secondary to perianal Crohn's disease or acquired immune deficiency syndrome, and in patients with severe anorectal sepsis. They are most commonly used in patients with perianal Crohn's disease that is symptomatic, does not respond to medical therapy, and whose fistula tracts encompass an appreciable amount of the sphincter mechanism (**Fig. 6**).[74,75] In a study by Williams and colleagues[74] 22 patients with Crohn's disease who met these conditions had draining setons placed in deep fistula tracts, thus converting the tracts to simple, drained fistulas with minimal symptoms. Three of the patients healed following removal of the seton. Nine patients required further treatment, but did not require a proctectomy.

In some instances, the combination of a fistulotomy and seton has been used. The theory is that a staged fistulotomy employing the use of a seton decreases the rate of incontinence postoperatively compared with the use of a fistulotomy or a cutting seton alone.[68,76,77] Durgan and colleagues[77] performed a prospective study on 10 patients with high extrasphincteric fistulas using a combination approach. First a partial fistulotomy was completed, and then 4 or 5 setons were placed through the fistula tract. The setons were sequentially tightened every 10th day. By doing this it was possible to drain the tracts and cut slowly through the remaining sphincter musculature. Twenty percent of the patients were incontinent to flatus postoperatively compared with more than 60% as found in other studies.[71] Other investigators do not believe a combination approach is beneficial. Zbar and colleagues[78] evaluated 34 patients and compared

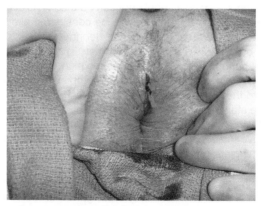

**Fig. 6.** The postoperative appearance of a draining seton using a vessel loop.

the combination approach with the use of a cutting seton alone. Eighteen patients were treated with a combined technique and 16 were treated with a cutting seton. The internal anal sphincter muscle was repaired after it was incised, and this was followed by placement of a seton through the intersphincteric space. No difference was found between the 2 groups in healing time, recurrence rates, or incontinence rates.

As mentioned earlier, incontinence is still common with the use of setons. It is rarely seen with noncutting setons because their function is primarily to drain, not to incise the anal sphincters.[16] Incontinence has been attributed to several factors, including hard and gutter-shaped scars in the anal canal, loss of sphincter function, and loss of anal canal sensation.[71] Patients may experience incontinence to flatus, liquid stool, or solid stool at varying levels, with different effects on their quality of life. Not all studies identify specifically the type of incontinence patients are experiencing, nor do they differentiate transient postoperative incontinence from long-term dysfunction. In addition, many studies refer simply to major and minor incontinence without defining them. Minor incontinence is defined as persistent incontinence to gas or occasionally liquid stool. Major incontinence refers to inability to control the passage of formed stool or frequently liquid stool. Isbister and Sanea[70] performed a retrospective review of 47 patients who had cutting setons placed for complex fistulas. Their postoperative incontinence rate was 36.2% for gas, 8.5% for liquid stool, and 2.3% for solid stool. Before seton placement 14.9% of their study group were incontinent to gas or liquid stool. One fistula recurrence was reported. An additional study reported a minor incontinence rate of 63% with a 6% recurrence rate.[71]

Although the risk of an impairment in continence is high with seton fistulotomy, this technique is used for complex, hard-to-treat fistulas that recur more frequently with sphincter-sparing methods including fibrin glue and fistula plugs.

## FISTULOTOMY

Fistulotomy is still considered the standard by many surgeons for low, simple anal fistulas, such as submucosal, intersphincteric, and low trans-sphincteric fistulas (**Fig. 7**).[67,79] According to 'The practice parameters for the treatment of perianal abscess and fistula-in-ano,' completed by Whiteford and colleagues[79] in 2005, fistulotomies may be used to treat simple anal fistulas in cryptoglandular disease and simple, low Crohn's fistulas that are symptomatic. Their definition of simple includes a fistula tract that crosses less than 30% to 50% of the external sphincter, is not anterior in women, has only 1 tract, is not recurrent, and is present in a patient with perfect continence. In addition, the patient should not carry a diagnosis of Crohn's disease or have received pelvic radiation for the fistula to be considered simple. Whiteford and colleagues[79] also recommended the use of tract debridement and fibrin glue injection for simple fistulas, because it is a benign treatment with no detrimental effects on further treatment, although the recurrence rates are higher than with fistulotomy. Fistulotomy can be used as a staged procedure for complex fistulas in conjunction with a seton according to the practice parameters.

Fistulotomy is the standard treatment for submucosal fistulas because there is no concern for incontinence and recurrence is low.[63] Controversy arises in the treatment of fistulas that involve the sphincter mechanism because of the potential for incontinence with nonsphincter-sparing methods. Most surgeons use fistulotomies for simple intersphincteric fistulas; however, some groups such as Tyler and colleagues[63] use fistulotomies only for submucosal fistulas. In all of their patients with sphincter involvement a seton is placed, followed by fibrin glue or a rectal advancement flap as a staged procedure.

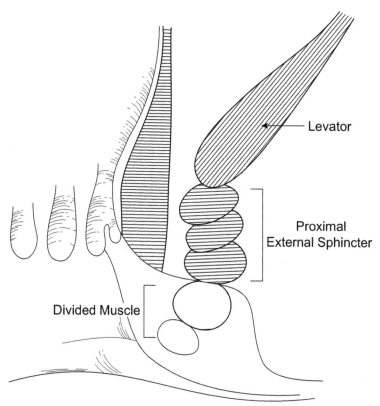

**Fig. 7.** Fistulotomy of a low trans-sphincteric fistula. (*From* Belliveau P. Anal fistula. In: Fazio VM, Church JM, Delaney CP, editors. Current therapy in colon and rectal surgery. 2nd edition. Philadelphia: Elsevier Mosby; 2005. p. 29; with permission.)

Other surgeons use fistulotomies more frequently and apply them to complex fistulas also. Perez and colleagues[80] have completed multiple studies looking at fistulotomies with primary sphincter reconstruction for complex fistulas. They conducted a prospective study with 16 patients who had recurrent high trans-sphincteric, suprasphincteric, or extrasphincteric fistulas. Each patient underwent a fistulotomy in which the internal and external sphincters were divided. All accessory tracts were excised. The internal and external anal sphincters were repaired using an overlapping technique. All patients who were incontinent preoperatively improved their continence score postoperatively (the Wexner grading scale was used) except for 1 female patient whose incontinence score was unchanged. Two patients (25%) developed new minor incontinence. The results were similar in a larger prospective study of 35 patients, in which 45% had recurrent disease preoperatively.[81] Perez and colleagues[60] also compared their method with advancement flaps. They completed a prospective randomized study of 55 patients with complex fistulas (high trans-sphincteric and suprasphincteric) and found no difference in the recurrence or incontinence rate between the 2 methods.

As mentioned earlier, the incontinence rate with fistulotomy is high and can vary greatly, with rates from 0% to 40% in low intersphincteric fistulas.[59,82] As a result, not only have new methods been developed to treat fistulas, such as fibrin glue and fistula plugs, but numerous studies have been undertaken to determine predisposing factors for incontinence. Toyonaga and colleagues[83] performed a prospective randomized study with 148 patients with intersphincteric fistulas and found that age, sex, previous surgery, duration of fistula, and location and level of the internal opening did not significantly influence incontinence postoperatively in patients undergoing a fistulotomy for treatment. In addition, low anal sphincter resting pressure and short anal canal length did not predispose patients to postoperative incontinence. These investigators found that low voluntary contraction pressure and multiple previous drainage procedures predisposed patients to postoperative incontinence. They recommend preoperative manometry for all patients, and avoidance of fistulotomy if the risk factors already mentioned were identified. Koperen and colleagues[59] performed a study of 179 patients in which gender, age, tertiary referral, prior fistula surgery, and smoking were not found to be risk factors. Other studies show conflicting results. Cavanaugh and colleagues[82] in a study of 110 patients found trans-sphincteric tracts and the extent of external sphincter involvement to be risk factors for postoperative incontinence after fistulotomy. In addition, Garcia-Aguilar and colleagues[84] determined female gender, previous surgery, high internal opening, and type of fistula surgery (procedures performed for high fistulas) were all risk factors for postoperative incontinence following a fistulotomy.

Gupta[85,86] conducted fistulotomies using radiofrequency ablation in an effort to decrease complications associated with conventional fistulotomy. In a study of 100 patients with low anal fistulas he compared conventional fistulotomy to radiofrequency fistulotomy and found those in the radiofrequency group had less gas incontinence (4 vs 12%). It is speculated that the reason for decreased incontinence is that there is less damage to the surrounding tissue because radiofrequency does not heat surrounding tissue. Similar results could be expected with the use of an ultrasonic dissector, although this has not been studied.

Recurrence has been reported to be lower with fistulotomy for low intersphincteric fistulas when compared with other methods, such as fibrin glue[36,59]; however, a long-term study conducted by Van der Hagen and colleagues[87] suggests that the recurrence rate is higher if follow-up of the patients is performed long enough. These investigators looked at the long-term (72 months) recurrence rates of fistulotomy for low perianal fistulas. Many studies follow patients up for 12 to 24 months, which for this study had a recurrence rate of 7% and 16%, respectively. These investigators noted at 72 months of follow-up the recurrence rate was 39%. Fifty-four percent of recurrences occurred in a new location, and patients with Crohn's disease were included in this trial. At 48 months, fistula had recurred in 60% of the patients with Crohn's disease included in the trial. Any study that includes inflammatory bowel disease patients in long-term follow-up will have a higher rate of recurrence compared with studies that do not. Although these data are useful, the elevated long-term recurrence rate seen in this study should be considered when selecting a method of treatment.

Although incontinence may be seen with low intersphincteric fistulotomy, most cases are minor (involving gas and occasionally liquid incontinence), but may still significantly affect the patient's lifestyle. Cavanaugh and colleagues[82] conducted a study to examination how postoperative incontinence affects the quality of life for these patients. They conducted a retrospective study of 110 patients that revealed that 64% of patients had at least occasional incontinence, with 14% reporting mild lifestyle restriction, 10% reporting moderate restriction, 9% reporting mild depression, and 4% reporting moderate depression. Moderate and severe embarrassment were reported by 5% and 1%, respectively.

Fistulotomy remains a major part of fistula treatment, despite the high rate of incontinence that may be seen postoperatively. It is an effective method of dealing with the disease, with the recurrence rates being much lower than those for sphincter-sparing methods. Although many patients experience minor incontinence that does not affect their lifestyle, it can have a severe effect on others.

## NEWER METHODS OF TREATMENT

The search for the optimal treatment of anal fistula continues because of disappointing success rates with sphincter-sparing options and high incontinence rates associated with sphincter dividing procedures. The ligation of the intersphincteric fistula tract (LIFT) procedure was first described in Thailand by Rojanasakul.[88] This is a procedure in which a small incision is made in the intersphincteric groove (much like an open internal sphincterotomy) just over where the fistula tract crosses from the internal to the external sphincter. The intersphincteric space is opened and the fistula tract is clearly defined and ligated with suture. Short-term results in 18 patients treated by the LIFT procedure and observed prospectively showed healing in all but 1 by a mean time of 4 weeks.[88] These results prompted the University of Minnesota Colorectal Surgery Group to adopt the technique and study it in the long term. Beals[89] presented results with the use of the LIFT technique at the 94th annual American College of Surgeons Clinical Congress and reported a 58% success rate in 31 patients followed for a mean time of 35 weeks. Time until failure ranged from 4 to 63 weeks with a median of 19 weeks. This result has prompted further investigation of this promising technique, and a trial comparing the LIFT technique with the collagen fistula plug is currently accruing patients.

Garcia-Olmo and colleagues[90] investigated the use of injected adipose-derived stem cells in the treatment of complex anal fistulas. Their idea was based on experience from plastic surgery of the use of these cells in tissue repair.[91] These investigators compared the use of injected fibrin glue with glue that contained 20 million units of adipose-derived stem cells in 49 patients with complex fistulas that were either cryptoglandular or related to Crohn's disease. Fistula healing was noted in 71% of the group treated with stem cells as opposed to only 16% healing in the group who received fibrin glue. There were no differences in adverse reactions between the groups and none appeared to be related to treatment with stem cells. A 17% recurrence rate was noted after 1 year of follow-up in the group treated with stem cells. Garcia-Olmo and colleagues concluded that fistula tract injection of adipose-derived stem cells was safe and effective in the treatment of this complex disease. Both of these techniques show promise and warrant further long-term, randomized investigation.

## SUMMARY

The surgical management of fistula-in-ano is driven by the amount of sphincter complex that is involved with the tract, and the potential coexistence of Crohn's disease. The preferred method of management is dictated by these factors. Sphincter-sparing methods have lower success rates than nonsphincter-sparing techniques, but come with little to no risk of fecal continence. The first line of treatment of this disease should focus on methods that do not require any sphincter division. These techniques do not prevent a more aggressive surgical approach if they fail. Submucosal fistulas can be treated by fistulotomy with little risk. Intersphincteric and low trans-sphincteric fistulas may be treated with fistulotomy as first-line management if the patient has perfect continence preoperatively, and the patient has no previous history of sphincter injury. Anterior fistulas in women must be approached with caution. It is to be hoped continued research will lead to improved success rates in sphincter-sparing options.

## REFERENCES

1. Loffler T, Welsch T, Muhl S, et al. Long-term success rate after surgical treatment of anorectal and rectovaginal fistulas in Crohn's disease. Int J Colorectal Dis 2009. [Epub ahead of print].
2. Abbas MA, Lemus-Rangel R, Hamadani A. Long-term outcome of endorectal advancement flap for complex anorectal fistulae. Am Surg 2008;74(10):921–4.
3. Hamadani A, Haigh PI, Liu IL, et al. Who is at risk for developing chronic anal fistula or recurrent anal sepsis after initial perianal abscess? Dis Colon Rectum 2009;52:217–21.
4. Ortiz H, Marzo M, de Miguel M, et al. Length of follow-up after fistulotomy and fistulectomy associated with endorectal advancement flap repair for fistula in ano. Br J Surg 2008;95(4):484–7.
5. Oliver I, Lavueva FJ, Piorez VF, et al. Randomized clinical trial comparing simple drainage of anorectal abscess with and without fistula tract treatment. Int J Colorectal Dis 2003;18(2):107–10.
6. Quah HM, Tang CL, Eu KW, et al. Meta-analysis of randomized clinical trials comparing drainage alone vs primary sphincter-cutting procedures for anorectal abscess-fistula. Int J Colorectal Dis 2006;21(6):602–9.
7. Aluwihar A. Finding the source of a fistula. Colorectal Dis 2005;7(5):528–9.
8. Erhan Y, Sakarya A, Aydede H, et al. A case of large mucinous adenocarcinoma arising in a long-standing fistula-in-ano. Dig Surg 2003;20(1):69–71.
9. Kim T, Chae G, Chung SS, et al. Faecal incontinence in male patients. Colorectal Dis 2008;10(2):124–30.
10. Lindsey I, Jones OM, Smilgin-Humphreys MM, et al. Patterns of fecal incontinence after anal surgery. Dis Colon Rectum 2004;47(10):1643–9.
11. Buchmann P, Keighley MR, Allan RN, et al. Natural history of perianal Crohn's disease. Ten-year follow up: a plea for conservatism. Am J Surg 1980;140(5):642–4.
12. Halme L, Sainio AP. Factors related to frequency, type and outcome of anal fistulas in Crohn's disease. Dis Colon Rectum 1995;35:55–9.
13. Jakobovits J, Schuster MM. Metronidazole therapy for Crohn's disease and associated fistulae. Am J Gastroenterol 1984;79:533–40.
14. Stringer EE, Nicholson TJ, Armstrong D. Efficacy of topical metronidazole (10 percent) in the treatment of anorectal Crohn's disease. Dis Colon Rectum 2005;48:970–4.
15. Sangwan YP, Schoetz DJ, Murray JJ, et al. Perianal Crohn's disease: results of local surgical treatment. Dis Colon Rectum 1996;39(5):529–35.
16. Faucheron J, Saint-Marc O, Guibert L, et al. Long-term seton drainage for high anal fistulas in Crohn's disease – a sphincter-saving operation? Dis Colon Rectum 1996;39:208–11.
17. Hanaver SB, Feagan BG, Lichtenstein GR, et al. Maintenance infliximab for Crohn's disease: the ACCENT I randomized trial. Lancet 2002;359:1541–9.
18. Present DH, Rutgerts P, Targan S, et al. Infliximab for the treatment of fistula in patients with Crohn's disease. N Engl J Med 1999;340:1398–405.
19. Sands BE, Anderson FH, Bernstein CN, et al. Infliximab maintenance for fistulizing Crohn's disease. N Engl J Med 2004;350:876–85.

20. Gaertner WB, Decanini A, Mellgren A, et al. Does infliximab infusion impact results of operative treatment for Crohn's perianal fistulas? Dis Colon Rectum 2007;50(11):1754–60.

21. Gonzalez-Ruiz C, Kaiser AM, Vukasin P, et al. Intraoperative physical diagnosis in the management of anal fistula. Am Surg 2006;72(1):11–5.

22. Ratto C, Grillo E, Parello A, et al. Endoanal ultrasound-guided surgery for anal fistula. Endoscopy 2005;37(8):722–8.

23. Buchanan GN, Williams AM, Bartram CI, et al. Potential clinical implications of directions of a trans-sphincteric anal fistula track. Br J Surg 2003;90(10): 1250–5.

24. Swinscoe MT, Ventakasubramanium AK, Jayne DG. Fibrin glue for fistula-in-ano: the evidence reviewed. Tech Coloproctol 2005;9(2):89–94.

25. Hjortrup A, Moesgaard F, Kjaergard J. Fibrin adhesive in the treatment of perineal fistulas. Dis Colon Rectum 1991;34:752–4.

26. Hammond TM, Grahn MF, Lunniss PJ. Fibrin glue in the management of anal fistulae. Colorectal Dis 2004;6(5):308–19.

27. de Parades V, Far HS, Etienney I, et al. Seton drainage and fibrin glue injection for complex anal fistulas. Colorectal dis 2008. [Epub ahead of print].

28. Ritchie RD, Sackier JM, Hodde JP. Incontinence rates after cutting seton treatment for anal fistula. Colorectal Dis 2008. [Epub ahead of print].

29. Dietz DW. Role of fibrin glue in the management of simple and complex fistula in ano. J Gastrointest Surg 2006;10(5):631–2.

30. Cintron JR, Park JJ, Orsay CP, et al. Repair of fistula-in-ano using fibrin adhesive. Long-term follow up. Dis Colon Rectum 2000;43:944–50.

31. Gisbertz SS, Sosef MN, Festen S, et al. Treatment of fistulas in ano with fibrin glue. Dig Surg 2005;22(1–2):91–4.

32. Maralcan G, Bakukonu I, Aybasti N, et al. The use of fibrin glue in the treatment of fistula-in-ano: a prospective study. Surg Today 2006;36(2):166–70.

33. Adams T, Yang J, Kondylis LA, et al. Long-term outlook after successful fibrin glue ablation of cryptoglandular transsphincteric fistula-in-ano. Dis Colon Rectum 2008;51(10):1488–90.

34. Sentovich SM. Fibrin glue for all anal fistulas. J Gastrointest Surg 2001;5(2): 158–61.

35. Sentovich SM. Fibrin glue for anal fistulas: long-term results. Dis Colon Rectum 2003;46(4):498–502.

36. Lindsey I, Smilgin-Humphreys MM, Cunningham C, et al. A randomized, controlled trial of fibrin glue vs conventional treatment for anal fistula. Dis Colon Rectum 2002;45(12):1608–15.

37. Zmora O, Neufeld D, Ziv Y, et al. Prospective, multicenter evaluation of highly concentrated fibrin glue in the treatment of complex cryptogenic perianal fistulas. Dis Colon Rectum 2005;7(5):528–9.

38. Patrlj L, Kocman B, Martinac M, et al. Fibrin glue-antibiotic mixture in the treatment of anal fistulae: experience with 69 cases. Dig Surg 2000;17(1): 77–80.

39. Witte ME, Klaase JM, Gerritsen JJ, et al. Fibrin glue treatment for simple and complex anal fistulas. Hepatogastroenterology 2007;54(76):1071–3.

40. Robb BW, Vogler SA, Nussbaum MN, et al. Early experience using porcine small intestinal submucosa to repair fistulas-in-ano. Dis Colon Rectum 2004;47: 565–660.

41. Johnson EK, Gaw JU, Armstrong D. Efficacy of anal fistula plug vs fibrin glue in closure of anorectal fistulas. Dis Colon Rectum 2006;49(3):371–6.

42. Ueno T, Pickett LC, de la Fuente SG, et al. Clinical application of porcine small intestinal submucosa in the management of infected or potentially contaminated abdominal defects. J Gastrointest Surg 2004;8:109–12.

43. Champagne BJ, O'Connor LM, Ferguson M, et al. Efficacy of anal fistula plug in closure of cryptoglandular fistulas: long-term follow-up. Dis Colon Rectum 2006; 49(12):1817–21.

44. Hammond TM, Lunniss PJ. Novel biomaterials in the management of anal fistulas. Dis Colon Rectum 2006;49(9):1463–4.

45. The Surgisis AFP anal fistula plug: report of a consensus conference. Colorectal Dis 2008;10(1):17–20.

46. O'Connor L, Champagne BJ, Ferguson MA, et al. Efficacy of anal fistula plug in closure of Crohn's anorectal fistulas. Dis Colon Rectum 2006;49(10):1569–73.

47. Ellis CN. Bioprosthetic plugs for complex anal fistulas: an early experience. J Surg Educ 2007;64(1):36–40.

48. Garg P. To determine the efficacy of anal fistula plug in the treatment of high fistula-in-ano: an initial experience. Colorectal Dis 2008. [Epub ahead of print].

49. Schwandner O, Stadler F, Dietl O, et al. Initial experience on efficacy in closure of cryptoglandular and Crohn's transsphincteric fistulas by the use of the anal fistula plug. Int J Colorectal Dis 2008;23(3):319–24.

50. Ky AJ, Sylla P, Steinhagen R, et al. Collagen fistula plug for the treatment of anal fistulas. Dis Colon Rectum 2008;51(6):838–43.

51. Thekkinkattil D, Botterill I, Ambrose S, et al. Efficacy of the anal fistula plug in complex anorectal fistulae. Colorectal Dis 2008. [Epub ahead of print].

52. Safar B, Jobanputra S, Sands D, et al. Anal Fistula Plug: intial experience and outcomes. Dis Colon Rectum 2009;52:248–52.

53. van Koperen PJ, D'Hoore A, Wolthuis AM, et al. Anal fistula plug for closure of difficult anorectal fistula: a prospective study. Dis Colon Rectum 2007;50(12): 2168–72.

54. Christoforidis D, Etzioni DA, Goldberg SM, et al. Treatment of complex anal fistulas with the collagen fistula plug. Dis Colon Rectum 2008;51(10):1482–7.

55. El-Gazzaz G, Zutshi M, Hull T. A retrospective review of chronic anal fistulae treated by anal fistulae plug. Colorectal Dis 2009. [Epub ahead of print].

56. Sonoda T, Hull T, Piedmonte MR, et al. Outcomes of primary repair of anorectal and rectovaginal fistulae using endorectal advancement flap. Dis Colon Rectum 2002;45:1622–8.

57. Golub RW, Wise WE, Kerner BA, et al. Endorectal mucosal advancement flap: the preferred method for complex cryptoglandular fistula-in-ano. J Gastrointest Surg 1997;1(5):487–91.

58. Uribe N, Million M, Minguez M, et al. Clinical and manometric results of endorectal advancement flaps for complex anal fistula. Int Colorectal Dis 2007;22(3):259–64.

59. Koperen P, Wind J, Bemelman W, et al. Long-term functional outcome and risk factors for recurrence after surgical treatment for low and high perianal fistulas of cryptoglandular origin. Dis Colon Rectum 2008;51:1475–81.

60. Perez F, Arroyo A, Serrano P, et al. Randomized clinical and manometric study of advancement flap versus fistulotomy with sphincter reconstruction in the management of complex fistula-in-ano. Am J Surg 2006;192:34–40.

61. Ellis CN, Clark S. Fibrin glue as an adjuvant to flap repair of anal fistulas: a randomized, controlled study. Dis Colon Rectum 2006;49(11):1736–40.

62. van Koperen PJ, Wind J, Bemelman WA, et al. Fibrin glue and transanal rectal advancement flap for high transsphincteric perianal fistulas; is there any advantage? Int J Colorectal Dis 2008;23(7):697–701.

63. Tyler K, Aarons C, Sentovich S. Successful sphincter-sparing surgery for all anal fistulas. Dis Colon Rectum 2007;50:1535–9.

64. Ho KS, Ho YH. Controlled, randomized trial of island flap anoplasty for treatment of trans-sphincteric fistula-in-ano: early results. Tech Coloproctol 2005;9(2):166–8.

65. van der Hagen SJ, Baeten CG, Soeters PB, et al. Staged mucosal advancement flap for the treatment of complex anal fistulas: pretreatment with noncutting setons and in case of recurrent multiple abscesses a diverting stoma. Colorectal Dis 2005;7(5):513–8.

66. Dubsky PC, Stift A, Friedl J, et al. Endorectal advancement flaps in the treatment of high anal fistula of cryptoglandular origin: full-thickness vs. mucosal-rectum flaps. Dis Colon Rectum 2008;51(6):852–7.

67. Towsend C, Beauchamp R, Evers B, editors. Sabiston textbook of surgery: the biological basis of modern surgical practice. 18th edition. Philadelphia: Saunders Elsevier; 2008. p. 1447–9.

68. Vasilevsky C, Gordon P. Results of treatment of fistula-in-ano. Dis Colon Rectum 1985;28(4):225–31.

69. Lawes DA, Efron JE, Abbas M, et al. Early experience with the bioabsorbable anal fistula plug. World J Surg 2008;32(6):1157–9.

70. Isbister WH, Sanea NA. The cutting seton: an experience at King Faisal Specialist Hospital. Dis Colon Rectum 2001;44:722–7.

71. Hamalainen KJ, Sainio AP. Cutting seton for anal fistulas: high risk of minor control defects. Dis Colon Rectum 1997;40:1443–7.

72. Ho KS, Tsang C, Seow-Choen F, et al. Prospective randomized trial comparing ayurvedic cutting seton and fistulotomy for low fistula-in-ano. Tech Coloproctol 2001;5:137–41.

73. Mentes BB, Oktemer S, Tezcaner T, et al. Elastic one-stage cutting seton for the treatment of high anal fistulas: preliminary results. Tech Coloproctol 2004;8: 159–62.

74. Williams JG, Rothenberger DA. Fistula-in-ano in Crohn's disease: results of aggressive surgical treatment. Dis Colon Rectum 1991;34:378–84.

75. Person B, Wexner S. Management of perianal Crohn's disease. Current treatment options. Gastroenterology 2005;8:197–209.

76. McCourtney JS, Finlay IG. Cutting seton without preliminary internal sphincterotomy in management of complex high fistula-in-ano. Dis Colon Rectum 1996;39:55–8.

77. Durgun V, Perek A, Kapan M, et al. Partial fistulotomy and modified cutting seton procedure in the treatment of high extrasphincteric perianal fistula. Dig Surg 2002;19:56–8.

78. Zbar AP, Ramesh J, Beer-Gabel M, et al. Conventional cutting vs. internal anal sphincter-preserving seton for high trans-sphincteric fistula: a prospective randomized manometric and clinic trial. Tech Coloproctol 2003;7:89–94.

79. Whiteford M, Kilkenny J, Hyman N, et al. Practice parameters for the treatment of perianal abscess and fistula-in-ano (revised). Dis Colon Rectum 2005;48: 1337–42.

80. Perez F, Arroyo A, Serrano P, et al. Prospective clinical and manometric study of fistulotomy with primary sphincter reconstruction in the management of recurrent complex fistula-in-ano. Int J Colorectal Dis 2006;21:522–6.

81. Perez F, Arroyo A, Serrano P, et al. Fistulotomy with primary sphincter reconstruction in the management of complex fistula-in-ano: prospective study of clinical and manometric results. J Am Coll Surg 2005;200:897–903.

82. Cavanaugh M, Hyman N, Osler T. Fecal incontinence severity index after fistulotomy: a predictor of quality of life. Dis Colon Rectum 2002;45:349–53.

83. Toyonaga T, Matsushima M, Kiriu T, et al. Factors affecting continence for fistulotomy for intersphincteric fistula-in-ano. Int J Colorectal Dis 2007;22:1071–5.

84. Garcia-Aguilar J, Belmone C, Wong D, et al. Anal fistula surgery: factors associated with recurrence and incontinence. Dis Colon Rectum 1996;39:723–9.

85. Gupta P. Anal fistulotomy with radiofrequency. Dig Surg 2004;21:72–3.

86. Gupta P. Radiosurgical fistulotomy: an alternative to conventional procedure in fistula in ano. Curr Surg 2003;60:524–8.

87. van der Hagen S, Baeten C, Soeters P, et al. Long-term outcome following mucosal advancement flap for high perianal fistulas and fistulotomy for low perianal fistulas. Recurrent perianal fistulas: failure of treatment or recurrent patient disease? Int J Colorectal Dis 2006;21:784–90.

88. Rojanasakul A. Total anal sphincter saving technique for fistula-in-ano: the ligation of intersphincteric fistula tract. J Med Assoc Thai 2007;90(3):581–6.

89. Beals JK. Novel surgical correction of intersphincteric perianal fistulas preserves anal sphincter. Presented at American College of Surgeons 94th Annual Clinical Congress. October 15, 2008.

90. Garcia-Olmo D, Herreros D, Pascual I, et al. Expanded adipose-derived stem cells for the treatment of complex perianal fistula: a Phase II clinical trial. Dis Colon Rectum 2009;52:79–86.

91. De Ugarte DA, Ashjian PH, Elbarbary A, et al. Future of fat as raw material for tissue regeneration. Ann Plast Surg 2003;50(2):215–9.

# Rectovaginal Fistula

Bradley J. Champagne, MD[a,b,*], Michael F. McGee, MD[c,d,e]

**KEYWORDS**

- Rectovaginal fistula • Crohn's disease • Etiology • Evaluation

The dramatic psychosocial impact that a rectovaginal fistula (RVF) has on a woman's life cannot be overstated. The patient's self-esteem and intimate relationships can be drastically altered. Furthermore, this condition commonly occurs in the background of another disabling disease state, such as Crohn's disease or malignancy.

The management involves an organized and detailed workup to accurately make the diagnosis and then implement the appropriate treatment. Only a combination of advanced imaging, physical examination, and clinical experience will afford the surgeon the opportunity to precisely identify the location and cause of this problem. There is no level I evidence for the appropriate management of RVFs. The most common causes, diagnostic tests, and available surgical treatments encountered are outlined in this article. The choice of repair depends on various patient and disease factors and basic surgical tenets.

## ETIOLOGY

A fistula is an abnormal communication between 2 epithelialized surfaces. RVFs are defined as perianal lesions that arise from a penetrating ulceration of the anal canal or rectum into the vagina.[1] Most RVFs arise from obstetric and vaginal trauma; however, inflammatory bowel disease (IBD), radiation proctitis, and pelvic infection are other causes.

### Obstetric and Vaginal Trauma

Obstetric trauma is the cause of up to 88% of RVFs,[2] occurring in 0.1% of vaginal deliveries in Western countries.[3] Fistula formation typically occurs as a result of a high-grade perineal body laceration caused during delivery. In Western counties,

[a] Division of Colorectal Surgery, University Hospitals Case Medical Center, Case Western Reserve University, 11100 Euclid Avenue, Cleveland, OH 44106-5047, USA
[b] University Hospitals Case Medical Center, Case Western Reserve University, 11100 Euclid Avenue, Cleveland, OH 44106-5047, USA
[c] Department of Surgery, University Hospitals Case Medical Center, Case Western Reserve University, 11100 Euclid Avenue, Cleveland, OH 44106-5047, USA
[d] Metrohealth Medical Center, Case Western Reserve University, USA
[e] Louis Stokes Wade Park Veterans Affairs Medical Center, USA
* Corresponding author. Department of Surgery, University Hospitals Case Medical Center, Case Western Reserve University, 11100 Euclid Avenue, Cleveland, OH 44106-5047.
*E-mail address:* brad.champagne@uhhospitals.org (B.J. Champagne).

Surg Clin N Am 90 (2010) 69–82
doi:10.1016/j.suc.2009.09.003
0039-6109/09/$ – see front matter © 2010 Published by Elsevier Inc.

surgical.theclinics.com

primiparity, midline episiotomies, increasing birth weight, and the use of vaginal forceps are the risk factors associated with severe perineal lacerations.[4] Often such lacerations are recognized and primarily repaired at the time of childbirth. Unrecognized deep tears or inadequate healing generates a persistent aberrant connection between the rectum and vagina, allowing passage of gas, mucus, and stool to the vagina. In developing nations with limited access to obstetric care, protracted obstructed delivery results in stillbirth with vaginal wall and perineal body pressure necrosis that leads to RVF formation. RVFs are endemic in sub-Saharan Africa and South Asia, with an estimated incidence of 50,000 to 100,000 new cases annually and a suggested prevalence of 2 million.[5,6] Vaginal trauma induced by retained foreign bodies, such as pessaries,[7–10] sexual objects,[11] and coitus can result in RVF.[12,13]

### IBD and Other Inflammatory Disorders

Fistulizing Crohn's disease (FCD) is an idiopathic, chronic, unremitting disease characterized by transmural inflammation of the gastrointestinal tract, and it is the second leading cause of RVF.[14] In general, the cumulative incidence of all perianal fistulas in Crohn's disease is 50% after age 20 years, and up to 9% of these are RVFs.[15] Other reports estimate that up to 10% of women with Crohn's disease will develop an RVF.[16] The incidence of Crohn's RVF is thought to be proportionate to the frequency and severity of large-bowel inflammation.[17] Rarely, RVF with ulcerative colitis has been reported.[18] Other autoimmune disorders, such as Behçet disease, have been associated with RVFs.[19,20]

### Radiation

Radiation therapy is an important component of multimodality therapy for several pelvic malignancies and can ultimately result in RVF. Adjuvant external beam radiotherapy is commonly used for the treatment of high-risk cervical cancer, high-grade endometrial cancer with lymph node metastases, and advanced vulvar and vaginal cancers. Radiation is acutely cytotoxic to targeted cells and causes chronic, lingering obliterative endarteritis to targeted tissues, resulting in chronic inflammation and ischemia. Occurrence of RVF in this ischemic and inflammatory environment is well described.[21,22] Interstitial brachytherapy, which relies on surgical implanted radioactive seeds to deliver more exacting doses of radiotherapy, is also a nidus for RVF formation.[23] Topical formalin, which is commonly used to treat bleeding from collateral radiation proctitis, is thought to be a rare cause of RVF formation.[24]

### Cancer

Primary anorectal, perineal, and pelvic cancers, with or without surgery or radiation, can cause RVF. Invasive tumor growth can erode into luminal structures, such as the vagina or rectum, allowing fistulization. The added combination of neoadjuvant radiation and surgery to remove cancer in this region render postoperative tumor beds particularly vulnerable to late RVF.

### Postoperative RVF

Postoperative iatrogenic complications are common causes of RVF. Previous anorectal, vaginal, or low pelvic surgery can lead to injury and abnormal healing that ultimately results in fistulization, especially in the posthysterectomy woman. Overall, the incidence of RVF after operative treatment for low rectal cancer is reported to be 0.9% to 10%.[25–28] Low and very low anterior proctosigmoidectomy, use of the double-stapled technique, and combined resection of the uterus and/or partial vaginectomy during proctectomy are identified as risk factors for the development of

RVF. Protective diverting ostomies in the setting of rectal cancer construction do not completely ameliorate fistula risk, as RVF can occur in up to 11% of patients despite complete enteric diversion.[27]

RVF is a reported complication of new anorectal procedures using specialized endorectal stapling devices, such as the procedure for prolapse and hemorrhoids[29–32] and stapled transanal rectal resection procedure[32–35] for obstructive defecation syndrome. In addition, contemporary urogynecologic procedures, such as transvaginal and perineal mesh placement for pelvic organ prolapse[36–39] and rigid vaginal dilatation, are reported to cause RVF.[40]

### Infection

Various pelvic, perianal, and urogenital infectious processes can lead to erosive inflammation and RVF. Abscesses arising from the crypts of Morgagni, Bartholin gland abscesses,[41] and diverticulitis can cause intense inflammation that culminates in a fistulous tract with the vagina. Typically, diverticular RVF occurs between the rectosigmoid junction and vaginal cuff in the setting of prior hysterectomy. Infections, such as tuberculosis, lymphogranuloma venereum, human papilloma virus, human immunodeficiency virus, cytomegalovirus, and schistosomiasis are infrequent causes of RVF.[42–47]

## ANATOMIC CLASSIFICATION

RVFs are further subclassified according to anorectal anatomic landmarks. RVFs with rectal origins proximal to the anorectal sphincter complex are considered "high" RVFs. Transphincteric fistulas, or more commonly "low" RVFs or "anovaginal" fistulas, originate distally from within the anal sphincter complex. The distinction between low and high RVFs is of paramount importance because the operative strategy for each entity varies.

## EVALUATION
### History and Physical Examination

Typically, women presenting to a clinic with undiagnosed RVF primarily complain of stool, gas, or odorous mucopurulent discharge per vagina. Occasionally, this may be confused with rectal incontinence by the patients or referring physician. Alternatively, dyspareunia, perineal pain, and recurrent vaginal infections may be heralding symptoms. Before examination, a careful and thorough history must be sought regarding medical, surgical, and obstetric history. Patients should be questioned thoroughly regarding Crohn's disease symptomology, and constitutional symptoms, such as recent weight loss and fatigue, should be assessed in screening consideration of malignancy. Obtaining past medical records specific to obstetric and surgical procedures may prove helpful, as many patients are unaware of the rationale and nature of past operations. Review of recent screening colonoscopy and gynecologic pelvic examinations, complete with histopathologic results, should be performed. A preexamination assessment of the patient's continence should also be performed, paying particular attention to the frequency and severity of any previous incontinence episodes.

After an appropriate basic physical examination, special consideration should be paid to extraintestinal signs consistent with that of Crohn's disease. Inguinal lymphadenopathy should be assessed. Inspection of the perineum and perianal areas should seek evidence of abscesses, fistulas, or scars that indicate prior perianal inflammation. Lighted vaginal speculum examination should seek to identify vulvar, vaginal, or cervical abnormalities as tolerated by the patient. Pelvic inflammatory disease must be excluded. Tender, inflamed, and infected tissue may require thorough examination under anesthesia. Particular attention should be focused on the posterior wall (ie, rectovaginal septum), as RVF orifice sizes range from microscopic to massive defects. Not all RVFs are seen on examination, so one must reject skepticism in a woman with proven risk factors and maintain a high index of suspicion during workup.

Visual inspection of the anoderm should follow pelvic examination, noting unusual findings, such as atypical fissures or mucosal irregularities. Irregular masses may be palpated on digital rectal examination. RVFs are often felt as an irregular mass arising from the rectovaginal septum on bimanual examination. A qualitative assessment of sphincter tone is important during digital rectal examination, as baseline continence affects surgical treatment options. Clinic-based anoscopy and rigid proctoscopy are necessary adjuncts during the initial workup of RVF. The entire rectum and anal canal should be inspected for mucosal irregularities, stricture, or active proctitis. Full colonoscopy may be necessary to exclude the presence of synchronous foci of inflammation or neoplasias.

If the suspicion for RVF is high but remains elusive on examination, a more thorough examination under anesthesia may be performed (**Fig. 1**).

### Radiography

For newly diagnosed patients without history of prior fistula, IBD, or obstetric trauma, pelvic malignancy must be considered as a potential cause. Moreover, in patients with known malignancy, regional recurrence must be considered as the cause of new RVF. In these cases, initial workup should include computed tomography (CT) of the abdomen and pelvis to exclude malignancy.

When thorough physical examination and examination under anesthesia fail to localize a fistula of high clinical suspicion, specialized diagnostic imaging can be helpful. Standard endoanal ultrasound can be used to locate internal openings and to define sphincter anatomy of anorectal fistula and RVF with 7% to 73% accuracy.[48–50] In women with obstetric injuries, performing an ultrasound is a routine part of the workup to evaluate for a sphincter defect. The addition of hydrogen peroxide contrast injected into the tract increases diagnostic accuracy to about 48% to 73%.[48,50] Magnetic resonance imaging (MRI) has a high sensitivity in demonstrating soft-tissue abnormalities and is recommended for the diagnosis of infection and fluid collection in the perianal area. MRI is more accurate in diagnosing anorectal fistula and RVF than surgical examination, ultrasound, and digital rectal examination,[48] with accuracy approaching 100%.[51] A study nearly 2 decades ago found 60% accuracy in diagnosing RVF with early generation CT scanners; the accuracy of modern-day multislice scanners in localizing RVF is unknown.[52] Contrast studies with basic fluoroscopic equipments are available at most institutions; however, vaginography and proctography have relatively low sensitivity at 79% and 35%, respectively.[53,54]

## MEDICAL TREATMENT OF CROHN'S RVF

Treatment of RVF is largely surgical; however, medical therapy does have a role in the treatment of Crohn's RVF. For Crohn's RVF, a thorough understanding of medical management of FCD is compulsatory because most patients are already treated with immunomodulation at the time of surgical referral.

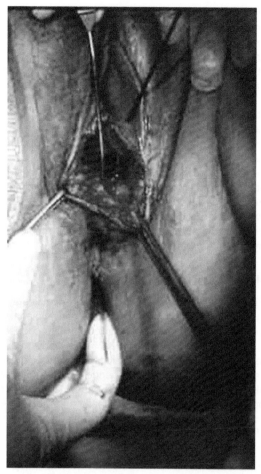

**Fig. 1.** RVF with probe placed through the tract. (*Courtesy of* Ann Lowry, MD, St Paul, MN.)

Present and colleagues[55] first reported the effects of infliximab in FCD in 1999, showing short-term fistula closure of 46% in a group of enterocutaneous Crohn's fistulas. But no RVFs were included in this sentinel study. A meta-analysis examining the efficacy of anti–tumor necrosis factor $\alpha$ therapy (infliximab and newer agents such as adalimumab, certolizumab) in 776 patients in 10 prospective randomized studies showed an overall success rate of less than 50% in FCD. Sands and colleagues[56] later published post hoc subset analysis of the ACCENT II (A Crohn's disease Clinical trial Evaluating infliximab in a New long-term Treatment regimen in patients with fistulizing Crohn's disease) trial of 25 women with Crohn's RVF. In nearly 1-year follow-up, treatment with infliximab closed about 60.4% of fistula initially, but long-term closure rates decreased to 36% by 14 weeks. Poritz and colleagues[57] reported that 54% of infliximab-treated patients ultimately required surgery for various external Crohn's fistulas (including RVF). In 2004, Parsi and colleagues[58] reported a 78% closure rate for all external Crohn's fistulas but only 14% total closure rate for Crohn's RVF at 4- to 6-week follow-up. Ricart and colleagues[59] from the Mayo Clinic reported a 60% nonresponse rate and a 33% complete healing rate of RVF and pouch-vaginal fistulas treated with infliximab at a median follow-up of 34 weeks. In the same study, non-RVF fistulas had higher success rates with infliximab (49% successful closure and only 39% nonresponders).

There is no clear explanation for lower rates of healing in RVF when compared with other anorectal fistulas that are treated with infliximab, but some hypothesize that the relatively thin, nonmuscular, and poorly vascularized rectovaginal septum is prone to healing delays.[17] The high costs of infliximab, which can exceed $16,000 USD annually for maintenance[60] or £1335 GBP/dose[61] ($2,238 USD as of June 2009), may render it a nonoptimal first-line treatment for FCD. Despite great excitement within the gastroenterologic community for all types of enterocutaneous fistulas, infliximab clearly has lesser long-term efficacy in the RVF subset.

Before the infliximab era, several older medical therapies existed and still sustain a role in the treatment of selected patients with FCD. Other immunomodulators, such as corticosteroids, azathioprine, 6-mercaptopurine,[62] and cyclosporine,[63,64] have been used with varying success to treat FCD. Local therapies, such as warm sitz baths, supplemental dietary fiber, and antidiarrheal medications, may provide minor relief from symptoms but are not curative measures.

## SURGICAL TREATMENT OF RVF

Despite advances in medical therapy, surgery remains the mainstay of RVF treatment, and like many surgical diseases, proper timing is essential in planning an operation for RVF. After preoperative preparation, the surgeon must choose from transanal, perineal, transvaginal, or an abdominal approach. This decision and the overall plan and success depend on several factors. The location, cause, quality of surrounding tissue, history of repair, and degree of incontinence dictate which approach is taken. In the following discussion, the most common cause, obstetric/traumatic RVFs, is addressed first and separately from Crohn's disease and radiation-related fistulas.

### Obstetric/Traumatic Injury

#### Transanal repair
The first report on the use of an anterior rectal advancement flap in a posttraumatic RVF was described by Noble[65] in 1902 and then modified by Laird[66] in 1948. The transanal approach is ideally performed for low fistulas in patients without coexisting incontinence and is favored by most colorectal surgeons because of familiarity and theoretical physics. Proponents of the transanal repair advocate theoretical benefits attributed to repairing the high-pressure inflow of the RVF. Various techniques have been described, but the principles of this procedure are relatively consistent.

Before the procedure, patients receive a full mechanical bowel preparation. The patients are then placed in the prone jackknife position and proctoscopy with irrigation is performed. The vagina, perineum, and anoderm are then prepared with antiseptic solution. Exposure can be the limiting factor for this approach and can be enhanced with effacement sutures or the Lone Star retractor.

Before making an incision, a momentary pause and mental outline of the ideal width and length of the flap should be considered. The base of the flap proximally should measure at least twice its width at the apex. This potential outline of the margins of the flap can then be created with the monopolar cautery. When the mucosa is injected with dilute epinephrine and the flap is raised, the anatomy is altered, and surgeons typically err on the side of safety resulting in a pedicle of tissue that is too delicate or thin. This can cause ischemia and does not provide enough integrity to the flap to prevent recurrence. A bivalve retractor is typically inserted, and the flap is raised by making a curvilinear incision around the dentate line comprising of one-third of the anal canal circumference. Ideally, the flap consists of mucosa, submucosa, and at least part of the circular muscle fibers. It is raised in the cephalad direction for a minimum length of 5 cm, and dissection can stop when the flap can easily cover the fistula tract without tension after the distal portion including the defect has been excised. Next, the fistulous tract is cored out, and any visible defect in the laterally placed sphincter complex or rectovaginal septum is sutured. The flap is then advanced and sutured in place. The authors prefer to anchor the center and most cephalad portion of the underside of the flap first with interrupted 2-0 absorbable sutures and then continue caudally. A Hill-Ferguson retractor is then placed as the lateral sides of the flap are secured with 3-0 absorbable suture in a running fashion. The vaginal side is left open.

Previous studies reporting outcomes of the endorectal advancement flap are plagued with heterogenous patient groups and significant variations in technique. This has undoubtedly led to the wide range of success rates in larger studies. Nonetheless, without any contrary level I evidence, it is still the preferred approach for traumatic low RVF without coexisting incontinence.

### Perineal

This approach should be used in women with coexisting incontinence, a sphincter defect, or a history of a failed transanal or transvaginal approach. Various techniques have been described but can generally be divided into perineoproctotomy followed by layered closure or a true transperineal approach without complete fistulotomy. These procedures are technically more demanding and have a higher risk of functional impairment but have realized great overall success.

Patients undergo a similar preoperative preparation as outlined earlier but are placed in a modified lithotomy position. A fistula probe is inserted through the defect, and the overlying skin, subcutaneous tissue, sphincter muscle, and rectal and vaginal walls are divided after being injected with local anesthesia with epinephrine. This creates a perineal cloaca and affords excellent exposure. After the fistula tract is excised and any epithelialized tissue is debrided, the layers within the defect and perineum are carefully identified. This can be more cumbersome in patients who have had previous repairs or have significant scar tissue and fibrosis from previous infection or primary closure at the time of delivery. The rectal mucosa is then separated from the sphincter complex and closed in 2 layers. The vaginal mucosa is then dissected and also closed primarily. The external and internal sphincters are then mobilized laterally within each ischiorectal fossa to allow for an overlapping sphincteroplasty. A small penrose drain is placed, and the skin is closed with interrupted sutures in a vertical fashion to help lengthen the perineal body. Patients are hospitalized for a short period for pain control and wound management.

The straight transperineal approach without fistulotomy involves making a circumanal right-angled[67] or H-shaped[68] incision in the perineal body. Through this incision, a similar layered repair is performed, but a levatorplasty is also added in most cases.

Success rates for both procedures range from 85% to 100%,[14,67–69] and there are no studies to date comparing the 2 approaches. Surgeon experience, preference, and personal outcomes should dictate which procedure is implemented.

### Transvaginal

Proponents of the transvaginal approach argue that this method offers the following advantages: (1) no perineal wound is created, (2) no anal or perineal deformity is produced, (3) no sphincter division is required, (4) sphincteroplasty can be performed simultaneously, (5) the technique incorporates a layer of intact tissue, (6) exposure is better, (7) the flap has redundant blood supply without tension, and (8) only minor morbidities have been reported.[70] However, the high-pressure side and primary opening are not addressed directly, theoretically increasing the risk of long-term failure.

An incision is commonly made between the mucosa of the posterior vaginal wall and perineal skin, and a vaginal flap is raised from apex to the base. The fistula is identified and excised, and the rectal defect is closed in 2 layers. The levator ani muscles are approximated without the need for lateral dissection. Finally, the vaginal mucosal flap is advanced over the defect and anchored to the skin with absorbable sutures.

There are few large series reporting long-term results of this approach. Cassadesus and colleagues[70] reported their 5-year results with this technique and achieved a 75% primary closure rate.

## CROHN'S DISEASE

IBD is the second most common cause of RVF. There are no prospective randomized trials for the surgical management of Crohn's-related RVF. The approach in patients with Crohn's disease is dependent on the current disease activity and location, the degree of infection, the presence of a synchronous sphincter defect, and the overall impact on quality of life. All acute abscesses and secondary tracks need to be definitively drained with setons before repair is considered. Furthermore, if the severity of the disease proximally exceeds the morbidity of the fistula, it must be primarily addressed. Surgical approaches range from local repairs with or without diversion to permanent stomas and proctectomy as the most definitive option.

### Local Repairs

Rectal advancement flaps can be used for Crohn's RVF when the fistula is low, the rectum is relatively spared, and there is no significant anal stenosis. The procedure is described earlier in the section on traumatic RVF, but consideration is given to a temporary diverting stoma. Patients with poor tissue quality, who are on high-dose immunosuppressive medication may benefit from a temporary diverting stoma. There are no prospective studies comparing repair with and without diversion, but overall results in retrospective series are improved with diversion.[71,72] Bauer and colleagues[71] reported a 92.3% cure rate with diversion and a transvaginal approach. The levator muscle was reconstructed between primary closure of the vaginal and mucosal layers, and all patients were diverted.

In patients with extensive stenosis and anal ulcerations, an advancement sleeve flap removing all of the diseased tissue in the anal canal can be performed. Marchesa and colleagues[73] reported 60% success with this procedure in 13 patients as an alternative to proctectomy. In severely symptomatic patients with anal and rectal disease who are not emotionally ready to accept proctectomy, perineal approaches can also be considered. In the authors' practice, this approach involves a layered repair as described earlier and usually the placement of a biologic mesh. Delayed wound healing of the perineal body should be expected with this technique, and temporary diversion may promote closure.

### Diversion

The indications for a temporary stoma for Crohn's RVF remain nebulous. It provides temporary relief and may facilitate healing of complex repairs, but there are no data to support its effect on long-term outcome. A laparoscopic loop ileostomy can be created with little morbidity in these settings and may prepare the patient mentally for proctocolectomy if needed in the future.

### Proctectomy

Proctectomy is the most definitive surgical option for Crohn's RVF in the presence of persistent severe proctitis and other failed repairs. If medical management has been optimized and the quality of life from the fistula and concomitant disease is poor, this is the best option. Delayed perineal wound healing should again be expected postoperatively.

## CARCINOMA AND RADIATION

RVFs from gynecologic and rectal malignancy or radiation for these tumors typically are considered high or existing above the sphincter mechanism. The first step in treating fistulas arising from a malignancy is to address respectability. Typically, the resection includes an en-block resection of the fistula, and in unresectable situations diverting stomas can improve quality of life.

Radiation-induced fistulas also begin with an extensive workup for recurrent cancer. This typically requires an examination under anesthesia, with biopsy and pelvic MRI.

In the absence of recurrent cancer, radiation-induced fistulas can be approached abdominally, locally, or with diversion. There are several variants of each, with little evidence to support 1 method over the next, but the location and extent of radiation injury usually determine the most prudent approach. Before surgery, the extent of radiation injury, including the compliance of the rectum, needs to be addressed. Compliance can be addressed with manometry and subjectively with attempted insulation during endoscopy.

### Local: Transvaginal/Transperineal

Considering the poor quality of the rectum and concomitant inflammation and edema of tissue planes, these repairs are typically performed in conjunction with a diverting stoma. The diverting stoma can be performed simultaneously or several months before the repair, depending on the amount of contamination and tissue integrity. If the vaginal mucosa is uninvolved with radiation and if the fistula is not higher than the apex of the vaginal vault, a vaginal flap can be raised. This is followed by closure of the rectal site of the fistula, anterior placation of the levator ani muscle, and then closure of the vaginal mucosa. This repair is significantly enhanced by transposition of nonirradiated tissue between the 2 suture lines. The Martius technique incorporates subcutaneous tissue and the bulbocavernosus muscle from 1 of the labia majora. When a transperineal incision is made, the sartorius and gracillis muscles can readily be used by creating a tunnel beneath the vaginal mucosa. As mentioned earlier, after the fistula is debrided and the rectum is closed, the interposition muscle is inserted and sutured to the contralateral ischial tuberosity.[14,74] Successful closure with these procedures ranges up to 80%.[75]

### Transabdominal

This approach is preferable for severely strictured or ulcerated disease in the absolute absence of recurrent malignancy, when local repairs have failed or are not technically feasible. The patient must also be highly motivated and understand the high morbidity of the procedure compared with a diverting stoma alone. The preoperative workup includes a pelvic MRI and the placement of ureteric stents. After the rectum is resected down to the anal canal, there are numerous reconstructive options. The preferred approach is to perform a coloanal J reservoir with hand-sewn anastomosis and obligatory use of a diverting ileostomy. Other methods described in small series that are beyond the scope of this article include nonresectional onlay techniques and bypasses, Soave procedure, and combined abdominotranssacral reconstruction.

### Diversion

Creating a laparoscopic or open diverting colostomy is still the safest option that also significantly improves quality of life. This is unquestionably the preferred procedure in patients with unresectable recurrent or primary malignancy and in patients with multiple comorbidities. Most of these procedures can be performed laparoscopically. A traditional cut-down incision suitable for a stoma is created at the premarked site, and pneumoperitoneum is created with a nondissecting balloon trocar to hold insufflation. The camera is inserted through this port, and two 5-mm trocars are then inserted through the right mid and lower quadrant to facilitate mobilization of the sigmoid colon.

## MISCELLANEOUS
### Bioprosthetics

During the last decade, biologic mesh and other configurations have become popular for the treatment of anorectal fistulas and RVFs. Ellis[76] reported 81% and 86% success rates with a bioprosthetic sheet and bioprosthetic plug, respectively, for the treatment of RVFs. This cohort of 34 patients included patients with Crohn's disease. Ongoing prospective studies are needed to strengthen the widespread implementation of these products, but the early results in this series are encouraging.

## SUMMARY

The diagnostic challenges imposed by RVFs are only superseded by the difficulty of achieving successful long-term repair. Obstetric and traumatic fistulas can usually be approached by the transanal or transperineal route, depending on the presence of incontinence. Reasonable outcomes can be expected in these patients who typically have normal rectal and vaginal tissue in close proximity to the defect. Radiation-induced and Crohn's-related fistulas are particularly more problematic because of the inherent poor tissue quality. A systemic workup is mandatory, and surgical approaches include abdominal and local repairs for these commonly high rectovaginal defects. There is a paucity of data to support specific techniques and the need for diversion in the management of RVFs. Hopefully, ongoing studies will help produce an universally accepted algorithm that may enhance long-term outcomes. Current investigations with interposition flaps, stem cell injections, and biologics are also ongoing to help improve the treatment success of this difficult problem.

## REFERENCES

1. Sandborn WJ, Fazio VW, Feagan BG, et al. AGA technical review on perianal Crohn's disease. Gastroenterology 2003;125:1508–30.
2. Senatore PJ Jr. Anovaginal fistulae. Surg Clin North Am 1994;74:1361–75.
3. Venkatesh KS, Ramanujam PS, Larson DM, et al. Anorectal complications of vaginal delivery. Dis Colon Rectum 1989;32:1039–41.
4. Angioli R, Gomez-Marin O, Cantuaria G, et al. Severe perineal lacerations during vaginal delivery: the University of Miami experience. Am J Obstet Gynecol 2000; 182:1083–5.

5. World Health Organization. Prevention and treatment of obstetric fistulae: report of a technical working group. Geneva: World Health Organization; 1989.
6. Murray C, Lopez A. World Health Organization: health dimensions of sex and reproduction. Geneva: World Health Organization; 1989.
7. Powers K, Grigorescu B, Lazarou G, et al. Neglected pessary causing a rectovaginal fistula: a case report. J Reprod Med 2008;53:235–7.
8. Kankam OK, Geraghty R. An erosive pessary. J R Soc Med 2002;95:507.
9. Arias BE, Ridgeway B, Barber MD. Complications of neglected vaginal pessaries: case presentation and literature review. Int Urogynecol J Pelvic Floor Dysfunct 2008;19:1173–8.
10. Hanavadi S, Durham-Hall A, Oke T, et al. Forgotten vaginal pessary eroding into rectum. Ann R Coll Surg Engl 2004;86:W18–9.
11. Ahmad M. Intravaginal vibrator of long duration. Eur J Emerg Med 2002;9:61–2.
12. Purwar B, Panda SN, Odogwu SO, et al. Recto-vaginal sex leading to colostomy and recto-vaginal repair. Int J STD AIDS 2008;19:57–8.
13. Singhal SR, Nanda S, Singhal SK. Sexual intercourse: an unusual cause of rectovaginal fistula. Eur J Obstet Gynecol Reprod Biol 2007;131:243–4.
14. Saclarides TJ. Rectovaginal fistula. Surg Clin North Am 2002;82:1261–72.
15. Schwartz DA, Loftus EV Jr, Tremaine WJ, et al. The natural history of fistulizing Crohn's disease in Olmsted County, Minnesota. Gastroenterology 2002;122:875–80.
16. Radcliffe AG, Ritchie JK, Hawley PR, et al. Anovaginal and rectovaginal fistulas in Crohn's disease. Dis Colon Rectum 1988;31:94–9.
17. Andreani SM, Dang HH, Grondona P, et al. Rectovaginal fistula in Crohn's disease. Dis Colon Rectum 2007;50:2215–22.
18. Zinicola R, Nicholls RJ. Restorative proctocolectomy in patients with ulcerative colitis having a recto-vaginal fistula. Colorectal Dis 2004;6:261–4.
19. Chawla S, Smart CJ, Moots RJ. Recto-vaginal fistula: a refractory complication of Behcet's disease. Colorectal Dis 2007;9:667–8.
20. Chung HJ, Goo BC, Lee JH, et al. Behcet's disease combined with various types of fistula. Yonsei Med J 2005;46:625–8.
21. Engle DB, Bradley KA, Chappell RJ, et al. The effect of laparoscopic guidance on gynecologic interstitial brachytherapy. J Minim Invasive Gynecol 2008;15:541–6.
22. Lee RC, Rotmensch J. Rectovaginal radiation fistula repair using an obturator fasciocutaneous thigh flap. Gynecol Oncol 2004;94:277–82.
23. Kasibhatla M, Clough RW, Montana GS, et al. Predictors of severe gastrointestinal toxicity after external beam radiotherapy and interstitial brachytherapy for advanced or recurrent gynecologic malignancies. Int J Radiat Oncol Biol Phys 2006;65:398–403.
24. Luna-Perez P, Rodriguez-Ramirez SE. Formalin instillation for refractory radiation-induced hemorrhagic proctitis. J Surg Oncol 2002;80:41–4.
25. Baran JJ, Goldstein SD, Resnik AM. The double-staple technique in colorectal anastomoses: a critical review. Am Surg 1992;58:270–2.
26. Rex JC Jr, Khubchandani IT. Rectovaginal fistula: complication of low anterior resection. Dis Colon Rectum 1992;35:354–6.
27. Kosugi C, Saito N, Kimata Y, et al. Rectovaginal fistulas after rectal cancer surgery: incidence and operative repair by gluteal-fold flap repair. Surgery 2005;137:329–36.
28. Nakagoe R, Sawai T, Tuji T, et al. Successful transvaginal repair of a rectovaginal fistula developing after double-stapled anastomosis in low anterior resection: report of four cases. Surg Today 1999;29:443–5.

29. Angelone G, Giardiello C, Prota C. Stapled hemorrhoidopexy. Complications and 2-year follow-up. Chir Ital 2006;58:753–60.

30. Cirocco WC. Life threatening sepsis and mortality following stapled hemorrhoidopexy. Surgery 2008;143:824–9.

31. Chang S, Hulme-Moir M. New Zealand's early experience in stapled haemorrhoidopexy. N Z Med J 2006;119:U1880.

32. Pescatori M, Gagliardi G. Postoperative complications after procedure for prolapsed hemorrhoids (PPH) and stapled transanal rectal resection (STARR) procedures. Tech Coloproctol 2008;12:7–19.

33. Bassi R, Rademacher J, Savoia A. Rectovaginal fistula after STARR procedure complicated by haematoma of the posterior vaginal wall: report of a case. Tech Coloproctol 2006;10:361–3.

34. Gagliardi G, Pescatori M, Altomare DM, et al. Results, outcome predictors, and complications after stapled transanal rectal resection for obstructed defecation. Dis Colon Rectum 2008;51:186–95.

35. Pescatori M, Dodi G, Salafia C, et al. Rectovaginal fistula after double-stapled transanal rectotomy (STARR) for obstructed defaecation. Int J Colorectal Dis 2005;20:83–5.

36. Caquant F, Collinet P, Debodinance P, et al. Safety of trans vaginal mesh procedure: retrospective study of 684 patients. J Obstet Gynaecol Res 2008;34:449–56.

37. Dwyer PL, O'Reilly BA. Transvaginal repair of anterior and posterior compartment prolapse with Atrium polypropylene mesh. BJOG 2004;111:831–6.

38. Hilger WA, Cornella JL. Rectovaginal fistula after posterior intravaginal slingplasty and polypropylene mesh augmented rectocele repair. Int Urogynecol J Pelvic Floor Dysfunct 2006;17:89–92.

39. Margulies RU, Lewicky-Gaupp C, Fenner DE, et al. Complications requiring reoperation following vaginal mesh kit procedures for prolapse. Am J Obstet Gynecol 2008;199:648.e1–4.

40. Hoffman MS, Wakeley KE, Cardosi RJ. Risks of rigid dilation for a radiated vaginal cuff: two related rectovaginal fistulas. Obstet Gynecol 2003;101:1125–6.

41. Hamilton S, Spencer C, Evans A. Vagino-rectal fistula caused by Bartholin's abscess. J Obstet Gynaecol 2007;27:325–6.

42. Lynch CM, Felder TL, Schwandt RA, et al. Lymphogranuloma venereum presenting as a rectovaginal fistula. Infect Dis Obstet Gynecol 1999;7:199–201.

43. Kunin J, Bejar J, Eldar S. Schistosomiasis as a cause of rectovaginal fistula: a brief case report. Isr J Med Sci 1996;32:1109–11.

44. Lebourthe F, Baur P, Calvy H. [Eight cases of rectovaginal fistula of lymphogranulomatous origin treated according to the technic of Musset and Cottrell]. Mem Acad Chir (Paris) 1963;89:823–6 [in French].

45. Lock MR, Katz DR, Samoorian S, et al. Giant condyloma of the rectum: report of a case. Dis Colon Rectum 1977;20:154–7.

46. Schuman P, Christensen C, Sobel JD. Aphthous vaginal ulceration in two women with acquired immunodeficiency syndrome. Am J Obstet Gynecol 1996;174:1660–3.

47. Ng FH, Chau TN, Cheung TC, et al. Cytomegalovirus colitis in individuals without apparent cause of immunodeficiency. Dig Dis Sci 1999;44:945–52.

48. Sudol-Szopinska I, Jakubowski W, Szczepkowski M. Contrast-enhanced endosonography for the diagnosis of anal and anovaginal fistulas. J Clin Ultrasound 2002;30:145–50.

49. Choen S, Burnett S, Bartram CI, et al. Comparison between anal endosonography and digital examination in the evaluation of anal fistulae. Br J Surg 1991;78:445–7.

50. Poen AC, Felt-Bersma RJ, Eijsbouts QA, et al. Hydrogen peroxide-enhanced transanal ultrasound in the assessment of fistula-in-ano. Dis Colon Rectum 1998;41:1147–52.
51. Dwarkasing S, Hussain SM, Hop WC, et al. Anovaginal fistulas: evaluation with endoanal MR imaging. Radiology 2004;231:123–8.
52. Kuhlman JE, Fishman EK. CT evaluation of enterovaginal and vesicovaginal fistulas. J Comput Assist Tomogr 1990;14:390–4.
53. Giordano P, Drew PJ, Taylor D, et al. Vaginography–investigation of choice for clinically suspected vaginal fistulas. Dis Colon Rectum 1996;39:568–72.
54. Bird D, Taylor D, Lee P. Vaginography: the investigation of choice for vaginal fistulae? Aust N Z J Surg 1993;63:894–6.
55. Present DH, Rutgeerts P, Targan S, et al. Infliximab for the treatment of fistulas in patients with Crohn's disease. N Engl J Med 1999;340:1398–405.
56. Sands BE, Blank MA, Patel K, et al. Long-term treatment of rectovaginal fistulas in Crohn's disease: response to infliximab in the ACCENT II Study. Clin Gastroenterol Hepatol 2004;2:912–20.
57. Poritz LS, Rowe WA, Koltun WA. Remicade does not abolish the need for surgery in fistulizing Crohn's disease. Dis Colon Rectum 2002;45:771–5.
58. Parsi MA, Lashner BA, Achkar JP, et al. Type of fistula determines response to infliximab in patients with fistulous Crohn's disease. Am J Gastroenterol 2004; 99:445–9.
59. Ricart E, Panaccione R, Loftus EV, et al. Infliximab for Crohn's disease in clinical practice at the Mayo Clinic: the first 100 patients. Am J Gastroenterol 2001;96:722–9.
60. Lichtenstein GR. Incorrect cost of infliximab in fistulizing Crohn's disease. Gastroenterology 2004;127:691–2.
61. Lindsay J, Punekar YS, Morris J, et al. Health-economic analysis: cost-effectiveness of scheduled maintenance treatment with infliximab for Crohn's disease–modelling outcomes in active luminal and fistulizing disease in adults. Aliment Pharmacol Ther 2008;28:76–87.
62. Present DH, Korelitz BI, Wisch N, et al. Treatment of Crohn's disease with 6-mercaptopurine. A long-term, randomized, double-blind study. N Engl J Med 1980;302:981–7.
63. Hanauer SB, Smith MB. Rapid closure of Crohn's disease fistulas with continuous intravenous cyclosporin A. Am J Gastroenterol 1993;88:646–9.
64. Present DH, Lichtiger S. Efficacy of cyclosporine in treatment of fistula of Crohn's disease. Dig Dis Sci 1994;39:374–80.
65. Noble GH. A new operation for complete laceration of the perineum designed for the purpose of eliminating danger of infection from the rectum. Trans Am Gynecol Soc 1902;27:357–63.
66. Laird DR. Procedures used in the treatment of complicated fistulas. Am J Surg 1948;76:701–8.
67. Chew SB, Rieger NR. Transperineal repair of obstetric-related anovaginal fistula. Aust N Z J Obstet Gynaecol 2004;44:68–71.
68. Senagore AJ. Treatment of acquired anovaginal and rectovaginal fistulas. Semin Colon Rectal Surg 1990;1:219–23.
69. Corman ML. Colon and rectal surgery. 5th edition. Philadelphia: JB Lippincott; 1998.
70. Cassadesus D, Villasana L, Sanchez IM, et al. Treatment of rectovaginal fistula: a 5 year review. Aust N Z J Obstet Gynaecol 2006;46:49–51.
71. Bauer JJ, Sher ME, Jaffin H, et al. Transvaginal approach for repair of rectovaginal fistulae complicating Crohn's disease. Ann Surg 1991;213:151–8.

72. Hull TL, Fazio VW. Surgical approaches to low anovaginal fistulas in Crohn's disease. Am J Surg 1997;173:95–8.
73. Marchesa P, Hull TL, Fazio VW. Advancement sleeve flaps for the closure of ano-vaginal fistula in Crohn's disease. Ann R Coll Surg Engl 1998;85:1695–8.
74. Ward MW, Morgan BG, Clark CG. Treatment of persistent perineal sinus with vagina fistula following proctocolectomy in Crohn's disease. Br J Surg 1982;6:228–9.
75. Boronow RC. Repair of the radiation induced vaginal fistula utilizing the Martius technique. World J Surg 1986;10:237.
76. Ellis N. Outcomes after repair of rectovaginal fistulas using bioprosthetics. Dis Colon Rectum 2008;51:1084–8.

# Anorectal Crohn's Disease

Robert T. Lewis, MD[a], David J. Maron, MD[b],*

**KEYWORDS**

- Crohn's • Abscess • Fistula • Stricture • Fistulotomy
- Advancement flap

Although Burrill Crohn's[1] sentinel description of his eponymous disease was published in 1932, Bissell[2] first described the associated perianal manifestations. Crohn[3] himself published similar findings in 1938. Granulomatous perianal disease was well known even earlier, but was most commonly caused by intestinal tuberculosis. In 1921, however, 17 years before the formal description of the disease, Gabriel[4] described patients with granulomatous perianal disease without signs of tuberculosis.

Patients with Crohn's disease often develop anal manifestations of their disease. Perianal Crohn's disease may present with fissures, skin tags, ulcers, strictures, abscesses, or fistulae. Treatment of these conditions can be complicated, and a full understanding of the etiology and all potential therapeutic options is therefore critical for success.

## EPIDEMIOLOGY

Reports of the prevalence of perianal involvement in patients with Crohn's disease have varied greatly, but the most current population-based series (from Sweden and Minnesota) have found that anorectal involvement is seen in 14% to 38% of patients,[5–7] with isolated perianal disease seen in only 5%.[8] Crohn's disease is typically grouped into 3 categories based on the segment of intestine involved: isolated ileal disease occurs in 30% of patients, ileocolic disease in 50%, and colonic disease in 20%.[9] The prevalence of perianal manifestations increases as the disease progresses distally. In patients with ileocolic Crohn's disease, only 15% develop fistulae, but fistulae occur in 92% of patients with Crohn's disease involving the colon and rectum.[7] In most cases, bowel involvement precedes perianal disease,[10] but as many as 4 in 10 patients can experience perianal symptoms before intestinal involvement manifests.[11] There does not seem to be a predilection for age, with between 13% and 62% of children and adolescents with Crohn's disease experiencing perianal manifestations[6,12,13]; however, a younger age of onset increases the odds of developing perianal disease over time.[14,15] A study of 1126 patients with Crohn's disease

[a] Department of Surgery, University of Pennsylvania Health System, Philadelphia, PA, USA
[b] Division of Colon and Rectal Surgery, University of Pennsylvania Health System, 39th & Market Streets, WS266, Philadelphia, PA 19104, USA
* Corresponding author.
*E-mail address:* david.j.maron@uphs.upenn.edu (D. J. Maron).

Surg Clin N Am 90 (2010) 83–97
doi:10.1016/j.suc.2009.09.004
0039-6109/09/$ – see front matter © 2010 Elsevier Inc. All rights reserved.

surgical.theclinics.com

found proximal disease is more common in whites (Odds ratio 1.8), and whites are less likely than Hispanics and African Americans to have perianal manifestations (OR 0.58)[16]; similar results were seen by Cross and colleagues.[17] The presence of perianal disease is associated with a more disabling natural history,[18] with increased extraintestinal manifestations[19] and greater steroid resistance.[20] Perianal Crohn's disease is often recurrent, with 35% to 59% of patients relapsing within 2 years.[21] More than 80% of patients require surgery, and as many as 20% require proctectomy.[5,7]

Patients with Crohn's disease have a known increased risk of colon cancer.[22] Large studies have failed to find a significantly higher incidence of rectal cancer,[23,24] but have shown an increased risk for squamous cell carcinoma and adenocarcinoma of the anus in patients with anorectal involvement.[25,26] Active disease and long duration of disease are risk factors,[27,28] and although the resultant tumors seem to be no more aggressive than those in patients without Crohn's disease, they are more likely to be diagnosed at an advanced stage.[29] Some investigators have therefore recommended that patients at high risk (including patients with extensive colitis, bypassed loops, diversion, refractory perianal disease, strictures, and primary sclerosing cholangitis) undergo cancer surveillance annually starting 15 years after diagnosis.[25]

## SPECIFIC CONDITIONS

The type of anorectal lesions with which a patient may present vary (**Table 1**).

### Skin Tags

Skin tags are present in 40% to 70% of patients with Crohn's disease,[30,31] and can vary in size, shape, and character.[6] These tags are often associated with either lymphedema or recurrent fissures and fistulae.[32] They are usually asymptomatic, soft, and mobile, but can become inflamed, hard, and painful during a Crohn's flare (**Fig. 1**).[33] Careful examination should be performed to prevent mismanagement, as they frequently can be difficult to differentiate from hemorrhoids.[34]

Skin tags are persistent, but benign; a study of 37 patients with skin tags found that tags were still present in 25 patients (68%) at 10 years.[31] Surgical excision should be

| Table 1 | |
| :--- | :--- |
| Perianal lesions in 202 consecutive patients[30] | |
| **Lesion Type** | **Number of Patients (%)** |
| Skin tag | 75 (37) |
| Fissure | 38 (19) |
| Low fistula | 40 (20) |
| High fistula | 12 (6) |
| Rectovaginal fistula | 6 (3) |
| Perianal abscess | 32 (16) |
| Ischiorectal abscess | 8 (4) |
| Intersphincteric abscess | 7 (3) |
| Supralevator abscess | 6 (3) |
| Anorectal stricture | 19 (9) |
| Hemorrhoids | 15 (7) |
| Anal ulcer | 12 (12) |
| Total | 110 (54) |

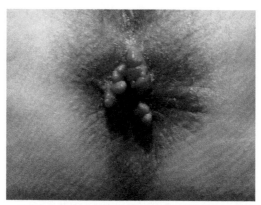

**Fig. 1.** Perianal skin tags in Crohn's disease. (*Courtesy of* Scott R. Steele, MD, Tacoma, WA.)

avoided unless they interfere with hygiene or are persistently symptomatic,[35] as there is an increased risk for delayed wound healing.[30]

### Hemorrhoids

Hemorrhoids are present in only 7% of patients with Crohn's disease,[30] which is lower than the estimated prevalence of 24% in the general population.[36] Although often asymptomatic, symptoms of hemorrhoids can be exacerbated by the severe diarrhea of Crohn's disease. Surgical intervention is generally avoided, because of the significantly high rate of delayed wound healing, inflammation, infection, and stenosis.[37] In highly selective patients without any active anorectal Crohn's manifestations, however, hemorrhoidectomy can be successful in up to 88% of patients, either with simple hemorrhoidectomy[33] or elastic banding.[6]

### Fissures

Fissures are present in up to 19% of patients with Crohn's disease.[30] In contrast to idiopathic anal fissures, which are almost always located in the midline, fissures in patients with Crohn's disease can be eccentrically located in up to 20%.[31,38] Painful fissures in a patient with Crohn's disease should prompt an examination for underlying abscess or fistula, although these examinations frequently fail to find any underlying sepsis, as 40% to 85% of all fissures in patients with Crohn's disease present with pain.[39]

These fissures are potentially challenging to treat. The first line of treatment should be medical management (including nitroglycerin paste, calcium channel blockers, and botulinum toxin[40]); these treatments are successful in up to 80% of cases.[34] In the case of nonhealing symptomatic fissure, proctitis should be ruled out. In patients with persistent fissures without proctitis, Fleshner found that 7 of 8 (88%) patients healed after sphincterotomy,[39] whereas 9 of 35 (26%) patients who received medical treatment only eventually developed abscesses or fistulae. However, in the presence of proctitis surgery should be avoided.[41]

### Anal Ulcer

Twelve percent of patients with Crohn's disease present with large, cavitating anal or rectal ulcers.[30] Anorectal pain is common, with 56% of patients reporting severe and unremitting pain, and 35% reporting dyschezia.[42] Local treatment, including debridement and intralesional corticosteroid injection can be effective, but patients often ultimately require proctectomy.[43]

### Stricture

Stricture is believed to occur as a consequence of chronic inflammation or fistula in either the anus (34%) or the rectum (50%). These strictures can present as short anal strictures, or long tubular strictures involving varying lengths of the rectum.[44] Symptoms are typically functional: difficulty with defecation, tenesmus, incontinence, or urgency.[6] In the absence of symptoms, no treatment is necessary.[41] If symptomatic, anal dilatation with a single finger or a coaxial balloon is effective,[45] but may be complicated by delayed wound healing in 47% of patients. Most patients with anal or rectal strictures have concomitant proctitis, and up to 43% require proctectomy.[44] The presence of strictures is a documented risk factor for both proctectomy and diversion,[46] however the use of diversion can result in progressive stenosis and retention of rectal fluid resulting in further illness.[47]

### Abscess/Fistulae

Abscess and fistula are the most common presentations of anorectal Crohn's disease. Twenty-six percent of patients present with an abscess, frequently complex (inter-sphincteric, supralevator, or ischiorectal), and an additional 29% present with a fistula.[30] A thorough examination must be performed before treatment is initiated, with special attention to establishing the presence or absence of rectal inflammation. Any collection should be immediately drained. Beyond this point, various options are available for the treatment of fistulae. Fistulae can be classified as simple (superficial, inter-, or trans-sphincteric fistula below the dentate line, with a single opening and no anorectal stricture or abscess), or complex (trans-, supra-, or extrasphincteric fistula above the dentate line, or a fistula with multiple external openings, associated abscess, or stricture, or rectovaginal fistula).[6] A combined medical and surgical approach offers the best chance for success.[48–50]

### Diagnosis/evaluation

Many manifestations of anorectal Crohn's disease are readily observed on a thorough physical examination, and a tissue biopsy documenting noncaseating granulomas is only occasionally necessary.[9] Fistulae associated with Crohn's disease, however, require more than a digital rectal examination to accurately assess the extent of the perianal disease. An examination under anesthesia (EUA) has traditionally been considered the gold standard, but a prospective study by Schwartz and colleagues[51] in 34 patients found that EUA had an accuracy of only 90% when compared with EUA combined with anal endoscopic ultrasound (EUS) and pelvic magnetic resonance imaging (MRI). This same study found that accuracy was 100% when any 2 of the 3 procedures were performed.

Fistulography has been shown to have an accuracy of 16% to 50%,[52,53] and is not routinely recommended. Differentiating fistulae and resolving structures of the pelvic floor using computed tomography (CT) scanning, although commonly performed, can be difficult.[54] One study found CT scanning had a sensitivity of only 24% in the diagnosis of fistula-in-ano,[55] and the investigators recommended that CT should not be routinely used in the characterization of anorectal disease.

Several studies have found endoanal ultrasound to be inferior to pelvic MRI in the diagnosis of perianal disease.[51,56,57] With the use of three-dimensional reconstruction of two-dimensional images, however, some investigators have shown that the results of EUS are comparable with MRI, with excellent patient tolerance.[58,59] The use of hydrogen peroxide injection in the fistula tract during EUS substantially improves accuracy.[60] EUS has also been used to document resolution and improvement in fistulae after treatment.[61,62]

Pelvic MRI is the preferred imaging modality in the classification of fistulizing perianal disease. It has been shown to have an accuracy of 90% when classifying fistulae and 97% when delineating complex abscesses.[56,63] Moreover, surgical management may be altered in 10% to 20% of patients by the addition of MRI to EUA, and this increases to up to 40% in patients with Crohn's disease.[64,65] In patients with complex perianal Crohn's disease, therefore, it is the authors' practice to combine a pelvic MRI with EUA and rigid proctoscopy to evaluate for rectal inflammation.

Once the anorectal disease is delineated, evaluation for proximal Crohn's disease with endoscopy and small bowel radiography should also be considered. A study of 5491 patients with Crohn's disease found an association between proximal fistulizing disease and perianal fistulae.[66] Some investigators have found that treatment of proximal disease may assist in the resolution of anorectal symptoms,[5,67] however, other investigators did not observe improvements in their series.[68,69] Most experts do not recommend operative intervention on the proximal bowel solely to improve anorectal disease.[35,43]

### Abscess/perineal sepsis

Abscess presents with pain, swelling, and fluctuance on rectal examination, and is believed to form by extension of a cryptoglandular infection or obstruction of a perianal fistula. Abscesses can be present in any plane (superficial, intersphincteric, ischiorectal, or supralevator), but regardless of location require prompt surgical incision and drainage, and treatment of systemic symptoms with broad-spectrum antibiotics.[6,35] Many investigators advocate placing a drain or partially dividing the sphincters to facilitate drainage, but these have not been shown to improve outcomes.[70,71] EUS has also been used with success to guide the drainage of deep or complex abscesses.[72]

In the presence of a fistula, a noncutting seton made of an inert material can be placed to prevent recurrence and facilitate drainage, with healing or improvement seen in 79% to 100% of patients.[73–78] Setons can be left in place long-term without consequence, and removal without definitive therapy results in recurrence of the fistula in 20% to 80% of cases.[76,79,80] In patients with persistent sepsis, a temporary diverting stoma can be effective in up to 80% of patients. However, these stomas are rarely reversed; only 4 of 18 (22%) patients underwent reversal in one study.[81]

### Medical treatment

Once a fistula is characterized and any concomitant abscess controlled, combined definitive medical and surgical therapy should be initiated. Medication options include antibiotics (such as metronidozole and ciprofloxacin), immunosuppressives (6-mercaptopurine and azathioprine, cyclosporine, and tacrolimus), and immunomodulators (infliximab and adalimumab).

Antibiotics have been shown to be effective as a bridge to immunosuppressive therapy,[82] with 70% to 95% of patients experiencing a positive clinical response within 6 to 8 weeks.[83,84] Symptoms often worsen when antibiotics are discontinued or decreased,[85] however, and fewer than 50% of patients experience healing of the fistula on antibiotic therapy alone.[86]

Definitive therapy must include immunosuppression or immunomodulation. A recent meta-analysis of 5 randomized controlled trials examined the efficacy of 6-mercaptopurine (6-MP) and azathioprine and showed that 54% of treated patients experienced fistula healing versus only 21% of controls.[87] Cyclosporine has also been shown to have a rapid effect in up to 83% of patients when given intravenously,[88,89] but the effect is not durable when patients are transitioned to oral cyclosporin or therapy is discontinued.[90] Tacrolimus has also shown efficacy in a randomized controlled trial, resulting in improvement in 43% of patients versus 8% in the placebo arm.[91]

Infliximab, a monoclonal antibody to tumor necrosis factor, has proven to be particularly effective in the treatment of perianal fistulae in Crohn's disease. One randomized trial of 92 patients showed efficacy with induction therapy; a 50% reduction in the number of draining fistulas was seen in 68% of patients treated with infliximab versus 26% of patients treated with placebo.[92] A second randomized trial documented a longer time to recurrence of fistulae (40 weeks with infliximab therapy vs 14 weeks with placebo), and treatment with infliximab resulted in less need for surgery and fewer hospitalizations.[93] Rectovaginal fistulae have a poorer response to infliximab therapy, with only 14% to 30% of patients showing a response.[92,94,95] Another anti-TNF antibody, adalimumab, has a similar safety profile to infliximab[96] and similar efficacy in a randomized controlled trial. Complete fistula closure occurred at 1 year in 39% of patients treated with adalimumab versus 13% of the placebo arm,[97] and these results have been shown to be durable at 2 years.[98]

### Surgical treatment

Fistulotomy offers the best chance for definitive treatment of perianal fistulas. Several series have examined the effect of fistulotomy in patients with low perianal fistula, with most reporting healing rates between 80% and 100%.[6] When the investigators specifically noted the absence of rectal inflammation, results were even better, with healing in 22/24 (95%) of patients, and recurrence in only 4/24 (15%).[71,99,100] However, a study that specifically noted active proctitis at the time of surgery documented a healing rate of only 27%.[101]

Although fistulotomy may be applicable to patients with low simple fistulas, patients with complex fistulas or fistulas involving a significant portion of the anal sphincter complex are at risk of iatrogenic injury to the sphincter.[102] In an effort to avoid sphincter damage, newer therapies using fibrin glue and anal fistula plugs have been developed.[103] Success using fibrin glue has been mixed, with 60% to 78% of simple fistulae healed, but only 14% to 50% of complex fistulae healed in patients without Crohn's disease.[104] Long-term success in closure of fistulae is seen in only 31% to 57% of patients with Crohn's disease.[105,106] In contrast, use of a collagen anal fistula plug may be promising. One prospective study of 20 patients found that the plug healed 80% of fistulae in patients with Crohn's disease[107] and 85% of fistulae in the general population.[108] Other investigators have seen less promising results.[109]

A high perianal fistula, branched ramifying tracts, associated abscess, or multiple external openings define more complex fistulae.[6] First-line therapy is infliximab, which, as mentioned earlier, has had excellent results in this population in multiple, randomized controlled trials.[92,93] Combined surgical therapy with temporary placement of a loose seton at the time of induction has resulted in healing in 47% to 67% of cases.[49,110]

Fistulotomy is not recommended in patients with complex perianal fistulae, as previous series have found nonhealing and incontinence in 40% to 60% of patients, many of whom eventually required proctectomy.[101,111] A loose seton can be left indefinitely, however, without significant effect on continence.[112] In the absence of proctitis, a transanal advancement flap may be a good option. In this procedure, the internal fistula opening is excised, and the mucosa, submucosa, and circular muscle mobilized as an island, which is then placed over the fistula tract. Some series have reported healing in as many as 89% of patients, but a disappointing rate of recurrence, as high as 50%.[113–115] A transanal sleeve advancement flap has also been shown to result in healing in 62% of cases, with a recurrence rate of 38%.[116] The combined use of infliximab and transanal advancement flap was shown to improve rates of healing[117] and decrease time to healing.[118] In the presence of proctitis, no surgical intervention is recommended; medical therapy should be continued until there is adequate resolution of proctitis. The authors' typical treatment algorithm is shown in **Fig. 2**.

Crohn's disease is the second most common cause of rectovaginal fistula.[119] The initial treatment does not vary from other complicated fistulae, although, as noted earlier, infliximab does not have the same response rate in this population.[120] Rectal advancement flaps are effective, with 54% to 71% healing,[121,122] and similar results are seen using rectal sleeve advancement flaps.[121,123] Although most investigators advocate repair of the fistula on the side of high pressure (rectum), others have achieved similar results with a vaginal advancement flap.[124]

## SPECIAL SITUATIONS
### Proctectomy

In patients in whom more conservative medical and surgical therapy fails, or in the presence of aggressive and unrelenting rectal disease, proctectomy may be appropriate. In published series, proctectomy is required in 10% to 20% of patients with perianal disease.[6] Proctectomy can be complicated by poor wound healing and

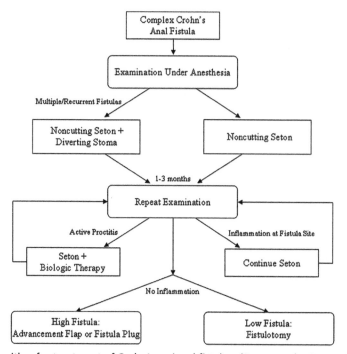

**Fig. 2.** Algorithm for treatment of Crohn's perianal fistulae. (*From* van der Hagen SJ, Baeten CG, Soeters PB, et al. Anti-TNF-alpha [infliximab] used as induction treatment in case of active proctitis in a multistep strategy followed by definitive surgery of complex anal fistulas in Crohn's disease: a preliminary report. Dis Colon Rectum 2005;48(4):758–67; with permission.)

perineal sinus formation in up to 25% to 50% of patients.[125,126] A gracilis flap[127] or diversion[126,128] can be used to help combat these complications.

### Anorectal Crohn's Disease After Restorative Proctocolectomy

Ileal pouch anal anastomosis (IPAA) is the procedure of choice for continent reconstruction in patients with ulcerative colitis requiring a total proctocolectomy.[129] However, this procedure results in poor outcomes in patients with Crohn's disease.[130–132] Pouches fail in 36% to 55% of patients with Crohn's disease, most commonly because of leaking at the anastomosis.[133,134] Differentiation between ulcerative colitis and Crohn's disease can be very challenging,[135] and in a series of 551 patients who underwent IPAA for presumptive ulcerative colitis, 3% were eventually diagnosed with Crohn's disease.[134]

Patients typically present with symptoms consistent with poor pouch function, chronic pouchitis,[136] or late (more than 1 month after IPAA) fistulizing pelvic or perianal disease.[137] Endoscopy showing ulcerations in the afferent limb has been shown to be helpful in diagnosis.[138,139] Azathioprine combined with infliximab improved pouch-perineal fistulae in 85% of patients in 1 small series,[140] and also shows promise as monotherapy.[141,142] Local advancement flaps can improve as many as 50% of cases with perianal fistulae,[143] but 3% to 6% of patients require pouch excision and permanent ileostomy, which can result in good long-term outcomes.[144]

### SUMMARY

Crohn's disease remains an incurable chronic illness with frequent relapses. Management of anorectal manifestations can pose an enormous challenge, as seen by the myriad of therapies that have been attempted. A thorough preoperative workup characterizing the nature of the disease is extremely important, and combined medical and surgical therapy offers the best route to durable remission. Surgeons should strive to minimize intervention as much as possible, although realizing that there is real benefit of definitive surgical treatment in carefully selected patients. Up to 20% of patients with perianal Crohn's disease eventually require proctectomy.

### REFERENCES

1. Crohn BB, Ginzberg L, Oppenheimer GD. Regional ileitis: a pathologic and clinical entity. JAMA 1932;99:1323.
2. Bissell AD. Localized chronic ulcerative ileitis. Ann Surg 1934;99(6):957–66.
3. Penner A, Crohn BB. Perianal fistulae as a complication of regional ileitis. Ann Surg 1938;108(5):867–73.
4. Gabriel WB. Results of an experimental and histological investigation in seventy-five cases of rectal fistulae. Proc R Soc Med 1921;14:156–61.
5. Hellers G, Bergstrand O, Ewerth S, et al. Occurrence and outcome after primary treatment of anal fistulae in Crohn's disease. Gut 1980;21(6):525–7.
6. Sandborn WJ, Fazio VW, Feagan BG, et al. AGA technical review on perianal Crohn's disease. Gastroenterology 2003;125(5):1508–30.
7. Schwartz DA, Loftus EV Jr, Tremaine WJ, et al. The natural history of fistulizing Crohn's disease in Olmsted County, Minnesota. Gastroenterology 2002;122(4): 875–80.
8. Lockhart-Mummery HE. Symposium. Crohn's disease: anal lesions. Dis Colon Rectum 1975;18(3):200–2.
9. McClane SJ, Rombeau JL. Anorectal Crohn's disease. Surg Clin North Am 2001; 81(1):169–83, ix.

10. Williams DR, Coller JA, Corman ML, et al. Anal complications in Crohn's disease. Dis Colon Rectum 1981;24(1):22–4.
11. Gray BK, Lockhart-Mummery HE, Morson BC. Crohn's disease of the anal region. Gut 1965;6(6):515–24.
12. Markowitz J, Daum F, Aiges H, et al. Perianal disease in children and adolescents with Crohn's disease. Gastroenterology 1984;86(5 Pt 1):829–33.
13. Palder SB, Shandling B, Bilik R, et al. Perianal complications of pediatric Crohn's disease. J Pediatr Surg 1991;26(5):513–5.
14. Cosnes J, Cattan S, Blain A, et al. Long-term evolution of disease behavior of Crohn's disease. Inflamm Bowel Dis 2002;8(4):244–50.
15. Roberts PL, Schoetz DJ Jr, Pricolo R, et al. Clinical course of Crohn's disease in older patients. A retrospective study. Dis Colon Rectum 1990;33(6):458–62.
16. Nguyen GC, Torres EA, Regueiro M, et al. Inflammatory bowel disease characteristics among African Americans, Hispanics, and non-Hispanic Whites: characterization of a large North American cohort. Am J Gastroenterol 2006; 101(5):1012–23.
17. Cross RK, Jung C, Wasan S, et al. Racial differences in disease phenotypes in patients with Crohn's disease. Inflamm Bowel Dis 2006;12(3):192–8.
18. Beaugerie L, Seksik P, Nion-Larmurier I, et al. Predictors of Crohn's disease. Gastroenterology 2006;130(3):650–6.
19. Rankin GB, Watts HD, Melnyk CS, et al. National Cooperative Crohn's Disease Study: extraintestinal manifestations and perianal complications. Gastroenterology 1979;77(4 Pt 2):914–20.
20. Gelbmann CM, Rogler G, Gross V, et al. Prior bowel resections, perianal disease, and a high initial Crohn's disease activity index are associated with corticosteroid resistance in active Crohn's disease. Am J Gastroenterol 2002;97(6):1438–45.
21. Makowiec F, Jehle EC, Starlinger M. Clinical course of perianal fistulas in Crohn's disease. Gut 1995;37(5):696–701.
22. Mahmoud N, Rombeau JL, Ross HM, et al. Colon and rectum. PA. In: Townsend CM, Beauchamp RD, Evers BM, et al, editors. Sabiston Textbook of Surgery. Philadelphia: Saunders; 2004. p. 1401.
23. Gillen CD, Walmsley RS, Prior P, et al. Ulcerative colitis and Crohn's disease: a comparison of the colorectal cancer risk in extensive colitis. Gut 1994; 35(11):1590–2.
24. Ekbom A, Helmick C, Zack M, et al. Increased risk of large-bowel cancer in Crohn's disease with colonic involvement. Lancet 1990;336(8711):357–9.
25. Sjodahl RI, Myrelid P, Soderholm JD. Anal and rectal cancer in Crohn's disease. Colorectal Dis 2003;5(5):490–5.
26. Ky A, Sohn N, Weinstein MA, et al. Carcinoma arising in anorectal fistulas of Crohn's disease. Dis Colon Rectum 1998;41(8):992–6.
27. Connell WR, Sheffield JP, Kamm MA, et al. Lower gastrointestinal malignancy in Crohn's disease. Gut 1994;35(3):347–52.
28. Weedon DD, Shorter RG, Ilstrup DM, et al. Crohn's disease and cancer. N Engl J Med 1973;289(21):1099–103.
29. Vermeire S, Van Assche G, Rutgeerts P. Perianal Crohn's disease: classification and clinical evaluation. Dig Liver Dis 2007;39(10):959–62.
30. Keighley MR, Allan RN. Current status and influence of operation on perianal Crohn's disease. Int J Colorectal Dis 1986;1(2):104–7.
31. Buchmann P, Keighley MR, Allan RN, et al. Natural history of perianal Crohn's disease. Ten year follow-up: a plea for conservatism. Am J Surg 1980;140(5): 642–4.

32. Ingle SB, Loftus EV Jr. The natural history of perianal Crohn's disease. Dig Liver Dis 2007;39(10):963–9.

33. Wolkomir AF, Luchtefeld MA. Surgery for symptomatic hemorrhoids and anal fissures in Crohn's disease. Dis Colon Rectum 1993;36(6):545–7.

34. Steele SR. Operative management of Crohn's disease of the colon including anorectal disease. Surg Clin North Am 2007;87(3):611–31.

35. Singh B, McC Mortensen NJ, Jewell DP, et al. Perianal Crohn's disease. Br J Surg 2004;91(7):801–14.

36. Nelson RL, Abcarian H, Davis FG, et al. Prevalence of benign anorectal disease in a randomly selected population. Dis Colon Rectum 1995;38(4):341–4.

37. Jeffery PJ, Parks AG, Ritchie JK. Treatment of haemorrhoids in patients with inflammatory bowel disease. Lancet 1977;1(8021):1084–5.

38. Sweeney JL, Ritchie JK, Nicholls RJ. Anal fissure in Crohn's disease. Br J Surg 1988;75(1):56–7.

39. Fleshner PR, Schoetz DJ Jr, Roberts PL, et al. Anal fissure in Crohn's disease: a plea for aggressive management. Dis Colon Rectum 1995;38(11):1137–43.

40. Madoff RD, Fleshman JW. AGA technical review on the diagnosis and care of patients with anal fissure. Gastroenterology 2003;124(1):235–45.

41. Singh B, George BD, Mortensen NJ. Surgical therapy of perianal Crohn's disease. Dig Liver Dis 2007;39(10):988–92.

42. Siproudhis L, Mortaji A, Mary JY, et al. Anal lesions: any significant prognosis in Crohn's disease? Eur J Gastroenterol Hepatol 1997;9(3):239–43.

43. Strong SA. Perianal Crohn's disease. Semin Pediatr Surg 2007;16(3):185–93.

44. Linares L, Moreira LF, Andrews H, et al. Natural history and treatment of anorectal strictures complicating Crohn's disease. Br J Surg 1988;75(7):653–5.

45. Alexander-Williams J, Allan A, Morel P, et al. The therapeutic dilatation of enteric strictures due to Crohn's disease. Ann R Coll Surg Engl 1986;68(2):95–7.

46. Galandiuk S, Kimberling J, Al-Mishlab TG, et al. Perianal Crohn's disease: predictors of need for permanent diversion. Ann Surg 2005;241(5):796–801 [discussion: 801–2].

47. Williamson ME, Hughes LE. Bowel diversion should be used with caution in stenosing anal Crohn's disease. Gut 1994;35(8):1139–40.

48. Regueiro M, Mardini H. Treatment of perianal fistulizing Crohn's disease with infliximab alone or as an adjunct to exam under anesthesia with seton placement. Inflamm Bowel Dis 2003;9(2):98–103.

49. Topstad DR, Panaccione R, Heine JA, et al. Combined seton placement, infliximab infusion, and maintenance immunosuppressives improve healing rate in fistulizing anorectal Crohn's disease: a single center experience. Dis Colon Rectum 2003;46(5):577–83.

50. Schwartz DA, White CM, Wise PE, et al. Use of endoscopic ultrasound to guide combination medical and surgical therapy for patients with Crohn's perianal fistulas. Inflamm Bowel Dis 2005;11(8):727–32.

51. Schwartz DA, Wiersema MJ, Dudiak KM, et al. A comparison of endoscopic ultrasound, magnetic resonance imaging, and exam under anesthesia for evaluation of Crohn's perianal fistulas. Gastroenterology 2001;121(5):1064–72.

52. Kuijpers HC, Schulpen T. Fistulography for fistula-in-ano. Is it useful? Dis Colon Rectum 1985;28(2):103–4.

53. Weisman RI, Orsay CP, Pearl RK, et al. The role of fistulography in fistula-in-ano. Report of five cases. Dis Colon Rectum 1991;34(2):181–4.

54. Yousem DM, Fishman EK, Jones B. Crohn disease: perirectal and perianal findings at CT. Radiology 1988;167(2):331–4.

55. Schratter-Sehn AU, Lochs H, Vogelsang H, et al. Endoscopic ultrasonography versus computed tomography in the differential diagnosis of perianorectal complications in Crohn's disease. Endoscopy 1993;25(9):582–6.
56. Buchanan GN, Halligan S, Bartram CI, et al. Clinical examination, endosonography, and MR imaging in preoperative assessment of fistula in ano: comparison with outcome-based reference standard. Radiology 2004;233(3):674–81.
57. Lunniss PJ, Barker PG, Sultan AH, et al. Magnetic resonance imaging of fistula-in-ano. Dis Colon Rectum 1994;37(7):708–18.
58. West RL, Dwarkasing S, Felt-Bersma RJ, et al. Hydrogen peroxide-enhanced three-dimensional endoanal ultrasonography and endoanal magnetic resonance imaging in evaluating perianal fistulas: agreement and patient preference. Eur J Gastroenterol Hepatol 2004;16(12):1319–24.
59. West RL, Zimmerman DD, Dwarkasing S, et al. Prospective comparison of hydrogen peroxide-enhanced three-dimensional endoanal ultrasonography and endoanal magnetic resonance imaging of perianal fistulas. Dis Colon Rectum 2003;46(10):1407–15.
60. Poen AC, Felt-Bersma RJ, Eijsbouts QA, et al. Hydrogen peroxide-enhanced transanal ultrasound in the assessment of fistula-in-ano. Dis Colon Rectum 1998;41(9):1147–52.
61. Ardizzone S, Maconi G, Colombo E, et al. Perianal fistulae following infliximab treatment: clinical and endosonographic outcome. Inflamm Bowel Dis 2004; 10(2):91–6.
62. Spradlin NM, Wise PE, Herline AJ, et al. A randomized prospective trial of endoscopic ultrasound to guide combination medical and surgical treatment for Crohn's perianal fistulas. Am J Gastroenterol 2008;103(10):2527–35.
63. Schaefer O, Lohrmann C, Langer M. Assessment of anal fistulas with high-resolution subtraction MR-fistulography: comparison with surgical findings. J Magn Reson Imaging 2004;19(1):91–8.
64. Beets-Tan RG, Beets GL, van der Hoop AG, et al. Preoperative MR imaging of anal fistulas: does it really help the surgeon? Radiology 2001;218(1):75–84.
65. Buchanan GN, Halligan S, Williams AB, et al. Magnetic resonance imaging for primary fistula in ano. Br J Surg 2003;90(7):877–81.
66. Sachar DB, Bodian CA, Goldstein ES, et al. Is perianal Crohn's disease associated with intestinal fistulization? Am J Gastroenterol 2005;100(7):1547–9.
67. Heuman R, Bolin T, Sjodahl R, et al. The incidence and course of perianal complications and arthralgia after intestinal resection with restoration of continuity for Crohn's disease. Br J Surg 1981;68(8):528–30.
68. Marks CG, Ritchie JK, Lockhart-Mummery HE. Anal fistulas in Crohn's disease. Br J Surg 1981;68(8):525–7.
69. Orkin BA, Telander RL. The effect of intra-abdominal resection or fecal diversion on perianal disease in pediatric Crohn's disease. J Pediatr Surg 1985;20(4): 343–7.
70. Pritchard TJ, Schoetz DJ Jr, Roberts PL, et al. Perirectal abscess in Crohn's disease. Drainage and outcome. Dis Colon Rectum 1990;33(11):933–7.
71. Sohn N, Korelitz BI, Weinstein MA. Anorectal Crohn's disease: definitive surgery for fistulas and recurrent abscesses. Am J Surg 1980;139(3):394–7.
72. Giovannini M, Bories E, Moutardier V, et al. Drainage of deep pelvic abscesses using therapeutic echo endoscopy. Endoscopy 2003;35(6):511–4.
73. Williams JG, Rothenberger DA, Nemer FD, et al. Fistula-in-ano in Crohn's disease. Results of aggressive surgical treatment. Dis Colon Rectum 1991; 34(5):378–84.

74. Halme L, Sainio AP. Factors related to frequency, type, and outcome of anal fistulas in Crohn's disease. Dis Colon Rectum 1995;38(1):55–9.
75. Sangwan YP, Schoetz DJ Jr, Murray JJ, et al. Perianal Crohn's disease. Results of local surgical treatment. Dis Colon Rectum 1996;39(5):529–35.
76. Faucheron JL, Saint-Marc O, Guibert L, et al. Long-term seton drainage for high anal fistulas in Crohn's disease–a sphincter-saving operation? Dis Colon Rectum 1996;39(2):208–11.
77. Pearl RK, Andrews JR, Orsay CP, et al. Role of the seton in the management of anorectal fistulas. Dis Colon Rectum 1993;36(6):573–7 [discussion: 577–9].
78. Thornton M, Solomon MJ. Long-term indwelling seton for complex anal fistulas in Crohn's disease. Dis Colon Rectum 2005;48(3):459–63.
79. Buchanan GN, Owen HA, Torkington J, et al. Long-term outcome following loose-seton technique for external sphincter preservation in complex anal fistula. Br J Surg 2004;91(4):476–80.
80. Eitan A, Koliada M, Bickel A. The use of the loose seton technique as a definitive treatment for recurrent and persistent high trans-sphincteric anal fistulas: a long-term outcome. J Gastrointest Surg 2009;13(6):1116–9.
81. Edwards CM, George BD, Jewell DP, et al. Role of a defunctioning stoma in the management of large bowel Crohn's disease. Br J Surg 2000;87(8):1063–6.
82. Dejaco C, Harrer M, Waldhoer T, et al. Antibiotics and azathioprine for the treatment of perianal fistulas in Crohn's disease. Aliment Pharmacol Ther 2003;18(11–12):1113–20.
83. Bernstein LH, Frank MS, Brandt LJ, et al. Healing of perineal Crohn's disease with metronidazole. Gastroenterology 1980;79(3):599.
84. Turunen UM, Farkkila MA, Hakala K, et al. Long-term treatment of ulcerative colitis with ciprofloxacin: a prospective, double-blind, placebo-controlled study. Gastroenterology 1998;115(5):1072–8.
85. Brandt LJ, Bernstein LH, Boley SJ, et al. Metronidazole therapy for perineal Crohn's disease: a follow-up study. Gastroenterology 1982;83(2):383–7.
86. Jakobovits J, Schuster MM. Metronidazole therapy for Crohn's disease and associated fistulae. Am J Gastroenterol 1984;79(7):533–40.
87. Pearson DC, May GR, Fick GH, et al. Azathioprine and 6-mercaptopurine in Crohn disease. A meta-analysis. Ann Intern Med 1995;123(2):132–42.
88. Hinterleitner TA, Petritsch W, Aichbichler B, et al. Combination of cyclosporine, azathioprine and prednisolone for perianal fistulas in Crohn's disease. Z Gastroenterol 1997;35(8):603–8.
89. Egan LJ, Sandborn WJ, Tremaine WJ. Clinical outcome following treatment of refractory inflammatory and fistulizing Crohn's disease with intravenous cyclosporine. Am J Gastroenterol 1998;93(3):442–8.
90. Gurudu SR, Griffel LH, Gialanella RJ, et al. Cyclosporine therapy in inflammatory bowel disease: short-term and long-term results. J Clin Gastroenterol 1999;29(2):151–4.
91. Sandborn WJ, Present DH, Isaacs KL, et al. Tacrolimus for the treatment of fistulas in patients with Crohn's disease: a randomized, placebo-controlled trial. Gastroenterology 2003;125(2):380–8.
92. Present DH, Rutgeerts P, Targan S, et al. Infliximab for the treatment of fistulas in patients with Crohn's disease. N Engl J Med 1999;340(18):1398–405.
93. Sands BE, Anderson FH, Bernstein CN, et al. Infliximab maintenance therapy for fistulizing Crohn's disease. N Engl J Med 2004;350(9):876–85.

94. Parsi MA, Lashner BA, Achkar JP, et al. Type of fistula determines response to infliximab in patients with fistulous Crohn's disease. Am J Gastroenterol 2004; 99(3):445–9.
95. Ricart E, Panaccione R, Loftus EV, et al. Infliximab for Crohn's disease in clinical practice at the Mayo Clinic: the first 100 patients. Am J Gastroenterol 2001; 96(3):722–9.
96. Schiff MH, Burmester GR, Kent JD, et al. Safety analyses of adalimumab (HUMIRA) in global clinical trials and US postmarketing surveillance of patients with rheumatoid arthritis. Ann Rheum Dis 2006;65(7):889–94.
97. Colombel JF, Sandborn WJ, Rutgeerts P, et al. Adalimumab for maintenance of clinical response and remission in patients with Crohn's disease: the CHARM trial. Gastroenterology 2007;132(1):52–65.
98. Colombel JF, Schwartz DA, Sandborn WJ, et al. Adalimumab for the treatment of fistulas in patients with Crohn's disease. Gut 2009;58(7):940–8.
99. Hobbiss JH, Schofield PF. Management of perianal Crohn's disease. J R Soc Med 1982;75(6):414–7.
100. Morrison JG, Gathright JB Jr, Ray JE, et al. Surgical management of anorectal fistulas in Crohn's disease. Dis Colon Rectum 1989;32(6):492–6.
101. Nordgren S, Fasth S, Hulten L. Anal fistulas in Crohn's disease: incidence and outcome of surgical treatment. Int J Colorectal Dis 1992;7(4):214–8.
102. Alexander-Williams J, Steinberg DM, Fielding JS, et al. Proceedings. Perianal Crohn's disease. Gut 1974;15(10):822–3.
103. Lindsey I, Smilgin-Humphreys MM, Cunningham C, et al. A randomized, controlled trial of fibrin glue vs. conventional treatment for anal fistula. Dis Colon Rectum 2002;45(12):1608–15.
104. Swinscoe MT, Ventakasubramaniam AK, Jayne DG. Fibrin glue for fistula-in-ano: the evidence reviewed. Tech Coloproctol 2005;9(2):89–94.
105. Vitton V, Gasmi M, Barthet M, et al. Long-term healing of Crohn's anal fistulas with fibrin glue injection. Aliment Pharmacol Ther 2005;21(12):1453–7.
106. Loungnarath R, Dietz DW, Mutch MG, et al. Fibrin glue treatment of complex anal fistulas has low success rate. Dis Colon Rectum 2004;47(4):432–6.
107. O'Connor L, Champagne BJ, Ferguson MA, et al. Efficacy of anal fistula plug in closure of Crohn's anorectal fistulas. Dis Colon Rectum 2006; 49(10):1569–73.
108. Champagne BJ, O'Connor LM, Ferguson M, et al. Efficacy of anal fistula plug in closure of cryptoglandular fistulas: long-term follow-up. Dis Colon Rectum 2006; 49(12):1817–21.
109. Ky AJ, Sylla P, Steinhagen R, et al. Collagen fistula plug for the treatment of anal fistulas. Dis Colon Rectum 2008;51(6):838–43.
110. Talbot C, Sagar PM, Johnston MJ, et al. Infliximab in the surgical management of complex fistulating anal Crohn's disease. Colorectal Dis 2005;7(2):164–8.
111. Matos D, Lunniss PJ, Phillips RK. Total sphincter conservation in high fistula in ano: results of a new approach. Br J Surg 1993;80(6):802–4.
112. Galis-Rozen E, Tulchinsky H, Rosen A, et al. Long-term outcome of loose-seton for complex anal fistula: a two-centre study of patients with and without Crohn's disease. Colorectal Dis 2009. [Epub ahed of print].
113. Makowiec F, Jehle EC, Becker HD, et al. Clinical course after transanal advancement flap repair of perianal fistula in patients with Crohn's disease. Br J Surg 1995;82(5):603–6.
114. Joo JS, Weiss EG, Nogueras JJ, et al. Endorectal advancement flap in perianal Crohn's disease. Am Surg 1998;64(2):147–50.

115. Robertson WG, Mangione JS. Cutaneous advancement flap closure: alternative method for treatment of complicated anal fistulas. Dis Colon Rectum 1998;41(7): 884–6 [discussion: 886–7].
116. Marchesa P, Hull TL, Fazio VW. Advancement sleeve flaps for treatment of severe perianal Crohn's disease. Br J Surg 1998;85(12):1695–8.
117. van der Hagen SJ, Baeten CG, Soeters PB, et al. Anti-TNF-alpha (infliximab) used as induction treatment in case of active proctitis in a multistep strategy followed by definitive surgery of complex anal fistulas in Crohn's disease: a preliminary report. Dis Colon Rectum 2005;48(4):758–67.
118. Gaertner WB, Decanini A, Mellgren A, et al. Does infliximab infusion impact results of operative treatment for Crohn's perianal fistulas? Dis Colon Rectum 2007;50(11):1754–60.
119. Andreani SM, Dang HH, Grondona P, et al. Rectovaginal fistula in Crohn's disease. Dis Colon Rectum 2007;50(12):2215–22.
120. Sands BE, Blank MA, Patel K, et al. Long-term treatment of rectovaginal fistulas in Crohn's disease: response to infliximab in the ACCENT II Study. Clin Gastroenterol Hepatol 2004;2(10):912–20.
121. Hull TL, Fazio VW. Surgical approaches to low anovaginal fistula in Crohn's disease. Am J Surg 1997;173(2):95–8.
122. Kodner IJ, Mazor A, Shemesh EI, et al. Endorectal advancement flap repair of rectovaginal and other complicated anorectal fistulas. Surgery 1993;114(4): 682–9 [discussion: 689–90].
123. Berman IR. Sleeve advancement anorectoplasty for complicated anorectal/ vaginal fistula. Dis Colon Rectum 1991;34(11):1032–7.
124. Sher ME, Bauer JJ, Gelernt I. Surgical repair of rectovaginal fistulas in patients with Crohn's disease: transvaginal approach. Dis Colon Rectum 1991;34(8): 641–8.
125. Cohen JL, Stricker JW, Schoetz DJ Jr, et al. Rectovaginal fistula in Crohn's disease. Dis Colon Rectum 1989;32(10):825–8.
126. Yamamoto T, Bain IM, Allan RN, et al. Persistent perineal sinus after proctocolectomy for Crohn's disease. Dis Colon Rectum 1999;42(1):96–101.
127. Rius J, Nessim A, Nogueras JJ, et al. Gracilis transposition in complicated perianal fistula and unhealed perineal wounds in Crohn's disease. Eur J Surg 2000; 166(3):218–22.
128. Yamamoto T, Allan RN, Keighley MR. Effect of fecal diversion alone on perianal Crohn's disease. World J Surg 2000;24(10):1258–62 [discussion: 1262–3].
129. Bach SP, Mortensen NJ. Revolution and evolution: 30 years of ileoanal pouch surgery. Inflamm Bowel Dis 2006;12(2):131–45.
130. Sagar PM, Dozois RR, Wolff BG. Long-term results of ileal pouch-anal anastomosis in patients with Crohn's disease. Dis Colon Rectum 1996;39(8): 893–8.
131. Reese GE, Lovegrove RE, Tilney HS, et al. The effect of Crohn's disease on outcomes after restorative proctocolectomy. Dis Colon Rectum 2007;50(2): 239–50.
132. Peyregne V, Francois Y, Gilly FN, et al. Outcome of ileal pouch after secondary diagnosis of Crohn's disease. Int J Colorectal Dis 2000;15(1):49–53.
133. Fazio VW, Tekkis PP, Remzi F, et al. Quantification of risk for pouch failure after ileal pouch anal anastomosis surgery. Ann Surg 2003;238(4):605–14 [discussion: 614–7].
134. MacRae HM, McLeod RS, Cohen Z, et al. Risk factors for pelvic pouch failure. Dis Colon Rectum 1997;40(3):257–62.

135. Melmed GY, Fleshner PR, Bardakcioglu O, et al. Family history and serology predict Crohn's disease after ileal pouch-anal anastomosis for ulcerative colitis. Dis Colon Rectum 2008;51(1):100–8.

136. Alexander F, Sarigol S, DiFiore J, et al. Fate of the pouch in 151 pediatric patients after ileal pouch anal anastomosis. J Pediatr Surg 2003;38(1):78–82.

137. Keswani RN, Cohen RD. Postoperative management of ulcerative colitis and Crohn's disease. Curr Gastroenterol Rep 2005;7(6):492–9.

138. Shen B, Remzi FH, Brzezinski A, et al. Risk factors for pouch failure in patients with different phenotypes of Crohn's disease of the pouch. Inflamm Bowel Dis 2008;14(7):942–8.

139. Wolf JM, Achkar J, Lashner BA, et al. Afferent limb ulcers predict Crohn's disease in patients with ileal pouch-anal anastomosis. Gastroenterology 2004; 126(7):1686–91.

140. Viscido A, Habib FI, Kohn A, et al. Infliximab in refractory pouchitis complicated by fistulae following ileo-anal pouch for ulcerative colitis. Aliment Pharmacol Ther 2003;17(10):1263–71.

141. Berrebi W, Chaussade S, Bruhl AL, et al. Treatment of Crohn's disease recurrence after ileoanal anastomosis by azathioprine. Dig Dis Sci 1993;38(8): 1558–60.

142. Colombel JF, Ricart E, Loftus EV Jr, et al. Management of Crohn's disease of the ileoanal pouch with infliximab. Am J Gastroenterol 2003;98(10):2239–44.

143. Ozuner G, Hull T, Lee P, et al. What happens to a pelvic pouch when a fistula develops? Dis Colon Rectum 1997;40(5):543–7.

144. Alexander F. Complications of ileal pouch anal anastomosis. Semin Pediatr Surg 2007;16(3):200–4.

# Condyloma and Other Infections Including Human Immunodeficiency Virus

Peter K. Lee, MD[a,c], Kirsten Bass Wilkins, MD, FACS, FASCRS[a,b],*

**KEYWORDS**

- Perianal sexually transmitted diseases • Human papillomavirus
- Anal intraepithelial neoplasia • High resolution anoscopy

Surgeons take care of many patients with sexually transmitted diseases (STDs). Populations at risk include men and women who engage in anal receptive intercourse. Immunosuppressed patients (human immunodeficiency virus [HIV], AIDS, transplant) are also at risk, as many presentations of STDs are the result of reactivation of latent disease. Prompt recognition of the signs and symptoms is necessary for timely diagnosis and optimal therapeutic outcomes. Central to the successful treatment of STDs is an accurate, detailed sexual history, including the documentation of anal intercourse, unprotected intercourse, history of sexual abuse or rape, and, in women, history of cervical or vulvar dysplasia. Because coinfection is frequent, a complete history of STDs, including HIV and hepatitis, should be elicited. Transplant patients, cancer patients, and patients with autoimmune diseases receiving immunosuppressive medications will also need to be identified. This article reviews the presentation and management of patients with perianal STDs, including those with HIV, as well as the evolving management of patients with anal intraepithelial neoplasia.

## NON-HUMAN PAPILLOMAVIRUS AND HUMAN PAPILLOMAVIRUS-RELATED SEXUALLY TRANSMITTED DISEASES

When approaching patients with STDs, it is helpful to first distinguish between non-human papillomavirus (HPV) and HPV-related diseases in terms of clinical diagnosis and treatment. Because so many STDs may present in the perianal area, it is often useful to categorize more common diseases based on usual clinical signs and symptoms. For non-HPV STDs, broad categories of clinical presentation include perianal ulceration, proctitis, proctocolitis, and enteritis (**Fig. 1**).

---

[a] UMDNJ-Robert Wood Johnson University Hospital, New Brunswick, NJ, USA
[b] 3900 Park Avenue, Suite 101, Edison, NJ 08820, USA
[c] 5965 E. Broad Street, Suite 120, Columbus, OH 43213, USA
* Corresponding author. 3900 Park Avenue, Suite 101, Edison, NJ 08820, USA.
*E-mail address:* kirstenbwilkins@gmail.com (K.B. Wilkins).

Surg Clin N Am 90 (2010) 99–112
doi:10.1016/j.suc.2009.09.005                    surgical.theclinics.com
0039-6109/09/$ – see front matter © 2010 Elsevier Inc. All rights reserved.

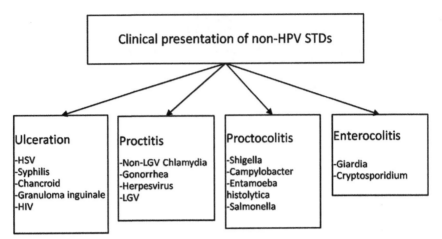

Fig. 1. Common causes of non-HPV sexually transmitted diseases. Refer to www.cdc.gov for an exhaustive review of sexually transmitted diseases.

## Non-Human Papillomavirus Sexually Transmitted Diseases

### Ulceration

The most common STDs to present with perianal ulceration include herpes, syphilis, chancroid, and granuloma inguinale. Depending on etiology, the ulcers may be painful or painless, and inguinal lymphadenopathy may be present. Genital ulceration facilitates the acquisition of HIV infection. Thus, it is paramount to perform HIV testing in these patients. Furthermore, in HIV-positive patients, decreasing CD4 counts is associated with more severe presentation of ulcers, facilitating the shedding and transmission of HIV particles.[1,2] Because coinfection is frequent, all patients should be evaluated for both syphilis and herpes.[3] At present, there is no Food and Drug Administration (FDA)-approved polymerase chain reaction (PCR) test for any of these organisms obtained from anal or rectal swabs. In general, diagnosis is made on clinical grounds and treatment is empiric. In addition, anoscopy and pelvic examination may be necessary to evaluate for extent of involvement, and possibly obtain cultures.

**Herpes simplex virus** The most common cause of genital ulcerations is herpes simplex virus-1 (HSV-1) and herpes simplex virus-2 (HSV-2), but the majority of anogenital infection is secondary to HSV-2. Approximately 22% of the population in the United States is seropositive for HSV-2.[3] HSV-2 may be responsible for perianal and genital ulceration as well as proctitis (see later discussion). Among HIV-positive individuals, HSV-1 or HSV-2 is the most common viral coinfection, with up to 95% of HIV-positive men who have sex with men (MSM) being seropositive for HSV-1 and/or HSV-2.[1,3,4]

Following viral inoculation, the virus enters the epithelial lining and is transported retrograde to the dorsal root ganglia of sensory nerves. The incubation period is approximately 2 to 12 days. At any time, the virus can be shed or reactivated by traveling back to the periphery via the sensory nerves. Infection is usually lifelong.[3] Reactivation and shedding of virus is increased in patients with decreased immune status.[4]

Genital herpes presents as painful skin vesicles that eventually coalesce and ulcerate. On initial infection, patients often have constitutional symptoms including fever, myalgias, and malaise. Clinical diagnosis should be confirmed with laboratory tests, including isolation of HSV in cell culture from specimens taken from vesicles. Unfortunately, cytologic examination of infected cells (Tzanck smear) is both insensitive and nonspecific.[3] Type-specific glycoprotein G-based serologic testing is available, however, given the lifelong nature of this disease, may not be useful in patients with known prior HSV infection.

Treatment should be directed toward controlling the symptoms of active episodes. For initial HSV-2 infection, antiviral therapy can consist of a 7- to 10-day oral course of acyclovir (400 mg by mouth 3 times a day or 200 mg by mouth 5 times daily), famciclovir (250 mg by mouth 3 times a day), or valacyclovir (1 g by mouth twice a day).[3] For recurrences, treatment can shorten the duration of episodes; however, patients need to begin therapy within 1 day of lesion onset in order for this to be effective. Options include the following: a 5-day course of acyclovir (400 mg by mouth 3 times a day or 800 mg by mouth twice a day), famciclovir (125 mg by mouth twice a day), or valacyclovir (1 g by mouth daily); a 3-day course of valacyclovir (500 mg by mouth twice a day); a 2-day course of acyclovir (800 mg by mouth 3 times a day); or a 1-day course of famciclovir (1 g by mouth twice a day). In addition, daily suppressive therapy has been shown to decrease the number of recurrences and has been shown to decrease transmission. Recommended regimens for suppressive therapy include acyclovir (400 mg by mouth twice a day), famciclovir (250 mg by mouth twice a day), or valacyclovir (500 mg or 1 g by mouth daily). In HIV-positive patients, regimens may be altered to include higher doses or prolonged duration of treatment for herpes as well as all STDs.[3]

**Syphilis** The causative organism of syphilis is *Treponema pallidum*. The clinical presentation of syphilis varies depending on the stage of presentation. Primary syphilis presents as a painful or painless ulcer, or chancre, at the infection site. Patients with atypical anal fissures should be evaluated for syphilis. In secondary syphilis, symptoms include a maculopapular rash of the trunk and extremities, lymphadenopathy, and condyloma lata in the perianal area. Tertiary syphilis is marked by neurologic or cardiac symptoms. Diagnostic testing includes darkfield examination or immunofluorescent testing of lesion exudates, as well as treponemal and non-treponemal (venereal disease research laboratory and rapid plasma reagin) serologic testing. Treatment depends on the stage of disease. For primary or secondary syphilis, treatment consists of a single dose of benzathine penicillin G (2.4 million units intramuscularly). For penicillin-allergic patients, alternative therapies include a 2-week course of doxycycline (100 mg by mouth twice a day) or tetracycline (500 mg by mouth 4 times a day). For tertiary syphilis without neurologic symptoms, a 3-week course of benzathine penicillin G (2.4 million units intramuscularly weekly) is recommended. For neurosyphilis, a 2-week course of aqueous crystalline penicillin G (18–24 million units intravenously daily) is recommended.[3]

**Chancroid** The causative organism of chancroid is *Haemophilus ducreyi*. Chancroid presents as a painful genital ulcer with concomitant inguinal lymphadenopathy. Unfortunately, this organism is difficult to culture, therefore the diagnosis is often based on clinical grounds alone. A patient with painful genital ulcers in conjunction with inguinal lymphadenopathy in whom syphilis and herpes have been excluded should raise the suspicion for chancroid.[3] Treatment consists of a single dose of azithromycin (1 g by mouth) or ceftriaxone (250 mg intramuscularly). Oral alternatives include a 3-day course of ciprofloxacin (500 mg by mouth twice a day) or a 7-day course of erythromycin (500 mg by mouth 3 times a day). Large ulcers may take as long as 2 weeks to heal; however, this should not prolong treatment.[3] Patients should be examined after 7 days and if there is no improvement; other diagnoses such as lymphogranu-loma venereum (LGV) may need to be considered and treated (see later discussion).

**Granuloma inguinale**  The causative organism of granuloma inguinale is *Klebsiella gran-ulomatis*. The disease is also referred to as donovanosis. Presentation includes the progressive development of painless ulcerations without inguinal lymphadenopathy. The lesions are vascular with extensive granulation tissue, which easily bleeds. Hyper-trophic, necrotic, and sclerotic variants of the disease also exist. This disease is rare in the United States, but it is endemic in the developing world. The organism is difficult to culture, but Donovan bodies may be seen on biopsy. First-line treatment consists of doxycycline (100 mg by mouth twice a day), and should continue for at least 3 weeks or until all lesions have healed. Second-line regimens include azithromycin (1 g by mouth weekly), ciprofloxacin (750 mg by mouth twice a day), erythromycin base (500 mg by mouth 4 times a day), or trimethoprim-sulfamethoxazole (160 mg/800 mg by mouth twice a day) for 3 weeks.[3]

**Human immunodeficiency virus**  HIV in and of itself may be associated with perianal ulcers that may be painful. These ulcers may be large and may look like atypical anal fissures, commonly presenting proximal to the dentate line. The best treatment for these ulcers typically is the institution of highly active antiretroviral therapy (HAART). As the patient's immune status improves (increasing CD4 counts and decreased viral loads), the ulcers and symptoms associated with them lessen. Surgical intervention should not generally be encouraged, especially if CD4 counts are very low, as wounds may worsen and are very slow to heal.[5]

### Proctitis

Proctitis is inflammation of the rectum. In a recent study of a San Francisco STD clinic, the most common origins of infectious proctitis in MSM were gonorrhea (30%), *Chla-mydia trachomatis* (19%), HSV-2 (16%), and syphilis (2%). In addition, there was a large number of patients in whom no cause was found (45%).[6] As with genital ulcers, proctitis secondary to STDs facilitates transmission of HIV due to breakdown of mucosal barriers. Thus, treatment of proctitis can reduce viral shedding. Patients typi-cally present with constipation, mucopurulent anal discharge, hematochezia, and tenesmus.[7] Workup for proctitis in high-risk populations should include all of the organisms listed previously in this paragraph. Physical examination should include anoscopy and rigid sigmoidoscopy to evaluate the extent of involvement and to obtain biopsies and cultures. Stool cultures with microscopic examination for ova and para-sites should also be routinely obtained. HIV testing should be performed if recent HIV status is unknown.[7]

**Chlamydia**  *Chlamydia trachomatis* (serovars A–K) is an obligate intracellular bacterium responsible for chlamydia proctitis. Patients typically report a bloody, mucopurulent discharge, tenesmus, and anal pain, but asymptomatic infection may occur.[7] Rectal inspection reveals friable, erythematous, and edematous mucosa. Organisms may be cultured from the discharge. Treatment is the same as for urethritis or vaginitis secondary to chlamydia, which consists of a single dose of azithromycin (1 g by mouth) or doxycycline (100 mg by mouth twice a day) for 7 days. Alternative single-agent regimens include a 7-day course of erythromycin base (500 mg by mouth 4 times a day), erythromycin ethylsuccinate (800 mg by mouth 4 times a day), ofloxacin (300 mg by mouth twice a day), or levofloxacin (500 mg by mouth daily).[8] Because co-infection with *Neisseria gonorrhoeae* is very common, empiric treatment of gonorrhea is also recommended.

**Gonorrhea** Gonorrhea is caused by *Neisseria gonorrhea,* a gram-negative diplo-coccus. Similar to chlamydia, patients report a mucopurulent discharge, tenesmus, and anal pain.[7] Inspection of the rectum reveals nonspecific erythema, edema, and friability. On anoscopic examination, gentle pressure on the crypts will produce a classic purulent discharge. Gram stains of rectal exudates may identify the gram-negative diplococcus and should be obtained.[9] Treatment is the same as for urethritis or vaginitis secondary to gonorrhea, and consists of a single dose of either ceftriaxone (125 mg intramuscularly) or cefixime (400 mg by mouth). Due to antibiotic resistance, fluoroquinolones are no longer recommended in the United States for the treatment of gonorrhea.[9] Because chlamydial coinfection is very common, empiric treatment of chlamydia should be instituted.

**Herpesvirus** The most common cause of viral proctitis is herpesvirus. Approximately 70% of herpes proctitis is secondary to HSV-2. Cytomegalovirus (CMV) is another herpesvirus that can produce proctitis in immunosuppressed patients. The initial infection from HSV-2 results from anoreceptive intercourse or oral-anal contact. In AIDS patients, decreased CD4 counts are associated with increased viral shedding.[4] Patients typically present with severe anorectal pain and tenesmus. Patients also complain of increased stool frequency and bloody mucoid discharge that may be confused with "diarrhea"; they may also complain of constipation, urinary retention, and impotence secondary to sacral radiculopathy. Anoscopy reveals diffuse mucosal erosions and erythema.[4] The proctitis is typically limited to the distal 10 cm of the rectum, whereas other pathogens may cause more proximal disease. Treatment consists of acyclovir (400 mg by mouth 5 times daily) and is associated with cessation of viral shedding in 80% of patients after 3 days of treatment.[4] In addition, given the frequency of coinfection, empiric treatment of gonorrhea and chlamydia is recommended.[6]

**Lymphogranuloma venereum** LGV is endemic in the developing world, but in recent years it has become a more commonly recognized cause of proctitis in Westernized countries, particularly in HIV-positive MSM. The causative organism of LGV is *C. tra-chomatis* (serovars L1, L2, or L3).[8,10] The initial presentation is anal ulceration at the site of inoculation, which often goes unrecognized. In later stages, it is characterized by painful inguinal or femoral lymphadenopathy known as buboes. However, 25% of patients develop anorectal symptoms exclusively without inguinal lymphadenopathy. This "anorectal syndrome" consists of acute proctocolitis in which there may be bloody, mucopurulent rectal discharge and narrowing on rectal examination. Flexible endoscopic examination demonstrates inflamed, hyperemic, and friable rectal mucosa that rarely extends proximal to the sigmoid colon.[10] Patients may also develop a chronic, progressive, inflammatory form of disease in which ulceration, strictures, and fistulae form in the anorectal region, which may mimic Crohn's disease.[10] Indeed, there have been case reports of LGV that have been misdiagnosed and treated ineffectively as Crohn's disease, due to clinical similarities. Again, this is a situation whereby an accurate sexual and social history leads to proper diagnosis and treatment. Diagnosis can be confirmed by culture or immunofluorescence identi-fication of *C. trachomatis* from lymph node aspirates or rectal swabs. However, treat-ment is typically started empirically. First-line treatment consists of a 3-week course of doxycycline (100 mg by mouth twice a day). Alternative treatment consists of a 3-week course of erythromycin base (500 mg by mouth 4 times a day).[8,11] It is important to differentiate LGV proctitis from non-LGV chlamydial proctitis, as the duration of treat-ment is different.

*Proctocolitis*
The organisms responsible for proctocolitis tend to be different from those that cause isolated proctitis. These organisms tend to be transmitted by the fecal-oral route, most commonly as food and waterborne illnesses, but they can also be spread directly by the oral-anal route. Etiologic agents include, but are not limited to, *Shigella*, *Campylobacter*, *Entamoeba histolytica*, *Salmonella*, and CMV. Patients typically present with small volume diarrhea, lower abdominal pain and mild hematochezia.[7] Physical examination should include anoscopy and rigid or flexible sigmoidoscopy, to evaluate the extent of involvement and obtain biopsy and cultures. Stool cultures with microscopic examination for ova and parasites should also be routinely obtained. Treatment of *Shigella*, *Salmonella*, and *Campylobacter* consists of a 7-day oral course of erythromycin (500 mg by mouth 4 times a day) or ciprofloxacin (250 mg by mouth twice a day). Treatment of *E. histolytica* consists of a 10-day course of metronidazole (750 mg by mouth 3 times a day) or tinidazole (2 g by mouth daily) followed by a 20-day course of iodoquinol (650 mg by mouth 3 times a day) to clear the entire gastrointestinal tract of organisms.

*Enteritis*
Patients with enteritis usually present with large-volume watery diarrhea and abdominal pain. Etiologic agents include *Giardia lamblia* and *Cryptosporidium*.[7] Endoscopic examination of the colon is usually normal in these cases unless there is coinfection with other pathogens. Workup should include stool samples for microscopic evaluation for trophozoites and cysts (*Giardia*) or oocysts (*Cryptosporidium*). These organisms may be difficult to see, therefore it may take multiple samples before they are identified. Immunoassays are available for both organisms and have been shown to be more sensitive than microscopic evaluation.[7] *Giardia* may also be isolated from duodenal biopsies. Treatment of giardiasis includes a 3-day course of metronidazole (2 g by mouth daily). Alternative treatments include a single dose of tinidazole (2 g by mouth) or a 5-day course of metronidazole (400 mg by mouth 3 times a day) for those who cannot tolerate the higher dose metronidazole. Some investigators have suggested that demonstration of cure of giardiasis requires 3 consecutive negative stool samples. Cryptosporidiosis is typically a self-limited illness in those with a competent immune system. In HIV-positive patients, treatment is focused on improving the overall immune status of the patient via HAART. Finally, as in all diarrheal disorders, fluid hydration should be assessed and properly maintained.

### Human Papilloma Virus-Related Sexually Transmitted Diseases

*Condyloma*
HPV is the most common STD. There are reports of up to 92% prevalence of HPV in HIV-positive MSMs. There are more than 80 serotypes. High-risk subtypes (most commonly 16, 18, 31, 35, and 58) are more commonly associated with high-grade dysplasia and cancer than low-risk subtypes (commonly 6, 11, 42, 43, and 44), which are associated with condyloma and low-grade dysplasia.[12,13]

Patients most commonly present with verrucous lesions, referred to as condyloma, in the perianal and intra-anal locations. These lesions tend to be relatively asymptomatic, and patients usually seek medical attention because they feel growths in the perianal area that may be associated with excess moisture in the area and occasionally a foul odor. One unusual variant of condyloma is Buschke-Lowenstein tumor, which represents a giant perianal condyloma accuminatum. Although dramatic in its clinical presentation, it is more commonly associated with low-risk HPV subtypes 6 and 11. Although clinically very aggressive with local tissue invasion and fistula forma-tion, the lesion is histologically benign.[14]

As with all STDs, a detailed sexual history is important. Physical examination should include anoscopy to identify intra-anal lesions. Biopsies should be taken of representa-tive lesions to confirm the diagnosis of condyloma and to exclude dysplasia or cancer. Specimens may be sent for HPV subtyping with PCR to categorize lesions as low-risk or high-risk for the progression to anal intraepithelial neoplasia (see later discussion).

Whereas some cases of condyloma may be cleared spontaneously by the patient's immune system, most cases require some form of treatment. The goal of treatment is to alleviate symptoms from the condyloma. However, of importance is that this treatment does not eradicate the underlying HPV infection. Therefore, recurrences are not uncommon after treatment and the disease is still transmissible. Both medical and surgical options are available for the management of condyloma. Medical treatments consist of topical agents that are used to ablate lesions. Common agents applied directly to the condyloma include podophyllin, bichloracetic acid, and trichloracetic acid. These agents are applied directly to the lesions with the wooden end of a cotton-tipped applicator, with precise attention being paid so that normal skin is not treated. The condyloma turns white on application of the aforementioned medica-tions as the proteins in the condyloma are coagulated. Podophyllin is limited to perianal use, and may be associated with the development of dysplasia after prolonged use. Patients should thoroughly wash the perianal area 8 hours after the podophyllin has been applied. Bichloracetic acid and trichloracetic acid may be used perianally as well as inside the anal canal. A novel agent that is administered by the patient is imiqui-mod. This is an immune modulator that enhances the proinflammatory cytokine response of the innate immune system via Toll-like receptor 7.[15] Imiquimod has achieved good results for perianal condylomas. The agent is supplied as a 5% cream that is applied perianally 3 times a week. The cream is applied at bedtime and washed off the following morning. Used consistently, the cream is associated with the develop-ment of perianal erythema and edema which, not uncommonly, limits the patient use.

Surgical treatment of condyloma consists of excision and biopsy of representative lesions followed by electrocautery or laser fulguration of affected areas. During fulgu-ration, extreme care is taken to produce only first-degree "burns" so as to prevent unnecessary scarring and distortion. When dealing with circumferential condyloma-tous disease extending into the anal canal, it is advisable to approach excision/fulgu-ration as staged procedures, leaving behind islands of intact mucosa, so as to reduce the risk of anal stenosis. Regardless of the surgical approach used, there is a fairly high chance of recurrent condyloma either from reactivation of persistent HPV or from new infections. Therefore, it is important to follow the patients closely so that recurrences can be addressed when the condylomatous burden is small.

Treatment of Buschke-Lowenstein tumor is also exclusively surgical, given the high risk of recurrence. The most common recommended treatment is wide local excision. Given the large size of these lesions, extensive wound defects may result and rota-tional flap coverage may be useful, although these wounds will heal by secondary intention.[14] It would be rare that an abdominoperineal resection or fecal diversion would be necessary in this particular setting. Sending off the entire specimen for pathologic evaluation is essential to rule out an underlying invasive squamous cell carcinoma.

### Anal intraepithelial neoplasia/anal cancer
Anal intraepithelial neoplasia (AIN) is regarded as a possible precursor lesion to anal squamous cell carcinoma. AIN's association with HPV has been well

described. The natural history of AIN remains poorly elucidated. However, high-risk individuals with AIN who are immunosuppressed (from AIDS or transplant medications) have a higher risk of progression to cancer.[12,16,17] There is a high association of cervical and anal dysplasia with high-risk HPV infection. Much about the management of AIN has been derived from the literature on cervical intraepithelial neoplasia (CIN) because they share HPV as the common etiologic agent; however, AIN and CIN appear to be clinically distinct entities.[13] One must be mindful that it has not yet been definitively proven that AIN is the precursor lesion to invasive anal squamous cell cancer or that aggressive treatment of AIN will prevent anal squamous cell cancer. However, there is a growing body of literature that supports the progression of AIN to invasive anal squamous cell cancer as well as the benefits of targeted treatment of AIN in certain high-risk populations, in particular HIV-positive MSMs (see later discussion).

**Pathology of anal intraepithelial neoplasia** On histological analysis the dysplastic epithelium appears thickened. The dysplasia begins at level of the basement membrane and progresses superficially. Dysplastic cells have a high nucleus-to-cytoplasmic ratio and do not "flatten" as they mature and migrate away from the basement membrane. There is an increased number of mitotic figures. With higher-grade AIN, more dysplastic features such as nuclear enlargement, irregularity, and hyperchromatism become more common.[13,16]

There are multiple grading schemes for AIN. AIN is categorized on the basis of histologic features, namely the thickness of epithelium that is dysplastic. This grading is analogous to the classification of cervical and vulvar intraepithelial neoplasia. AIN 1 refers to dysplasia that is confined to the lower third of the epithelium. In AIN 2, the dysplasia spreads to two-thirds the thickness of the epithelium. In AIN 3, from two-thirds to the entire thickness of epithelium is dysplastic. There seems to be agreement about what constitutes AIN 3; however, there continues to be controversy about the differentiation of AIN 1 and AIN 2.[18] Thus, another nomenclature has emerged: low-grade squamous intraepithelial lesion (LSIL) and high-grade squamous epithelial lesion (HSIL). AIN 1 is considered LSIL whereas AIN 2 and 3 are both HSIL. Some recommend the use of this nomenclature as it actually describes the behavior of disease and dictates the course of treatment. Whereas LSIL can regress spontaneously without treatment, HSIL may progress to anal carcinoma.[12,17]

**Association of human papilloma virus and anal cancer** HPV has been associated with most squamous cell cancers of the anogenital region (cervical, anal, vulvar). HPV DNA has been detected by PCR in up to 81% of patients with anal squamous cell cancer and 88% of patients with AIN.[19] Just as in cervical dysplasia and cancer, of the more than 80 subtypes of HPV, high-risk subtypes (most commonly 16, 18, 31, 35, and 58) are more commonly associated with high-grade dysplasia and cancer than low-risk subtypes (commonly 6, 11, 42, 43, and 44), which are associated with condyloma and low-grade dysplasia.[12,13] The high-risk subtypes have malignant transformation potential because of 2 viral oncogenes, E6 and E7. E6 binds p53, resulting in its degradation via ubiquitin pathway and preventing the cell from entering cell cycle arrest or apoptosis. E7 binds to retinoblastoma (Rb) tumor suppressor protein, allowing the cell to progress through the cell cycle and result in cell proliferation.[12,20–23] An additional protein, E2, allows HPV to attach to host chromatin and evade host cell detection.[12] Chronic high-risk HPV infection and integration into the host genome result in dysplastic changes.[24] The combination of cell proliferation and inability to enter cell cycle arrest or apoptosis if genetic errors have occurred leads to accumulation of mutations and nuclear instability, resulting in malignant transformation.

**Epidemiology and risk factors** Whereas the epidemiology of AIN is difficult to ascertain, work on population-based cancer registries has yielded information about anal cancer. Review of the National Cancer Institute's Surveillance, Epidemiology and End Results (SEER) program has found a prevalence rate of 1.28 per 100,000 for anal squamous cell carcinoma for the period 1998 to 2003.[25] Increasing rates correlated with increasing age. Hence, in the general population anal cancer is a rare disease. However, when one looks at a high-risk population, MSM, it is much more common. The Multicenter AIDS Cohort Study recently reported that incident anal cancer rates in MSM were 69 per 100,000 person-years in those who were HIV-positive and 14 per 100,000 person-years for those who were HIV-negative.[26] Although the degree of immunocompromise has been implicated in the development of anal cancer in HIV-positive MSM, the introduction of HAART has not resulted in a decrease in anal cancer.[26,27] In fact, the rate of anal cancer has increased from 30 per 100,000 person-years during the pre-HAART era to 137 per 100,000 person-years in the post-HAART period in subgroup analysis.[26] This increase may be due to the fact that HIV-positive patients are living longer from effective antiretroviral treatment. These patients continue to chronically harbor high-risk HPV infections, which then predispose them to dysplasia and possibly cancer. Several studies on the SEER database identified high number of sexual partners, history of anogenital warts, history of cervical cancer or CIN 3, smoking, anal intercourse, HIV positivity, and immunosuppression as risk factors for women developing anal cancer.[25,28,29] Of special mention are solid organ transplant patients on immunosuppressive medications. These medications have been associated with overall increases in other cancers, and this is also seen for anal cancer. In renal transplant patients, the prevalence of anal cancer was estimated to be about 14 per 100,000, about 10-fold higher than the general population.[30]

**Clinical presentation and diagnosis** AIN typically presents in the upper anal canal, anal transition zone, and the perianal skin. Squamous metaplasia of the anal transitional epithelium occurs in a fashion similar to cervical dysplasia.[16,17] Often there are no gross pathologic features, thus cytology and histology are required for diagnosis. AIN may be asymptomatic, symptomatic, or incidental (ie, found in routine hemorrhoidectomy specimens). Symptomatic patients may present with nonspecific anal irritation, and examination may reveal erythematous plaques with ulcerations or areas of lichenification on anoscopy or on perianal visual inspection.[16] Patients may present with severe perianal (within a 5 cm radius from the anal verge) pruritus ani that is unresponsive to standard medical therapy, and this should be biopsied to evaluate for AIN.[17,31]

Many patients, however, are asymptomatic and AIN is frequently first detected on screening via anal cytology. Whereas cytologic screening for cervical dysplasia by Pap smear is proven to decrease the incidence of cervical cancer, the same cannot be extrapolated for AIN and anal cancer at this point. Nonetheless, anal cytologic screening is being used by some physicians who care for high-risk patient populations (HIV-positive men and women, MSM, women with cervical/vulvar dysplasia, and transplant patients). Anal cytology is obtained by taking a blind smear of the anal transition zone by gently inserting a moistened Dacron swab 5 cm into the anal canal and taking circumferential samples while withdrawing the swab. The sample is then immersed in Thin Prep solution and sent for cytologic examination. The cells are described as normal, LSIL, HSIL, or atypical squamous cells of unknown significance (ASCUS). The sensitivity ranges from 47% to 90% and specificity ranges from 16% to

92% for detection of dysplasia. There has been no difference between patient-collected or clinician-collected samples.[17] Several trials have looked at the predictive values of cytology in different populations. It is generally agreed that in high-risk populations such as HIV-positive MSM, anal cytology as a screening modality is cost effective.[16,17]

Some have advocated high-resolution anoscopy (HRA) once a diagnosis of LSIL, HSIL, or ASCUS is obtained from cytology. HRA is analogous to colposcopy for the detection of cervical dysplasia in women who have abnormal Pap smears. HRA uses an anoscope as well as a colposcope or operating microscope. A gauze pad soaked in 3% acetic acid solution is inserted into the anus and removed after several minutes. The anal canal can then be inspected using the colposcope. Areas with ace-towhitening are then examined for abnormal vascular patterns such as punctuation and mosaicism, and targeted biopsies are performed of areas suspicious for HSIL. Lu-gol's iodine solution can also be applied, which stains normal tissues brown. Areas that do not stain with Lugol's appear yellow and correlate with areas of HSIL, and should be biopsied.[31,32] Correlation of biopsy results with anal cytology results has been variable.[17,33] Perianal skin can also be evaluated with this technique. Given a high rate of perianal disease in those referred for HRA for abnormal cytology, some recommend performing concurrent HRA evaluation of the perianal skin.[31]

**Treatment** The goal of treating HSIL is to prevent its progression to anal squamous cell carcinoma, although effectiveness of cancer prevention has not been proven with this approach. The traditional procedure for anal dysplasia was mapping of the perianal area and anal canal with or without frozen section, followed by wide local excision of biopsy-proven disease. Mapping often required at least 24 biopsies encompassing all 4 quadrants as well as the biopsy of suspicious areas.[34,35] Because HSIL may not have many gross features, wide excision to clear margins often resulted in large defects. Thus many patients required proximal diversion or extensive reconstructive procedures to heal, and many developed complications such as anal stenosis.[34] Despite this radical approach, the recurrence rate of HSIL was 11% to 23%.[34,35] Thus this highly morbid approach is beginning to fall out of favor.

Given that HSIL is a premalignant lesion, targeted ablative therapies may be effective and less morbid. HRA provides a good view of affected areas and provides an opportunity for directed therapy. Ablative procedures have been performed using a variety of techniques including electrocautery, laser, and infrared coagulation. Chang and colleagues[36] reported the first prospective series on electrocautery as an ablative technique. This series of 37 MSM patients with HSIL showed a recurrence rate of 79% after 12 months within the HIV-positive group and none in the HIV-nega-tive group. However, it may be difficult to differentiate between persistent disease and recurrent disease, as many patients have multifocal, extensive disease that is not always addressed at the initial treatment session. Infrared coagulation brings therapy from the operating room to the office. This technique was first reported by Goldstone and colleagues[37] in a series of 68 MSM patients with HSIL. These investigators reported an initial recurrence rate of HSIL of 65% (median time to recurrence 217 days). However, recurrences only required 1 or 2 further treatments such that the over-all cure rate was 72%. Pineda and colleagues[38] recently published the largest series of 241 patients with HSIL. In this study, the majority of patients had large-volume disease (>50% circumferential disease) and most were treated in stages (the first usually being in the operating room). Pineda and colleagues reported a 57% initial recurrence rate (mean time 19 months). Again, recurrences were small and were managed in the office with 1 subsequent treatment. The overall cure rate was 78%. Only 1.2% progressed to squamous cell carcinoma, and less than 4% required surgical intervention for complications such as bleeding, anal stenosis, or fissure.[38] In addition, perianal disease could be addressed concurrently.[31]

There are some who advocate expectant management or observation for those with HSIL. To support their position these investigators point to the unknown natural history and asymptomatic nature of HSIL, the slow rate of progression to cancer (historically 7%–11%), the good prognosis for anal squamous cell cancer if detected in early stages, and the high rate of postoperative pain after ablative procedures.[39–41] Watson and colleagues[41] followed 55 patients with HSIL of whom 8 (15%) progressed to squamous cell cancer. Only 2 patients required abdominoperineal resection. In another series, Devaraj and colleagues[39] followed 40 patients (70% with HSIL) of whom 3 (7.5%) progressed to cancer. None of these patients required abdominoperineal resection. Thus even if patients progressed to cancer, it seems that close surveillance every 6 months could detect progression to cancer and still detect it at an early stage without requiring major resection such as abdominoperineal resection.

Finally, imiquimod has emerged as a potential ablative therapy for HSIL. As previously discussed, imiquimod is frequently used for the treatment of condyloma. Imiquimod has recently been used for the treatment of LSIL and HSIL in a nonrandomized study, with regression rates of up to 78% in patients who were able to successfully complete the treatment regimen.[15] Similar to the treatment of condylomas, the limiting factor with patient compliance was erythema and burning from the drug itself, which frequently caused therapy cessation. In addition, intra-anal application is difficult unless imiquimod suppositories are available. In Europe, where these are available, Wieland and colleagues[15] have reported this as a safe and effective treatment of AIN. However, this has yet to be approved by the FDA in the United States.

In their own practice, the authors advocate the use of HRA and targeted therapy versus expectant management of AIN based on the overall risk of the individual patient. In high-risk patients (HIV-positive men and women, MSM, women who engage in anal intercourse, transplant patients, and women with a history of cervical

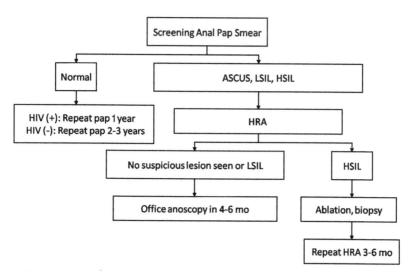

**Fig. 2.** Management of AIN in high-risk individuals. ASCUS, atypical squamous cells of uncertain significance; LSIL, low-grade squamous intraepithelial lesion; HSIL, high-grade squamous intraepithelial lesion; HRA, high-resolution anoscopy.

or vulvar dysplasia), acquisition of cytology via anal Pap smear is recommend. In patients with abnormal anal cytology, HRA and targeted biopsy and ablative therapy are performed for HSIL. Close surveillance is continued with HRA in 3 to 6 months. In patients with normal findings or LSIL on HRA, the authors advocate expectant management with careful perianal and anoscopic examination every 4 to 6 months in the office. If any gross lesions are evident, they are to be biopsied and treated accordingly (**Fig. 2**). In patients who are low risk and in whom dysplasia is found incidentally (ie, hemorrhoidectomy specimens), an expectant approach is also used.

## SUMMARY

Recognition of high-risk patients for STDs is important. STDs are a common public health problem and as such may be more common in a surgical practice than is believed. A detailed sexual history is paramount in the evaluation of a patient with a suspected STD, as there is a complex menu of treatments depending on the etiology. Although many laboratory tests exist for different organisms, the majority of diagnoses are still made clinically due to poor sensitivity and specificity of these tests. In addition, STDs need to be considered in the differential diagnosis of inflammatory bowel disease, as these diseases may mimic one another both clinically and pathologically. The reader is referred to the Web site, www.cdc.gov, for an excellent review of the diagnosis and treatment of STDs that is more exhaustive than the discussion in this article.

Finally, the recognition that a virus can be responsible for a cancer has profound significant public health implications. Screening and surveillance will become more focused and benefit a larger population as the natural history and connection of HPV with anal cancer is elucidated. With the development of an effective vaccine for cervical cancer already a reality, the day when anal squamous cell cancer can be prevented may be on the horizon.[42]

## REFERENCES

1. O'Farrell N, Morison L, Moodley P, et al. Genital ulcers and concomitant complaints in men attending a sexually transmitted infections clinic: implications for sexually transmitted infections management. Sex Transm Dis 2008;35(6): 545–9.
2. Wu JJ, Huang DB, Pang KR, et al. Selected sexually transmitted diseases and their relationship to HIV. Clin Dermatol 2004;22:499–508.
3. Centers for Disease Control and Prevention. Sexually transmitted diseases treatment guidelines. MMWR 2006;55(No.RR-11):14–30.
4. Lavery EA, Coyle WJ. Herpes Simplex Virus and the Alimentary Tract. Curr Gastroenterol Rep 2008;10:417–23.
5. Whitlow CB, Gottesman L. Sexually transmitted diseases. In: Wolff BG, Fleshman JW, Beck DE, et al, editors. The ASCRS textbook of colon and rectal surgery. New York: Springer Science+Business Media, LLC; 2007. p. 256–68.
6. Klausner JD, Kohn R, Kent C. Etiology of clinical proctitis among men who have sex with men. Clin Infect Dis 2004;38:300–2.
7. McMillan A, van Voorst Vader PC, de Vries HJ. The 2007 European Guideline (International Union against Sexually Transmitted Infections/World Health Organization) on the management of proctitis, proctocolitis, and enteritis caused by sexually transmissible pathogens. Int J STD AIDS 2007;18:514–20.
8. Centers for Disease Control and Prevention. Sexually transmitted diseases treatment guidelines. MMWR 2006;55(No.RR-11):38–42.

9. Centers for Disease Control and Prevention. Sexually transmitted diseases treatment guidelines. MMWR 2006;55(No.RR-11):42–9.

10. Ahdoot A, Kotler DP, Suh JS, et al. Lymphogranuloma venereum in human immunodeficiency virus-infected individuals in New York City. J Clin Gastroenterol 2006;40(5):385–90.

11. McLean CA, Stoner BP, Workowski KA. Treatment of lymphogranuloma venereum. Clin Infect Dis 2007;44:S147–52.

12. Welton ML, Sharkey FE, Kahlenberg MS. The etiology and epidemiology of anal cancer. Surg Oncol Clin N Am 2004;13:263–75.

13. Zbar AP, Fenger C, Efron J, et al. The pathology and molecular biology of anal intraepithelial neoplasia: comparisons with cervical and vulvar intraepithelial carcinoma. Int J Colorectal Dis 2002;17:203–15.

14. DeToma G, Cavallaro G, Bitonti A, et al. Surgical management of perianal giant condyloma accuminatum. Eur Surg Res 2006;38:418–22.

15. Wieland U, Brockmeyer NJ, Weissenborn SJ, et al. Imiquimod treatment of anal intraepithelial neoplasia in HIV-positive men. Arch Dermatol 2006;142:1438–44.

16. Shepherd N. Anal intraepithelial neoplasia and other neoplastic precursor lesions of the anal canal and perianal region. Gastroenterol Clin North Am 2007;36: 969–87.

17. Pineda CE, Welton ML. Controversies in the management of anal high-grade squamous intraepithelial lesions. Minerva Chir 2008;63:389–99.

18. Colquhoun P, Nogueras JJ, Dipasquale B, et al. Interobserver and intraobserver bias exists in the interpretation of anal dysplasia. Dis Colon Rectum 2003;46: 1332–8.

19. Varnai AD, Bollman M, Griefingholt H, et al. HPV in anal squamous cell carcinoma and anal intraepthelial neoplasia: impact of HPV analysis of anal lesions on diagnosis and prognosis. Int J Colorectal Dis 2006;21:135–42.

20. Fernandes-Brenna SM, Syrjanen KJ. Regulation of cell cycles is of key importance in human papilloma virus-associated cervical carcinogenesis. Sao Paulo Med J 2003;121:128–32.

21. Indinnimeo M, Cicchini C, Stazi A, et al. Human papillomavirus infection and p53 nuclear overexpression in anal canal carcinoma. J Exp Clin Cancer Res 1999;18: 47–52.

22. Lu DW, El-Mofty SK, Wang HL. Expression of p16, Rb, p53 proteins in squamos cell carcinomas of the anorectal region harboring human papilloma virus DNA. Mod Pathol 2003;16:692–9.

23. Palefsky JM, Holly EA, Hogeboom CJ, et al. Virologic, immunologic, and clinical parameters in the incidence and progression of anal squamous intraepithelia lesions in HIV-positive and HIV-negative men. J Acquir Immune Defic Syndr Hum Retrovirol 1998;17:314–9.

24. Bosch FX, Lorincz A, Munoz N, et al. The causal relation between human papilloma virus and cervical cancer. J Clin Pathol 2002;55:244–55.

25. Joseph DA, Miller JW, Wu X, et al. Understanding the burden of HPV associated anal cancers in the US. Cancer 2008;113(Supp 10):2892–900.

26. D'Souza G, Wiley DJ, Li X, et al. Incidence and epidemiology of anal cancer in the multicenter AIDS cohort study. J Acquir Immune Defic Syndr 2008;48(4):491–9.

27. Bower M, Powles T, Newsom-Davis T, et al. HIV-associated anal cancer: has highly active antiretroviral therapy reduced the incidence or improved the outcome? J Acquir Immune Defic Syndr 2004;37(5):1563–5.

28. Holly EA, Ralston ML, Darragh TM, et al. Prevalence and risk factors for anal squamous intraepithelial lesions in women. J Natl Cancer Inst 2001;93(11):843–9.

29. Daling JR, Madeleine MM, Johnson LG, et al. Human papilloma virus, smoking, and sexual practices in the etiology of anal cancer. Cancer 2004;101:270–80.
30. Patel HS, Silver AR, Northover JM. Anal cancer in renal transplant patients. Int J Colorectal Dis 2007;22:1–5.
31. Nahas CS, Lin O, Weiser MR, et al. Prevalence of perianal intraepithelial neoplasia in HIV-infected patients referred for high-resolution anoscopy. Dis Colon Rectum 2006;49:1581–6.
32. Jay N, Berry JM, Hogeboom CJ, et al. Colposcopic appearance of anal squamous intraepithelial lesions: relationship to histopathology. Dis Colon Rectum 1997;40:919–28.
33. Scott H, Khoury J, Moore BA, et al. Routine anal cytology screening for anal squamous intraepithelial lesions in an urban HIV clinic. Sex Transm Dis 2008;35(2): 197–202.
34. Margenthaler JA, Dietz DW, Mutch MG, et al. Outcomes, risk of other malignancies, and need for formal mapping procedures in patients with perianal Bowen's disease. Dis Colon Rectum 2004;47:1655–60.
35. Sarmiento JM, Wolff BG, Burgart LJ, et al. Perianal Bowen's disease: associated tumors, HPV, surgery and other controversies. Dis Colon Rectum 1997;40:912–8.
36. Chang GJ, Berry JM, Jay N, et al. Surgical treatment of high-grade squamous intraepithelial lesions: a prospective study. Dis Colon Rectum 2002;45:453–8.
37. Goldstone SE, Kawalek AZ, Huyett JW. IRC: a useful tool for treating anal squamous intraepithelial lesions. Dis Colon Rectum 2005;48:1042–54.
38. Pineda CE, Berry JM, Jay N, et al. High-resolution anoscopy targeted surgical destruction of anal high-grade squamous intraepithelial lesions: a ten-year experience. Dis Colon Rectum 2008;51:829–37.
39. Devaraj B, Cosman BC. Expectant management of anal squamous dysplasia with HIV. Dis Colon Rectum 2006;49:36–40.
40. Scholefield JH, Castle MT, Watson NF. Malignant transformation of high-grade anal intraepithelial neoplasia. Br J Surg 2005;92:1133–6.
41. Watson AJ, Smith BB, Whitehead MR, et al. Malignant progression of anal intra-epithelial neoplasia. ANZ J Surg 2006;76:715–7.
42. Garland SM, Hernandez-Avila M, Wheeler CM, et al. Quadrivalent vaccine against human papillomavirus to prevent anogenital diseases. N Engl J Med 2007;356:1928–43.

# Evaluation and Management of Pilonidal Disease

Ashley E. Humphries, MD, James E. Duncan, MD, FACS, FASCRS[a,b,]*

**KEYWORDS**

• Pilonidal sinus • Pilonidal disease • Evaluation • Management

## ETIOLOGY AND DIAGNOSIS

The history of pilonidal disease dates back to the early 1800s, and it continues to be a significant health issue today. Herbert Mayo was the first to describe a disease that involved a hair-filled cyst at the base of the coccyx in 1833.[1] In 1880, Hodge coined the name "pilonidal" from the Latin *pilus* that means hair and *nidus* that means nest.[2] During World War II, over 80,000 soldiers in the United States Army were hospitalized with the condition. It was termed "Jeep riders' disease" because a large number of soldiers who were being hospitalized for pilonidal disease rode in jeeps and long journeys on rough terrain were felt to cause the condition because of pressure on and irritation of the coccyx.[3]

Currently, pilonidal disease is a fairly common condition that affects many patients worldwide. In the United States alone, nearly 70,000 patients are diagnosed with this potentially morbid condition each year.[4] The disease itself and many of its treatments often result in time lost from work or school, and it burdens patients and caregivers with wound care and frequent trips to the office or hospital.

Initially thought to be congenital in origin,[2] pilonidal disease is now thought to be an acquired condition related to the presence of hair in the natal cleft.[5] This loose hair causes a foreign body reaction that leads to midline pit formation (**Fig. 1**).[6,7] Pilonidal disease can present as a simple cyst, an acute abscess with or without cellulitis, or a chronic draining sinus. Treatment, therefore, is also highly variable and can include observation and hair removal, incision and drainage, or excision with sometimes complex surgical reconstruction.

Diagnosis begins with a focused history and physical examination to include symptoms, risk factors, and presence of active infection. Patients may present with complaints of a tender, fluctuant sacrococcygeal mass in the case of secondary infection or may report midline drainage and discomfort in the case of a chronic sinus. On

[a] Department of Surgery, National Naval Medical Center, 8901 Wisconsin Avenue, Bethesda, MD 20889, USA
[b] Uniformed Services, University of The Health Sciences, Bethesda, MD, USA
* Corresponding author. Uniformed Services, University of The Health Sciences, Bethesda, MD, USA.
*E-mail address:* James.Duncan@med.navy.mil (J.E. Duncan).

Surg Clin N Am 90 (2010) 113–124
doi:10.1016/j.suc.2009.09.006
0039-6109/09/$ – see front matter. Published by Elsevier Inc.
surgical.theclinics.com

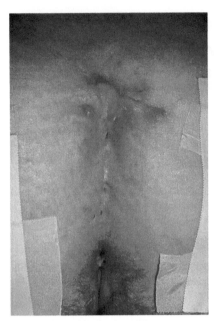

**Fig. 1.** Typical midline pits and underlying sinus tracts.

examination, the patient will almost always have the characteristic midline gluteal cleft pits located approximately 5 cm cephalad to the anus. Additionally, they may have a tracking sinus or multiple sinuses. Anorectal examination should be performed to rule out other disease processes. The differential for pilonidal disease is wide and includes perianal abscess, hidradenitis, skin furuncle, Crohn disease, and syphilitic, tubercular, and actinomycotic infection.[7,8] Risk factors for the development of pilonidal disease, although not found to be directly causative, should be considered: obesity, sedentary lifestyle, family history, hirsute body habitus, and trauma or irritation to the gluteal cleft skin. Lifestyle changes can be implemented if risk factors are identified.[4,9]

## MANAGEMENT OPTIONS: PRIMARY PILONIDAL DISEASE
### Nonoperative Management and Adjuncts to Operative Strategy

Because the cause of pilonidal sinus disease is widely attributed to hair follicle ingrowth and subsequent foreign body reaction, local hair control, whether by shaving or laser epilation, has been used as a primary treatment and as an adjunctive strategy.[5,6,8,10–14] Compared with various surgical techniques, shaving and improved hygiene have been demonstrated to decrease total hospital admission days and surgical procedures and has resulted in faster return to work or school.[15] The frequency and extent of shaving, however, has not been clarified, and, depending on rate of hair growth and hair volume, can affect the quality of life of the patient and caregiver. Laser epilation, therefore, has been examined on a smaller scale as an alternative to shaving in the treatment and adjunctive roles. The results of these studies are encouraging for recurrence prevention.[12–14]

Phenol or fibrin glue injection into the pilonidal sinus is an additional nonoperative adjunct to treatment. Both methods are typically used after all hair and debris have been removed or curetted from the sinus, and they help to eliminate granulation tissue and further debris formation. The injection is followed by hair control and strict hygiene. The use of phenol (1–2 mL of 80% phenol solution) causes an intense inflammatory reaction which destroys the epithelial lining, and care should be taken to protect surrounding skin. Pain is intense and may require inpatient admission for pain control but success rates have been reported to range from 60% to 95%.[16–18] Fibrin glue has been used similarly as an adjunctive treatment in chronic or recurrent sinuses and following various interventions. Success rates are high (90%–100% in small series) and morbidity is low.[19,20]

Cleansing and curettage of the midline pilonidal pits is an alternative treatment to excision, although primarily of historical value. Described in 1965 by Lord and Millar, this therapy involves brushing the sinus with a thin bottle brush to cleanse the sinus of hair and debris. This treatment is labor intensive and must be accompanied by continued strict hair removal and hygiene.[21]

Antibiotic use in pilonidal disease has a limited role. The most common organisms isolated in chronic pilonidal sinus are aerobes, whereas anaerobes such as bacteroides predominate in associated abscesses. Antibiotic therapy has been evaluated in the perioperative prophylactic, postoperative treatment, and topical roles. Preoperative, single-dose, intravenous antibiotic before excision of a chronic sinus has not been shown to decrease wound complications, healing, or recurrence, whereas varying courses of postoperative therapy have remained controversial. Overall, the use of antibiotics in this role has shown no benefit in reducing wound infection rates.[22–26] Topical therapy evaluated in the setting of pilonidal disease primarily involves antibiotic or abrasive solution-soaked sponge or dressing being packed into an abscess cavity or excised sinus. As with most outcomes of antibiotic use in this disease process, there is no conclusive evidence to support this practice because there has been no demonstrable benefit.[27,28] There has been no strong data to support antibiotic use in acute or chronic pilonidal disease, although expert opinion has suggested a role in the setting of cellulitis, underlying immunosuppression, or concurrent systemic illness.[6–8,10,29]

Asymptomatic, incidentally discovered pilonidal sinus is a rare presentation of this disease. A retrospective study, performed by Doll and colleagues,[30] evaluated the presence of hair and inflammation within asymptomatic pilonidal sinuses and found the presence of both in most cases. The conclusion of this study was that asymptomatic pilonidal sinus is actually subclinically inflamed and that hair and chronic inflammation are often present. However, prophylactic surgery in this small patient population did not demonstrate benefit over surgical intervention for symptomatic disease. Therefore, nonoperative strategies, such as hygiene, hair control, and observation, are recommended in this group.

### Operative Management

There are many options for the surgical management of chronic pilonidal disease. These options range widely and encompass simple excision with or without primary closure to complex flap reconstruction. Most advocate adjunctive hair removal and strict hygiene, and no single operative intervention has been proven superior to another in overall healing, time away from work, or recurrence.

Pilonidal disease can present acutely as an abscess with or without associated cellulitis. In the acute setting, the appropriate therapy is simple incision and drainage. The majority (approximately 60%) of those presenting with abscess at initial episode and treated in this way will heal without further intervention.[31] The remainder of patients will need a more definitive excision to address hypertrophic granulation tissue before closure. Even after complete healing, 10% to 15% of patients will have recurrence.[31] Curettage of the cavity at time of incision and drainage is controversial, and only one study has demonstrated greater complete healing (96% vs 79%) and lower incidence of recurrence (10% vs 54%) as compared with no curettage.[32] Another issue at acute presentation is whether to excise the midline pits at time of incision and drainage, the theoretical benefit being the elimination of future disease. This practice, however, has not been shown to increase rate of healing, decrease hospital stay, or decrease rate of recurrence.[33]

Pilonidal sinus excision with or without primary closure can be performed in many different ways. Complete sinus excision, which involves removal of the pilonidal sinus while sparing normal tissue, can be approached through a midline or lateral incision. For sinus removal through a midline approach, the wound can be primarily closed, marsupialized, or left open and allowed to heal by secondary intention (**Fig. 2**). Several studies have demonstrated faster median healing rates[22,34–38] and more rapid return to work with primary closure,[35,36] but they have also shown higher recurrence rates with this intervention as compared with healing by secondary intention.[39–41] Marsupialization entails suturing the skin edges to the wound base after debridement and acts to decrease the overall wound volume and prevent premature epithelialization. Should this repair break down, the wound can continue to heal by secondary intention without requiring further procedures. Comparison of primary closure versus marsupialization in healing time and recurrence remains conflicted.[7,10,41–43]

Incision from the midline, or lateral incision, is another alternative to sinus excision. Theoretical advantages include a richer blood supply; dryer, a less bacteria-rich environment; and less sheer with ambulation as compared with incision in the gluteal cleft. This approach has demonstrated faster healing time, decreased wound complications, and decreased recurrence rates.[44] One technique involves lateral incision with sinus cavity curettage and pit removal either separately or en bloc (**Fig. 3**), whereas an alternative approach is sinus removal through lateral incision with removal of the midline pits through this lateral incision (**Fig. 4**). Lateral incisions can be closed primarily, left open to heal by secondary intention (although a reported advantage of

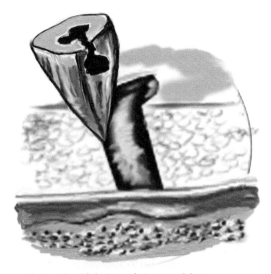

**Fig. 2.** Midline approach to pilonidal pit and sinus excision.

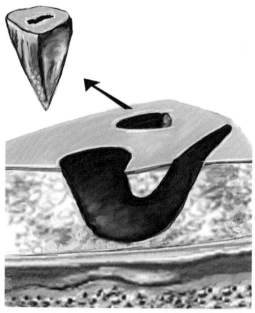

**Fig. 3.** Lateral incision and curettage with separate or en bloc pit excision.

the lateral approach is that this is typically avoided), or closed via flap reconstruction if the excision is extensive.[45–48]

There are many types of flap-based options that can be used in the treatment of chronic pilonidal disease. Often, chronic disease presents with complex or extensive sinus tracts, which, after excision, can leave a sizable defect. The theory behind flap-based reconstruction is to excise disease and cover the defect with healthy tissue that has rich blood supply.

The Karydakis flap involves midline excision of the pilonidal sinus tracts followed by soft tissue coverage in the form of mobilized fasciocutaneous tissue that is sutured laterally to the sacrococcygeal fascia to avoid midline tension. (**Fig. 5**) In his own

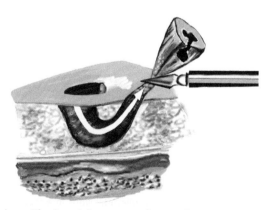

**Fig. 4.** Lateral incision with pit and sinus removal. A small incision around the pits allows en bloc removal with the underlying sinus through the lateral incision.

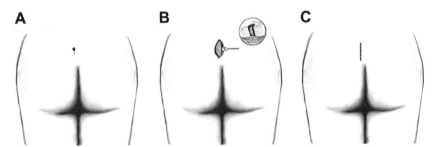

**Fig. 5.** Karydakis flap. (*A*) An off-midline incision is made and the sinus excised to the sacrococcygeal fascia. (*B*) Raise a full-thickness flap on one side. (*C*) Slide the flap to the opposite side and close primarily lateral to the midline.

review of more than 6000 cases, Karydakis[5] demonstrated a wound complication rate of 8% and recurrence rate of 2%. Subsequent studies have reproduced similar results.

The rhomboid or Limberg flap has similar principles to the Karydakis flap in that it involves midline excision of the pilonidal disease to the presacral fascia and involves fasciocutaneous coverage.[45,46,49,50] However, the flap in this instance is rotational and results in flattening of the gluteal cleft (**Fig. 6**). The potential downfall of this surgical option includes the large area of tissue mobilization, the increased risk of hematoma/seroma, and wound dehiscence, although these complications are rare (0%–6%).

An additional flap option is the Bascom, or cleft-lift, technique. This technique involves the excision of all diseased tissue with the creation of flap-based coverage lateral to the midline. This completely obliterates the cleft. A triangular incision is performed with the apex located above and lateral to the cleft apex, and all disease is excised. Hair and granulation tissue are debrided and a skin flap is raised toward the midline. Excess skin is then removed and the flap sutured closed over a drain (**Fig. 7**), Bascom and Bascom[51] reported healing rates in the 80% to 95% range and recurrence rates as low as 4%, confirmed by subsequent studies.[51–53]

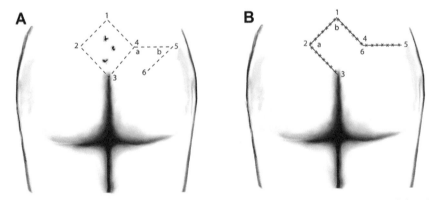

**Fig. 6.** Rhomboid (Limberg) flap. Excise the pilonidal sinus in a diamond shape. (*A*) Incise flap as demonstrated, including skin and subcutaneous tissue. (*B*) Rotate flap into place and close donor site primarily.

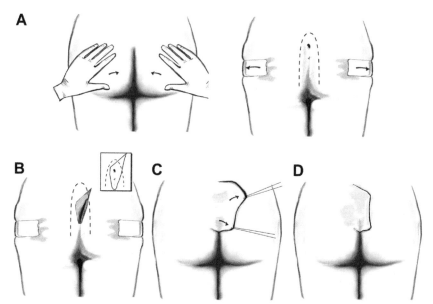

**Fig. 7.** Bascom (cleft-lift). (*A*) Mark the buttock contact lines and then tape the buttocks apart for visualization. (*B*) Excise the nonhealing wound or pilonidal pits/sinus tracts in a triangular shape off-midline. (*C*) Raise a skin flap to the previously marked line and release the tape. Position the skin flap. (*D*) Excise excess skin and close. A drain can be used.

Two additional local advancement flaps that have been used to provide tissue coverage in other areas of the body have also been applied to the management of pilonidal disease. The V-Y advancement flap is composed of skin, fat, and gluteal fascia and can cover defects 8 to 10 cm in size. This flap eliminates the gluteal cleft and can be used unilaterally or bilaterally. The final suture line is midline, which some consider a drawback, and drains are often used. (**Fig. 8**) Case series have demonstrated good

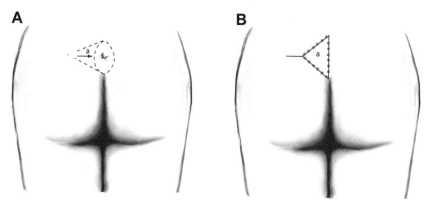

**Fig. 8.** V-Y advancement flap. Use an elliptical incision to excise pits and sinus tracts to the level of the sacrococcygeal fascia. Using the apices of the ellipse, extend the incision laterally in a V shape and include skin, fat and gluteal fascia in this flap. Advance the flap toward the midline and primarily close, creating a Y shape. This flap can be used unilaterally or bilaterally.

healing and minimal wound complication and recurrence rates.[54] Another local flap is the Z-plasty, which involves sinus excision and Z limbs that are marked at a 30-degree angle to the long axis of the wound. Flaps of skin and subcutaneous tissue are raised, transposed, and sutured, obliterating the gluteal cleft. (**Fig. 9**) Although this technique has been described in many studies, it is generally reported to have higher wound complication and recurrence rates.[55]

When larger, deeper wounds are encountered after excision, they may require more complex flap reconstruction. The gluteus maximus fasciocutaneous or myocutaneous rotational flap is an option in this setting. The flap is raised and rotated into place, thus filling the defect with vascular-rich tissue and obliterating the remaining dead space and gluteal cleft. (**Fig. 10**) Drawbacks to this procedure include longer operative duration, operative complexity, and higher morbidity with flap failure.[56]

Vacuum-assisted closure (V.A.C., Kinetic Concepts, Inc, San Antonio, TX, USA) devices use a negative pressure to wound beds and have been used for the management of various complex wounds and as adjuncts to skin grafting. This system has been used as the primary treatment following wide excision or as the bolstering mechanism for skin grafts following a wide excision.[57,58] These concepts have been extrapolated to include treatment of pilonidal disease at National Naval Medical Center, Bethesda, where a small, nonpublished series is examining the use of V.A.C. as a bridge to delayed primary closure (Forrest Sheppard, MD, Bethesda, personal

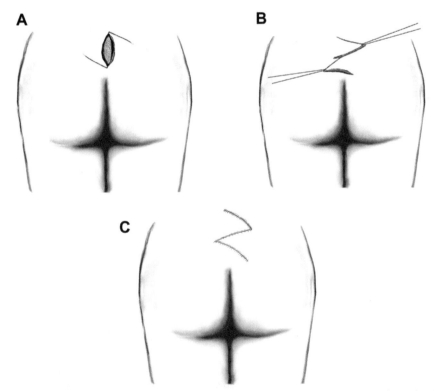

**Fig. 9.** Z-plasty. Excise the pilonidal pits and underlying sinuses using a midline elliptical incision. (*A*) Mark the Z limbs at a 30-degree angle from the apices of the excised ellipse. (*B*) Raise full-thickness flaps and transpose. (*C*) Primary wound closure.

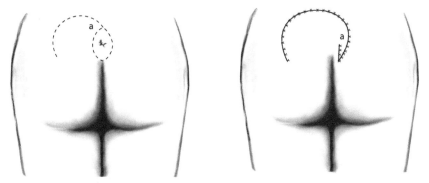

**Fig. 10.** Gluteus maximus fasciocutaneous or myocutaneous flap. Excise pilonidal pits and sinuses in the midline and rotate flap for off-midline coverage.

communication, May 2009). V.A.C. devices are well tolerated by patients and smaller home systems are readily available. A strong recommendation does not exist for V.A.C. application in pilonidal disease but may be considered in selected cases as primary or adjunctive therapy.

## MANAGEMENT OPTIONS: RECURRENT PILONIDAL DISEASE

Recurrence rates for pilonidal disease vary widely and have been reported to be as high as 50% following primary intervention, and as high as 10% to 30% after subsequent interventions.[10] These rates indicate that many patients will continue to have treatment failure despite the type of management chosen. The cause of these failures is not completely known, although wound complications at primary intervention were shown to be predictive.

Management of recurrent disease is similar to that of primary disease. Thorough examination should be performed and other processes excluded, such as inflammatory bowel disease, malignancy, and other differential diagnoses as discussed earlier. Recurrent disease treatment includes nonoperative adjuncts, such as hygiene and hair control. If an abscess is present, an incision and drainage should be performed and associated cellulitis treated with antibiotics. The operative strategy for recurrent disease varies widely, and, depending on the extent of disease, can range from wide excision with primary closure to the use of more complex flap closure.

## CARCINOMA IN PILONIDAL SINUS

Carcinoma arising from a pilonidal sinus is rare, occurring in approximately 0.1% of patients with chronic untreated or recurrent pilonidal disease. It is believed that the process involves the release of oxygen free-radicals by activated inflammatory cells, similar to carcinoma arising in other ulcerating and chronically inflamed disorders. The first case was reported by Wolff in 1900, and less than 100 cases have been reported in the literature since that time. The cell-type is usually well-differentiated squamous. These tumors will classically present as an ulcer with rapidly progressing fungating margins, and computed tomographic imaging is an often useful adjunct to determine extent of disease. Treatment is wide, en-bloc excision and often requires flap reconstruction or grafting. Involvement in locoregional lymph nodes is a poor prognostic indicator and, in the case of palpable inguinal lymph nodes, excision versus radiotherapy should be considered. Pilonidal sinus carcinoma behaves more aggressively than squamous cell carcinoma at other sites and recurrence rate approaches 50%. Adjunctive radiotherapy can decrease local recurrence but overall survival is poor.[59,60]

## SUMMARY

Pilonidal disease is a fairly common condition that is associated with significant morbidity. It exists in many forms: asymptomatic, acutely infected with associated cellulitis and abscess, and chronic in nature, presenting a management dilemma because of its location. There are a multitude of described interventions, surgical and nonsurgical, and, thus far, no treatment modality has proven to be superior. The general principles of therapy include good hygiene practices, hair control, and excision of all disease with primary closure or soft tissue coverage. Recurrence is not uncommon and may require extensive excision and flap closure. Malignancy arising in the setting of chronic pilonidal disease is extremely rare but should be considered when ulceration or fungating mass is present.

## REFERENCES

1. Mayo OH. Observations on injuries and diseases of the rectum. London: Burgess and Hill; 1833. p. 45–46.
2. Hodges RM. Pilonidal sinus. Boston Med Surg J 1880;103:485–6.
3. Buie L. Jeep disease. South Med J 1944;37:103.
4. Sondenaa K, Andersen E, Nesvik I, et al. Patient characteristics and symptoms in chronic pilonidal sinus disease. Int J Colorectal Dis 1995;10:39–42.
5. Karydakis GE. Easy and successful treatment of pilonidal sinus after explanation of its causative process. Aust N Z J Surg 1992;62:385–9.
6. Hull TL, Wu J. Pilonidal disease. Surg Clin North Am 2002;82:1169–85.
7. Nelson J, Billingham R. Pilonidal disease and hidradenitis suppurativa. In: Wolff BG, Fleshman JW, Beck DE, et al, editors. The ASCRS textbook of colon and rectal surgery. New York: Springer; 2007. p. 228–35.
8. Chinn BT. Outpatient management of pilonidal disease. Semin Colon Rectal Surg 2003;14:166–72.
9. da Silva JH. Pilonidal cyst: cause and treatment. Dis Colon Rectum 2000;43:1146–56.
10. Notaro JR. Management of recurrent pilonidal disease. Semin Colon Rectal Surg 2003;14:173–85.
11. Surrell JA. Pilonidal disease. Surg Clin North Am 1994;74:1309–15.
12. Lukish JR, Kindelan T, Marmon LM, et al. Laser epilation is a safe and effective therapy for teenagers with pilonidal disease. J Pediatr Surg 2009;44:282–5.
13. Conroy FJ, Kandamany N, Mahaffey PJ. Laser depilation and hygiene: preventing recurrent pilonidal sinus disease. J Plast Reconstr Aesthet Surg 2008;61:1069–72.
14. Schulze SM, Patel N, Hertzog D, et al. Treatment of pilonidal disease with laser epilation. Am Surg 2006;72:534–7.
15. Armstrong JH, Barcia PJ. Pilonidal sinus disease. The conservative approach. Arch Surg 1994;129:914–7.
16. Maurice B, Greenwood R. A conservative treatment of pilonidal sinus. BJS 1964;51:510–2.
17. Dogru O, Camci C, Aygen E, et al. Pilonidal sinus treated with crystallized phenol: an eight-year experience. Dis Colon rectum 2004;47:1934–8.
18. Hegge HG, Vos GA, Patka P, et al. Treatment of complicated or infected pilonidal sinus disease by local application of phenol. Surgery 1987;102:52–4.

19. Saleem MI, Al-Hashemy AM. Management of pilonidal sinus using fibrin glue: a new concept and preliminary experience. Colorectal Dis 2005;7:319–22.
20. Greenberg R, Kashtan H, Skornik Y, et al. Treatment of pilonidal sinus disease using fibrin glue as a sealant. Tech Coloproctol 2004;8:95–8.
21. Lord P, Millar M. Pilonidal sinus: a simple treatment. Br J Surg 1965;52:298–300.
22. Sondenna K, Nesvik I, Gullaksen F, et al. The role of cefoxitin prophylaxis in chronic pilonidal sinus treated with excision and primary suture. J Am Coll Surg 1995;180:157–60.
23. Sondenaa K, Nesvik I, Andersen E, et al. Bacteriology and complications of chronic pilonidal sinus treated with excision and primary suture. Int J Colorectal Dis 1995;10:161–6.
24. Lundhus E, Gjode P, Gottrup F, et al. Bactericidal antimicrobial cover in primary suture of perianal or pilonidal abscess. A prospective, randomized, double-blind clinical trial. Acta Chir Scand 1989;155:351–4.
25. Kronborg O, Christensen K, Zimmermann-Neilson C. Chronic pilonidal disease: a randomized trial with a complete 3-year follow-up. Br J Surg 1985;72:303–4.
26. Marks J, Harding K, Hughes L, et al. Pilonidal sinus excision- healing by open granulation. BJS 1985;72:637–40.
27. Vogel P, Lenz J. Treatment of pilonidal sinus with excision and primary suture using a local, absorbable antibiotic carrier. Results of a prospective randomized trial. Chirurg 1992;63:748–53.
28. Williams R, Wood R, Mason M, et al. Multicentre prospective trial of Silastic foam dressing in management of open granulating wounds. Br Med J 1981;282:21–2.
29. Hanley PH. Acute pilonidal abscess. Surg Gynecol Obstet 1980;150:9–11.
30. Doll D, Friederichs J, Boulesteix AL, et al. Surgery for asymptomatic pilonidal sinus disease. Int J Colorectal Dis 2008;23:839–44.
31. Jensen SL, Harling H. Prognosis after simple incision and drainage for a first-episode acute pilonidal abscess. Br J Surg 1988;75:60–1.
32. Vahedian J, Nabavizadeh F, Nakhaee N, et al. Comparison between drainage and curettage in the treatment of acute pilonidal abscess. Saudi Med J 2005; 26:553–5.
33. Matter I, Kunin J, Schein m, et al. Total excision versus non-resectional methods in the treatment of acute and chronic pilonidal disease. Br J Surg 1995;82:752–3.
34. Rao M, Zawislak W, Gilliland R. A prospective randomized trial comparing two treatment modalities for chronic pilonidal sinus. Oral. Int J Colorectal Dis 2001; 3(Supp1):102.
35. Khawaja HT, Bryan S, Weaver PC. Treatment of natal cleft sinus: a prospective clinical and economical evaluation. BMJ 1992;304:1282–3.
36. Hameed KK. Outcome of surgery for chronic natal cleft pilonidal sinus: A randomized trial of open compared with closed technique. Med Forum Monthly 2001;12:20–3.
37. Sondenaa K, Nesvik E, Soreide J. Recurrent pilonidal sinus after excision with closed or open treatment: final result of a randomized trial. Eur J Surg 1996; 162:237–40.
38. Sondenaa K, Andersen E, Soreide JA. Morbidity and short term results in a randomized trial of open compared with closed treatment of chronic pilonidal sinus. Eur J Surg 1992;158:351–5.
39. Mohamed HA, Kadry I, Adly S. Comparison between three therapeutic modalities for non-complicated pilonidal sinus disease. Surgeon 2005;3:73–7.
40. Miocinovic M, Horzic M, Bunoza D. The treatment of pilonidal disease of the sacrococcygeal region by the method of limited excision and open wound healing. Acta Med Croatica 1999;54:27–31.

41. Oncel M, Kurt N, Kement M, et al. Excision and marsupialization versus sinus excision for the treatment of limited chronic pilonidal disease: a prospective randomized trial. Tech Coloproctol 2002;6:165.

42. Al-Hassan HK, Francis IM, Neglen P. Primary closure or secondary granulation after excision of pilonidal sinus? Acta Chir Scand 1990;156:695–9.

43. Spivak H, Brooks P, Nussbaum M, et al. Treatment of chronic pilonidal disease. Dis Colon Rectum 1996;39:1136–9.

44. McCallum I, King PM, Bruce J. Healing by primary versus secondary intention after surgical treatment for pilonidal sinus. Cochrane Database Syst Rev 2007;(4):CD006213.

45. Abu Galala KH, Salam IM, Abu Samaan KR, et al. Treatment of pilonidal sinus by primary closure with a transposed rhomboid flap compared with deep suturing: a prospective randomized clinical trial. Eur J Surg 1999;165:468–72.

46. Akca T, Colak T, Ustunsoy B, et al. Randomized clinical trial comparing primary closure with the Limberg flap in the treatment of primary sacrococcygeal pilonidal disease. Br J Surg 2005;92:1081–4.

47. Berkem H, Topalloglu S, Ozel H, et al. V-Y advancement flap closures for complicated pilonidal sinus disease. Int J Colorectal Dis 2005;20:343–8.

48. Wright DM, Anderson JH, Molloy RG. A randomized trial of the Bascom procedure vs. primary closure for pilonidal sinus. Poster. Colorectal Dis 2001;3(1 Suppl 1):185.

49. Urhan M, Kucukel F, Topgul K, et al. Rhomboid excision and Limberg flap for managing pilonidal sinus: Results of 102 cases. Dis Colon Rectum 2002;45:656–9.

50. Topgul K, Ozdemir E, Kilic K, et al. Long-term results of Limberg flap procedure for treatment of pilonidal sinus: a report of 200 cases. Dis Colon Rectum 2003;46:1545–8.

51. Bascom J, Bascom T. Utility of the cleft lift procedure in refractory pilonidal disease. Am J Surg 2007;193:606–9.

52. Theodoropoulos GE, Vlahos K, Lazaris AC, et al. Modified Bascom's asymmetric midgluteal cleft closure technique for recurrent pilonidal disease: early experience in a military hospital. Dis Colon Rectum 2003;46:1286–91.

53. Abdelrazeq AS, Rahman M, Botterill ID, et al. Short-term and long-term outcomes of the cleft lift procedure in the management of nonacute pilonidal disorders. Dis Colon Rectum 2008;51(7):1100–6.

54. Schoeller T, Wechselberger G, Otto A, et al. Definite surgical treatment of complicated recurrent pilonidal disease with a modified fasciocutaneous V-Y advancement flap. Surgery 1997;121:258–63.

55. Hodgson W, Greenstein R. A comparative study between Z-plasty and incision and drainage or excision with marsupialization for pilonidal sinus. Surg Gynecol Obstet 1981;153:842–4.

56. Perez-Gurri JA, Temple WS, Ketcham AS. Gluteus maximus myocutaneous flap for treatment of recalcitrant pilonidal disease. Dis Colon Rectum 1984;27:262–4.

57. Leininger BE, Rasmussen TE. Experience with wound V.A.C. and delayed primary closure of contaminated soft tissue injuries in Iraq. J Trauma 2007;63(1):248–9.

58. Venturi MC, Attinger CE. Mechanism and clinical applications of the V.A.C. device: a review. Am J Clin Dermatol 2005;6(3):185–94.

59. Davis KA, Mock CN, Versaci A, et al. Malignant degeneration of pilonidal cysts. Am Surg 1994;60:200–4.

60. de Bree E, Zoetmulder F, Christodoulakis M, et al. Treatment of malignancy arising in pilonidal disease. Ann Surg Oncol 2001;8:60–4.

# Pruritus Ani: Etiology and Management

Katharine W. Markell, MD[a,b], Richard P. Billingham, MD[c,d],*

KEYWORDS

• Pruritus ani • Dermatologic • Itch

## DEFINITION

Pruritus ani is defined as a dermatologic condition characterized by an unpleasant itching or burning sensation in the perianal region.[1] It is a common complaint seen by primary care physicians and also in certain specialties such as dermatology and colorectal surgery. Appropriate management can be difficult and requires a detailed assessment looking for any 1 of the various causes.

## INCIDENCE AND CLASSIFICATION

The incidence of pruritus ani ranges from 1% to 5% in the general population. Men are more commonly affected than women with a 4:1 ratio,[2,3] and this condition is most common in the fourth to sixth decades of life.[4] Because patients with these symptoms generally attribute them to insufficient perianal hygiene or some rash or inflammation (which would respond to topical steroids or other agents), common attempts to alleviate the itching include vigorous washing with soap and washcloth, extended cleansing with dry toilet paper or "baby wipes," scratching with the fingernails, or the generous application of creams, ointments, or other substances, all of which generally exacerbate the symptoms. Pruritus ani is classified either as primary pruritus ani, also known as idiopathic pruritus ani, or as secondary pruritus ani. Primary or idiopathic pruritus is responsible for 50% to 90% of all cases of pruritus ani.[5] Because secondary causes are so uncommon, most physicians begin with a therapeutic trial of generic management for idiopathic pruritus ani, which is effective in more than 90% of patients. In those patients in whom the usual management strategy is not effective after 1 to 2 months, attention should be given to excluding the multiple potential causes of secondary pruritus ani. The causes of secondary pruritus ani can be divided into several broad categories: infectious, dermatologic, systemic disease, local irritants, and colorectal or anal causes (**Table 1**).[2,3]

[a] US Army Medical Corps, San Antonio, TX, USA
[b] Division of Colon and Rectal Surgery, Brooke Army Medical Center, San Antonio, TX, USA
[c] Swedish Colon & Rectal Clinic, 1101 Madison Street, Suite 500, Seattle, WA 98104, USA
[d] Department of Surgery, University of Washington, Seattle, WA, USA
* Corresponding author. Swedish Colon & Rectal Clinic, 1101 Madison Street, Suite 500, Seattle, WA 98104, USA.
*E-mail address:* rbham@u.washington.edu (R.P. Billingham).

Surg Clin N Am 90 (2010) 125–135
doi:10.1016/j.suc.2009.09.007
0039-6109/09/$ – see front matter © 2010 Elsevier Inc. All rights reserved.

surgical.theclinics.com

**Table 1**
**Causes of secondary pruritus ani**

| | | |
|---|---|---|
| 1. | Infectious | a. Bacterial<br>b. Fungal/yeast<br>c. Viral<br>d. Parasitic |
| 2. | Dermatologic | a. Psoriasis<br>b. Lichen planus, lichen simplex chronicus<br>c. Lichen sclerosus et atrophicus<br>d. Contact dermatitis<br>e. Atopic dermatitis<br>f. Local malignancy: Bowen and Paget disease |
| 3. | Systemic disease | a. Diabetes mellitus<br>b. Leukemia and lymphoma<br>c. Hepatic diseases (obstructive jaundice)<br>d. Thyroid disorders |
| 4. | Local irritants | a. Fecal contamination and moisture<br>b. Soaps<br>c. Diet<br>d. Topical or systemic medications |
| 5. | Colorectal and anal causes | a. Prolapse (internal hemorrhoids or rectal)<br>b. Fistula in ano<br>c. Fissures<br>d. Diarrhea |

## PRIMARY "IDIOPATHIC" PRURITUS ANI

After a thorough history and physical examination, when no other demonstrable cause can be found, this condition is termed primary or idiopathic pruritus ani. Washington Hospital Center classifies pruritus ani based on the physical features of the skin: stage 0 is normal skin, stage 1 is red and inflamed skin, stage 2 has lichenified skin (**Fig. 1**), and stage 3 has lichenified skin, coarse ridges, and often ulcerations (**Fig. 2**).[6] This particular condition can be chronic and very difficult to treat.

### Routine Therapy

The treatment of idiopathic pruritus ani focuses on reestablishing ideal anal hygiene and providing reassurance that there is no underlying condition causing the symptoms. Often this reassurance to the patient is just as effective in management of the disease as any other medicinal treatment.[6] Routine management begins with several simple steps. First, avoid using known irritants such as soaps, lotions, creams, perfumed powders, baby wipes, and any product with witch hazel. Second, avoid further trauma to the perianal skin. This means no scratching, not using dry toilet paper, and no vigorous scrubbing during showering. The authors recommend using moist toilet paper to gently blot the skin clean. Those who have difficulties with nocturnal scratching should wear a pair of light, soft, cotton gloves at night. Step 3 is to avoid moisture and keep the area dry. This means avoiding tight fitting, synthetic undergarments and using a small piece of cotton and/or a small amount of cornstarch, to help soak up any excess moisture. Using a hair dryer on a cool setting can be an excellent means of gently and thoroughly drying this area after cleansing. Lastly, patients should maintain regular bowel movements, normal in consistency with

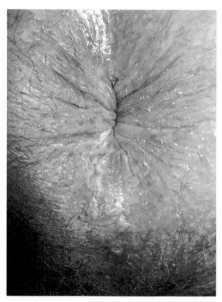

**Fig. 1.** Pruritus ani stage 2: notice the lichenified skin from chronic irritation. (*Courtesy of* C. Os Finne, St Paul, MN).

a high fiber diet and avoid excessive fluid intake.[7] If these measures fail other alternatives for treatment include topical steroids, capsaicin, and injected methylene blue.

### Topical Therapy

In the setting of proper anal hygiene, topical steroids have been shown to be a safe and effective treatment for pruritus ani. Using a weak topical steroid such as 1% hydrocortisone cream 2 to 3 times a day for a short period of time is effective in relieving the symptoms of pruritus. Al-Ghnaniem and colleagues[8] studied a group of patients with idiopathic pruritus ani using a pilot, double-blinded, randomized, placebo-controlled, crossover trial. For 2 weeks before treatment, patients filled out a daily visual analog score (VAS) for severity of itch and a weekly Dermatology Life Quality Index (DLQI) questionnaire. They were then examined and randomly assigned into the treatment arm (1% hydrocortisone in white soft paraffin) or the placebo group (white soft paraffin). This was followed by a 2-week period of washout and a final 2-week period of the opposite treatment. The VAS and DLQI questionnaires were repeated during the second week of each treatment. They were able to show a 68% reduction in VAS and 75% reduction in DLQI scores in the 1% hydrocortisone group when compared with the placebo group. The more potent steroids or prolonged use of steroids can lead to skin atrophy and sometimes worsen pruritus ani.[6,9]

Topical capsaicin is the only other treatment studied in a randomized fashion. The mechanism of capsaicin is not completely understood but evidence show a depressant effect in the synthesis, storage, transport, and release of substance "P", a neuropeptide that triggers the sensation of itching and burning pain.[10] Lysy and colleagues[10] performed a randomized, placebo-controlled, crossover trial that compared topical capsaicin (0.006%) with placebo (1% menthol) in a group of patients with chronic pruritus ani (defined as symptoms lasting more than 3 months). Of 44 patients, 31 (70%) had relief of their symptoms with capsaicin, 8 had no change in

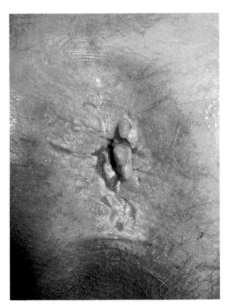

**Fig. 2.** Pruritus ani stage 3: notice the lichenified skin with ridges and ulcerations. (*Courtesy of* C. Os Finne, St Paul, MN).

symptoms, 1 had equal relief with capsaicin and placebo, and 4 withdrew from the study because of side effects. To maintain relief of symptoms, 29 of the 31 patients required at least a single daily application. They concluded that capsaicin is a safe and highly effective treatment option for severe, intractable idiopathic pruritus ani.

## Injectable Therapy

Intradermal injection of methylene blue has been described several times in the literature for intractable idiopathic pruritus ani. The presumed mechanism is destruction of nerve endings by methylene blue.[9] One of the earliest descriptions of this technique was by Eusebio and colleagues[11]; they described a series of patients over a 9.5-year period, who were treated for intractable pruritus ani with methylene blue injection. They performed this procedure in the operating room with intravenous sedation and began by injecting 30 to 40 mL of 0.25% bupivacaine (Marcaine) with 1:200,000 epinephrine mixed with equal volumes of 0.5% lidocaine (Xylocaine) into the intracutaneous and subcutaneous anoderm and perianal area. They then injected up to 30 mL of 0.5% methylene blue into the same areas using a 22- to 25-guage spinal needle. Although they claimed good results (21 out of 23 patients had either short-term or long-term relief), 3 patients developed full thickness skin necrosis and required surgical debridement. This complication is presumably due to the large volumes of fluid injected.

Mentes and colleagues[12] described a slightly different technique using injected methylene blue in a group of 30 patients with intractable idiopathic pruritus ani. They performed this procedure in their office using a sterile technique without anesthesia or sedation. The mixture consisted of 7 to 8 mL of 2% methylene blue mixed with equal volumes of 0.5% lidocaine (Xylocaine) such that a 1% methylene blue solution was created. Using a 22-guage needle this solution was injected intracutaneously and subcutaneously into the affected perianal area targeting the dermo-epidermal junction. Follow-up was for 1 month, 6 months, and then annually thereafter. A "rescue treatment" was offered to the patients 1 month after the first application if they had a partial but not complete response. At 1 month, 80% of patients were free of symptoms and 5 out of 30 had partial response. These 5 patients had a second injection or "rescue treatment" and 4 patients had complete relief of symptoms, increasing the response rate to 93.3%. Their results dropped slightly over time but still seem convincing with 77% of patients symptom free at 12 months after treatment. In their study, there were no major complications and no reported cases of skin necrosis. They attribute this to the use of much lesser volumes, 10 to 15 mL of total injected volume. The other important point is not to inject too superficially because that may also contribute to skin ulcerations and necrosis.

## SECONDARY PRURITUS ANI
### Infectious

Infection can be bacterial, viral, fungal, or parasitic in origin, but in general, infectious sources are rarely the cause of pruritus ani. Several different bacteria have been described as causative agents of pruritus ani. Beta-hemolytic streptococci, *Staphylococcus aureus* and *Corynebacterium minutissimum* have all been described as presenting with perianal itch and can last up to 1 year.[9] Beta-hemolytic streptococcal perianal dermatitis is most common in children from 6 months to 10 years of age, and according to Sheth and Schechtman,[13] 92% of these cases also had positive pharyngeal cultures for group A beta-hemolytic streptococcus, which suggests an autoinoculation. Typical presentation is a moist, bright, erythematous rash with distinct borders and no satellite lesions, that fails to respond to topical steroids. This can be quickly diagnosed with a rapid streptococcal test and should then be treated with oral penicillin.[13] Weismann and colleagues[14] described a series of adult patients (19 patients over a 12-month period) who were found to have beta-hemolytic streptococcus as a source of their pruritus ani. They found the course in adults to be prolonged and unlike the outcomes in children, beta-hemolytic streptococcus is often difficult to eradicate with a single, 10- to 14-day course of antibiotics. Baral[15] described a small group of patients with pruritus who underwent culture testing and 6 out of 7 patients' samples showed growth of *Staphylococcus aureus*. The patients were treated with systemic antibiotics and topical medications, with good success.

Erythrasma was initially thought to be a fungal infection, but in 1961, the organism responsible for this condition was identified as a gram-positive bacillus called *Corynebacterium minutissimum*.[16] This cutaneous infection involves intertriginous areas of the body: the groins, axillae, intergluteal folds, toe web spaces, and in women the inframammary creases.[16,17] Erythrasma has been reported to be the cause of pruritus ani in 1% to 18% of cases.[9] The classic skin findings are scaly, well-defined patches of initially reddish and then brownish colored lesions developing in the previously mentioned areas. Confirming a diagnosis of erythrasma is easily done, as these lesions show a characteristic coral-red fluorescence when examined with a Wood lamp. If the patient has recently showered, the fluorescence may not be detected because the porphyrin responsible for its fluorescence is water-soluble. If this is suspected, the patient should refrain from washing for 48 hours and then the perianal Wood lamp examination is repeated.[17] Bowyer and McColl[17] found 15 patients with erythrasma in a group of 81 patients presenting with pruritus ani. In all 15 patients, Wood lamp examination was positive in the groins, thighs, and toe web spaces but only 9 had fluorescence of the perianal region. This reinforces the importance of examining the classic sites involved in this condition. Erythrasma is treated with systemic antibiotics, classically with erythromycin 1 g per day in 4 divided doses for 10 days. Tetracycline is a second alternative.[16,17] Bowyer and McColl[17] also recommend topical therapy with betamethasone (Betnovate) lotion to the perianal region and half-strength Whitfield ointment to all other involved areas. With this combined systemic and topical therapy, they reported relief of symptoms in all 15 patients within 2 to 4 days of beginning treatment.

Fungal infections can account for 10% to 15% of pruritus ani infections[3,9] and although *Candida albicans* may be commonly cultured from the perianal region, according to Dodi and colleagues[18] it was only concomitant with pruritus ani in 27% of their patients. Although dermatophytes were found less frequently, they were always associated with pruritus and should always be considered pathogenic and treated appropriately.[9] *Candida* sp are infrequently pathogenic but should always be treated in patients who are immunosuppressed, diabetic, or recently treated with systemic steroids or antibiotics.[9] Many providers are fooled by the common physical findings of pruritus ani (erythema with distinct borders) and begin treatment for a candidal infection with antifungal creams. Again, it is important to remember, *Candida* is not commonly a pathogenic organism in the perianal region and its treatment can often worsen pruritus ani because the creams contribute to perianal moisture.

Several sexually transmitted diseases can present with pruritus ani, including herpes simplex, syphilis, gonorrhea, and condyloma accuminata. Parasitic infestations should also be excluded during the workup for pruritus ani. Some common offenders include *Enterobius vermicularis* (pinworms), *Sarcoptes scabei*, and *Pediculosis pubis*.[2] In children, pinworms are a common cause of pruritus ani; this occurs at night and is exacerbated after defecation. A cellophane tape test in the early morning hours identifies the adult worms and their eggs and confirms the diagnosis.[3]

### Dermatologic

Several dermatologic conditions may manifest with perianal symptoms and pruritus ani. These conditions include psoriasis, seborrheic dermatitis, atopic dermatitis, contact dermatitis, lichen planus, lichen sclerosus et atrophicus, lichen simplex chronicus, and local malignancies, including extramammary Paget and Bowen disease. Because many of these conditions do not show their classic appearance in the perianal region, accurate diagnosis depends on a thorough physical examination of the entire body.[6]

Psoriasis typically appears as well-demarcated, scaly, plaquelike lesions that are bright red in color. The lesion are commonly found on the scalp, elbows, knees, knuckles, and penis.[6] In the perianal region, however, the physical findings have been described as inverse psoriasis[3] and tend to be poorly demarcated, paler, non-scaling lesions.[6] Psoriasis is not a curable condition but symptoms can be kept a bay with 1% hydrocortisone cream.

Seborrheic dermatitis is an uncommon cause of pruritus ani, characterized by extensive, moist erythema in the perineum.[3] A thorough physical examination with special attention to the scalp, chest, ears, beard, and suprapubic area helps significantly in making this diagnosis. Treatment involves 2% sulfur with 1% hydrocortisone or miconazole lotion.[6]

Atopic dermatitis is a chronic inflammatory, pruritic disease of the skin, that is an allergic response to environmental allergens. Patients with this condition are also likely to have asthma, hay fever, and eczema. These lesions are typically dry, scaling lesions on the face, neck, dorsum of the hands, and popliteal and antecubital fossa and the mainstay of treatment is to identify the allergen if possible and avoid contact. In the perineum, one should avoid soaps because they can act as an irritant and worsen the symptoms.[6]

A careful history is important when assessing secondary pruritus ani, and should include questions about the use of any over-the-counter medications or home remedies. Contact dermatitis can result from several products including lanolin, neomycin, parabens, topical anesthetics from the "-caine" family, and certain toilet papers.[6] Bowyer and McColl[19] studied a group of 200 patients with pruritus ani and found multiple agents responsible for contact dermatitis presenting as pruritus ani. When divided into drug subgroups, 1 case was caused by antihistamines, 1 from topical antibiotics, 15 cases from topical antiseptics, and 23 patients developed contact dermatitis from topical local anesthetics. The typical appearance is extreme erythema with vesicles and macerated skin. The key to treatment is avoiding irritants and tight constricting undergarments, sitting in a warm sitz bath for comfort, and keeping the affected area dry at all other times; 1% hydrocortisone lotion is also helpful in management.[6]

Lichen planus is believed to be caused by an altered, cell-mediated immune response to some unknown source. This condition may be seen in patients with other disease processes of altered immunity, such as ulcerative colitis, lichen sclerosis, and myasthenia gravis. Lichen planus has also been seen in patients with hepatitis C infection, chronic active hepatitis, and primary biliary cirrhosis and these should be searched for if there is widespread lichen planus.[20] The cutaneous manifestations are shiny, flat-topped papules that are more darkly pigmented than the surrounding skin. These lesions begin on the volar aspects of the wrists and forearms. Genital involvement and mucous membrane involvement are common, and pruritus is common with genital involvement.[6] Wickham striae are intersecting gray lines that can be seen if mineral oil is applied to the plaques and help to establish the diagnosis. This is typically a self-limited disease resolving over 8 to 12 months, and the symptoms are treated with topical steroids or systemic steroids in very severe cases.[6,20]

Lichen sclerosus et atrophicus is a disease seen mainly in women with a 5:1 to 6:1 female to male ratio and involves the vulva and extends posteriorly to the perianal region.[3,6,21] The first phase of this condition begins as ivory-colored, atrophic papules that break down and expose underlying erythematous, raw tissue, which is intensely pruritic and painful. As this heals, the area is replaced by chronic inflammation, sclerosis, and atrophy of the affected area. On physical examination, one classically finds white patches in a figure-8 pattern around the vulva and anus. The clitoris and labia minora may be flattened as they become involved in the sclerosis phase.[3,6] If symptoms are present, treatment should be started with topical steroids and it is important to explain that the outward appearance may never change even if the symptoms are relieved.[21] Potent topical steroid creams, such as clobetasol, for a short course followed by less potent hydrocortisone cream are the mainstay of treatment. Retinoids and testosterone creams have also been described.[13,21] Because of the small risk of developing squamous cell carcinoma, all nonresponders or those with recurrent sclerosis should have a skin biopsy to rule out malignancy.[9]

Lichen simplex chronicus, also known as neurodermatitis, is a secondary skin manifestation that develops in an area of repetitive trauma from scratching or rubbing, which then leads to thickening and scaling of the skin, also known as lichenification. There may or may not be any underlying primary pathology.[22] An itch-scratch-itch cycle begins when a patient senses pruritus consciously or unconsciously at night. The patient begins scratching the area resulting in local irritation and more itching.[19] Pruritus is typically intermittent and worsens when a patient is quiet or still; it is much less noticeable during activity. Scratching the area provides temporary relief and once this cycle begins, it is extremely difficult to break. Management begins with topical steroids to decrease the inflammation and break the itch-scratch-itch cycle. Other described medicines include oral antihistamines, doxepin or capsaicin creams, and topical acetylsalicylic acid/dichloromethane or immunomodulators, such as tacrolimus, for those patients who are nonresponders to topical steroids.[22]

Although uncommon, pruritus ani can be a presenting symptom of local malignancy such as Paget and Bowen disease. Extramammary Paget disease (cutaneous adenocarcinoma in situ) is rare, but if found it may be indicative of an underlying carcinoma. The classic presentation is an erythematous, eczematoid plaque seen in the perianal region and this commonly occurs in the seventh decade. Treatment for this involves wide local excision and may require V-Y flaps and/or staged surgeries with split-thickness skin grafts. The recurrence rate is high and can occur up to a decade after initial excision, which makes long-term follow-up imperative.[6] Powell and Perry[23] presented a 53-year-old man with a 20-year history of pruritus ani that responded to local therapy but never completely resolved. Diagnostic workup revealed Paget disease with no evidence of underlying bowel malignancy and he subsequently underwent a wide local excision with grafting. Eight years later the itching returned and biopsies revealed recurrent Paget disease. Reexcision was performed and 7 years later at the time of their presentation the patient was disease free.

Bowen disease is the eponym for squamous cell carcinoma in situ of the anus, which is synonymous with high-grade anal intraepithelial neoplasia-III or high-grade squamous intraepithelial lesion. The purpose of this discussion is not to fully describe Bowen disease, but rather to highlight its importance in the differential diagnosis of a patient with pruritus ani.

### Systemic Diseases

There are several systemic diseases that may present with pruritus ani; diabetes mellitus is the most common. Other conditions include liver disease, lymphoma, leukemia, pellagra, vitamin A and D deficiencies, renal failure, iron-deficiency anemia, and hyperthyroidism.[2,3,9] If no obvious source for pruritus is found, then a more methodical search should be conducted to rule out these conditions as the possible cause.

### Local Irritants

Several irritants are known to cause pruritus ani. Although fecal contamination to some degree is universal, feces does not cause the same irritation on skin elsewhere on the body. People with colostomies do not complain of pruritus around their stoma. Therefore, the etiology of stool causing pruritus may simply be related to the increased wetness and maceration of the perianal skin. Other irritants include perianal wetness or moisture, tight or synthetic underclothing, soaps, abrasion by vigorous scrubbing or dry toilet paper, and certain medications, including quinidine, colchicine, and mineral oil.[2] There have been many claims about certain foods causing pruritus but there has been no substantiation of these claims, and therefore there is no evidence supporting avoidance of any particular food.[24] Excessive fluid intake affects the consistency of the stool and may cause diarrhea, which requires more wiping or cleansing, worsens fecal contamination, and worsens pruritus, so it is important to take a fluid history in someone who presents with pruritus ani in the setting of diarrhea.

### Colorectal and Anal

Many of the attributable colorectal and anal sources cause pruritus either by contributing to fecal contamination or by increasing perianal wetness and moisture. When managing pruritus ani, it is important to look for and treat these common anorectal problems first. The anorectal problems include conditions contributing to perianal wetness, prolapse of the rectum or internal hemorrhoids, anal fissures, anal fistulas, chronic diarrhea, chronic constipation, papillomas, polyps, and cancer.[3] Murie and colleagues[25] studied a group of patients with symptomatic, bleeding and/or prolapsing internal hemorrhoids, and they found these patients to have soiling and pruritus much more commonly than normal controls. They also found significant improvement in symptoms when these patients were treated with either rubber band ligation or excisional hemorrhoidectomy. This again supports the rationale of treating any obvious anorectal causes first and then if pruritus ani persists to proceed with a more methodical search for any other secondary causes of pruritus ani as discussed earlier.

## SUMMARY: APPROACH TO THE PATIENT

Pruritus ani is an uncommon problem overall, affecting 1% to 5% of the general population. When it does occur however, it is bothersome, can be life altering for the patient, and is difficult for the physician to manage.

During the initial visit for pruritus ani, it is important for the physician to take a detailed history (including fluid intake, frequency, and consistency of bowel movements) and a detailed past medical history to look for the common systemic diseases that can present with pruritus. Although these are less commonly the underlying cause, it is important to ask about them.

The physical examination during the first visit should be focused on finding and treating the common anorectal causes of pruritus. This may mean several visits to the office for rubber band ligation of prolapsing internal hemorrhoids or identifying and beginning treatment for anal fistulas and fissures. Although treatment ensues for the common anorectal causes, the physician must also stress good perianal hygiene, which means avoiding wetness and further trauma to the perianal region as described earlier. This is also a good time to begin treatment with a tiny amount of 1% hydrocortisone cream, which can help break the scratch-itch-scratch cycle. This should be applied sparingly, so as not to perpetuate the problem with chronic perianal moisture, and it should be followed by the use of cornstarch and/or a small amount of cotton left in place during the day. This is also the time to begin managing the balance of fluid and fiber intake to help alter and normalize stool consistency. The patient should attend follow-up in the office in 1 month.

If the patient continues to have pruritus at follow-up despite treatment of all anorectal causes, adequate perianal hygiene, and good stool consistency, then a more methodical search should ensue. At this visit a more detailed dermatologic history and physical examination should be performed looking for the common dermatologic causes. The potential infectious and dermatologic causes can be diagnosed with cultures and biopsies of the perianal skin and sometimes may require special examining tools, such as the Wood lamp to look for erythrasma. Having a dermatologist who can assist with diagnosis and management of the multiple, potential dermatologic causes can be helpful.

If this diligent search for secondary causes of pruritus reveals no obvious source, then idiopathic pruritus ani becomes the diagnosis of exclusion. As described earlier, this can often be managed with the same perianal hygiene measures and by reassuring the patient that there is no underlying malignancy. If these fail, the next step in management is injectable therapies. Methylene blue injected into the perianal subcutaneous tissues, as described earlier, seems to be the safest injectable method and can have long-lasting results.

**REFERENCES**

1. Billingham RP, Isler JT, Kimmins MH, et al. The diagnosis and management of common anorectal disorders. Curr Probl Surg 2004;33(7):586–645.
2. Hanno R, Murphy P. Pruritus ani: classification and management. Dermatol Clin 1987;5(4):811–6.
3. Zuccati G, Lotti T, Mastrolorenzo A, et al. Pruritus ani. Dermatol Ther 2005;18(4):355–62.
4. Mazier WP. Hemorrhoids, fissures, and pruritus ani. Surg Clin North Am 1994;74(6):1277–92.
5. Metcalf A. Anorectal disorders. Five common causes of pain, itching and bleeding. Postgrad Med 1995;98(5):81–4, 87–9, 92–4.
6. Gordon PH, Nivatvongs S. Perianal dermatologic disease. In: Gordon PH, editor. Principles and practice of surgery for the colon, rectum and anus. 3rd edition. New York: Informa Healthcare; 2007. p. 247–73.
7. Alexander-Williams J. Causes and management of anal irritation. Br Med J (Clin Res Ed) 1983;287(6404):1528.
8. Al-Ghnaniem R, Short K, Pullen A, et al. 1% Hydrocortisone ointment is an effective treatment of pruritus ani: a pilot randomized controlled crossover trial. Int J Colorectal Dis 2007;22(12):1463–7.
9. Siddiqi S, Vijay V, Ward M, et al. Pruritus ani. Ann R Coll Surg Engl 2008;90(6):457–63.
10. Lysy J, Sistiery-Ittah M, Israelit Y, et al. Topical capsaicin—a novel and effective treatment for idiopathic intractable pruritus ani: a randomized, placebo controlled, crossover study. Gut 2003;52(9):1323–6.
11. Eusebio EB, Graham J, Mody N. Treatment of intractable pruritus ani. Dis Colon Rectum 1990;33(9):770–2.
12. Mentes BB, Akin M, Leventoglu S, et al. Intradermal methylene blue injection for the treatment of intractable idiopathic pruritus ani: results of 30 cases. Tech Coloproctol 2004;8(1):11–4.
13. Sheth S, Schechtman AD. Itchy perianal erythema. J Fam Pract 2007;56(12):1025–7.
14. Weismann K, Sand Petersen C, Roder B. Pruritus ani caused by beta-haemolytic streptococci. Acta Derm Venereol 1996;76(5):415.
15. Baral J. Pruritus ani and *Staphylococcus aureus* [letter]. J Am Acad Dermatol 1983;9(6):962.
16. Sindhuphak W, MacDonald E, Smith EB. Erythrasma: overlooked or misdiagnosed? Int J Dermatol 1985;24(2):95–6.
17. Bowyer A, McColl I. Erythrasma and pruritus ani. Acta Derm Venereol 1971;51(6):444–7.
18. Dodi G, Pirone E, Bettin A, et al. The mycotic flora in proctological patients with and without pruritus ani. Br J Surg 1985;72(12):967–9.
19. Bowyer A, McColl I. A study of 200 patients with pruritus ani. Proc R Soc Med 1970;63(Suppl):96–8.
20. Chuang TY, Stitle L. Lichen planus. Emedicine website. Available at: http://emedcine.medscape.com/article/1123213-overview. Updated: April 18, 2008.
21. Meffert J. Lichen sclerosus et atrophicus. Emedicine website. Available at: http://emedicine.medscape.com/article/1123316-overview. Updated: January 29, 2009.
22. Hogan DJ, Mason SH, Bower SM. Lichen simplex chronicus. Emedicine website. Available at: http://emedicine.medscape.com/article/1123423-overview. Updated October 10, 2008.

23. Powell FC, Perry HO. Pruritus ani: could it be malignant? Geriatrics 1985;40(1): 89–91.
24. Friend WG. The cause and treatment of idiopathic pruritus ani. Dis Colon Rectum 1977;20(1):40–2.
25. Murie JA, Sim AJW, Mackenzie I. The importance of pain, pruritus and soiling as symptoms of haemorrhoids and their response to haemorrhoidectomy or rubber band ligation. Br J Surg 1981;68(4):247–9.

# Anal Stenosis

Mukta V. Katdare, MD, Rocco Ricciardi, MD, MPH*

**KEYWORDS**

• Anal stenosis • Stricture • Anoplasty • Advancement flap

## INTRODUCTION AND ETIOLOGY

Anal stenosis occurs when the normally pliable anoderm is replaced with fibrotic connective tissue leading to an abnormally tight and inelastic anal canal.[1] The stenotic segment may be localized to the proximal or distal anal canal, but often the irregularities are noted to be diffuse and circumferential involving the entire anal canal.[2] Several classification systems have been developed, but the method by Khubchandani[3] is the most useful in classifying anal stenosis as congenital, primary, or secondary. Congenital causes are generally secondary to developmental issues from imperforate anus or anal atresia. Alternatively, primary anal stenosis, which like congenital stenosis occurs early on in development, is most often related to senile or involutional stenosis. Most anal stenosis cases are secondary to surgical trauma, relating to hemorrhoidectomy, perianal lesion excision, fistulectomy, sphincteroplasty, fulguration of condyloma, or excision of a low rectal tumor. Other secondary causes include radiation therapy to the anorectum, other traumatic injuries to the perineum, chronic anorectal suppurative disease, inflammatory bowel disease, sexually transmitted infections, chronic laxative use, Paget disease, anal dysplasia, or chronic diarrhea.[2,3]

Given the number of surgical hemorrhoidectomies performed in the United States and the substantial anorectal mucosal trauma that is involved, hemorrhoidectomy is the most common cause of anal stenosis with an incidence ranging from 1.5% to 3.8%.[4] Overzealous hemorrhoidectomy may denude large areas of anoderm and rectal mucosa from the lining of the anal canal, resulting in scarring and progressive chronic stricture formation making the anus less pliable.[1] The underlying sphincter mechanism may also be damaged with hemorrhoidectomy, resulting in severe stenosis. Anal stenosis can occur following stapling procedures for hemorrhoids, especially with staple line dehiscence or when the stapler is placed too superficially in the anal canal leading to scarring.[5] In a series of 212 patients with anal stenosis, hemorrhoidectomy was identified as the underlying cause in 87.7% of cases.[2] Although the authors were unable to determine if overaggressive hemorrhoidectomy

No funding support for this article.

Department of Colon and Rectal Surgery, Lahey Clinic, 41 Mall Road, Burlington, MA 01805, USA

* Corresponding author.

*E-mail address:* rocco.ricciardi@lahey.org (R. Ricciardi).

doi:10.1016/j.suc.2009.10.002
0039-6109/09/$ – see front matter

surgical.theclinics.com

was the cause of stenosis, it is generally accepted that removal of large areas of ano-derm raises the risk of stenotic complications to the anus.

Patients with inflammatory bowel disease, particularly Crohn's disease, often report difficulty with anal stenosis. However, because of the liquid or semi-solid nature of their stools, some patients may remain asymptomatic without requiring surgical treat-ment. Given the significant perianal disease and poor wound healing, severe anal stenosis secondary to Crohn's disease poses a surgical treatment challenge, often leading to fecal diversion. In a study of 224 patients with anorectal complications of Crohn's disease, 65 patients presented with anal stenosis and 4 patients went on to develop anal stenosis during the study.[6] Most of these patients specifically indicated that anal stenosis was their only complaint. Of this total, only a small number required absolutely no surgical intervention; 16 patients underwent mechanical dilatation and 17 patients ultimately underwent proctectomy or diverting stoma within a mean follow-up of 19 months.[6]

## DIAGNOSIS

Patients with anal stenosis often complain of painful bowel movements, constipation, obstipation, narrow caliber of stool, tenesmus, diarrhea, fecal leakage, or bleeding.[1] Pain with defecation is the most frequent complaint followed by constipation and bleeding, but frequently there is an overlap of symptoms.[7] Constipation may be so severe that many patients begin to rely on laxatives, enemas, suppositories, and digital manipulation to aid in defecation, which can ultimately lead to more trauma, further aggravating their condition,[1,8] Diarrhea noted in these patients is often the result of chronic laxative use leading to "paraffin anus" or from fecal overflow secondary to impaction.[8]

Physical examination is obviously very important in making the diagnosis and iden-tifying the cause of anal stenosis, but often, anatomic findings may not directly corre-spond with the severity of symptoms. Inspection of the anal canal will reveal a narrowing of the anal opening with circumferential fissure formation seen from parting of the gluteal folds.[3] Visualization of cicatricial tissue may also reveal cauliflo-werlike lesions similar to those seen with anal condyloma or verrucous carcinoma. In addition to condyloma, the differential diagnosis for these lesions includes squamous dysplasia, ulcerated papillary lesions or squamous cell cancer.[8] A thorough history and physical examination will help in making the diagnosis, but the examination may need to be performed under general anesthesia because of the associated pain and discomfort. Apart from patient comfort and the ability to perform an adequate biopsy, another advantage of an examination under anesthesia is that it may allow the differentiation of an anatomic versus functional cause of the stenosis. With functional stenosis, the anus will relax under anesthesia whereas with an anatomic stenosis, the stricturing caused by scar tissue will only relax with forceful dilatation. During the examination, anoscopy or proctoscopy can help delineate the extent of anal scarring. Biopsy is typically not required but should be performed if squamous dysplasia or carcinoma is suspected.

Based on physical examination, anal stenosis may be classified by the severity of the stricture and by the level of involvement in the anal canal. When based on severity, anal stenoses are classified as mild, if the anal canal can be examined by a lubricated index finger or a medium Hill-Ferguson retractor; moderate, if insertion of the lubri-cated index finger or a medium Hill-Ferguson into the anal canal requires forceful dila-tation; and severe, if forceful dilatation is required to insert the little finger or a small Hill-Ferguson retractor.[2] Classification based on the level of involvement includes low (at least 0.5 cm distal to the dentate line), middle (0.5 cm distal and proximal to the dentate line), and high (0.5 cm above the dentate line).[1] Involvement of the entire length of the anal canal is unusual but has been seen in extreme cases.

## PREVENTING ANAL STENOSIS

Prevention of anal stenosis should be discussed before treatment is addressed. With all perineal procedures, the surgeon should practice meticulous dissection, aiming to avoid excessive undermining or excision of normal anoderm and not injure the sphincter musculature. For example, during hemorrhoidectomy, viable tissue bridges should be preserved to assure proper healing and less scarring. It is critical that the surgeon not attempt to remove all hemorrhoids, especially in the setting of an acute exacerbation of hemorrhoidal disease. Similar attention is necessary when performing excision of anal tags or low rectal lesions. At the completion of many anorectal operations, it is the authors' practice to assure easy passage of an operating anoscope or proctoscope.

## TREATMENT

Treatment of stenosis is based on the patient's symptoms and the impact of those symptoms on quality of life. Obviously, a patient who is seen for other reasons and is coincidently noted to have anal stenosis does not require treatment although the surgeon should be mindful of ruling out malignancy. A methodical approach that begins with nonoperative measures and progresses to more invasive options is best and is presented in the following paragraphs.

### Nonoperative Management

Mild stenosis whether due to functional or anatomic conditions can often be treated with dietary modifications, stool softeners, or "bulking agents." Attempts at anal dilatation in patients with mild stenosis and symptoms generally occurs with the natural stretch of a fecal bolus passing through the anal canal, but digital or mechanical anal dilatation may be required if patients begin having more difficulty with regular bowel movements. The patient often undergoes the first dilatation under anesthesia followed by regular dilatations with either a digit or a small plastic dilator. The described dilatation technique has been found to be particularly useful in those with mild-to-moderate anal stenosis due to Crohn's disease, previous radiation, or in those patients in whom surgery carries significant risk.[9] Small case series reveal that even patients with Crohn's disease treated with anal dilatation under anesthesia achieve good results.[2] In one study of 44 patients with anal stenosis secondary to Crohn's disease, 75% underwent mechanical dilatation and 43% eventually required proctectomy.[10] Similarly, Michelassi[6] reported that of 33 patients with Crohn's disease and anal stenosis, 16 patients underwent mechanical dilatation and 17 patients ultimately underwent proctectomy or diverting stoma.[6] These studies highlight the significant risk of loss of bowel continence in patients with Crohn's and anal stenosis; however, as mentioned earlier, some patients respond well to repeated dilatations. Despite these reported results, some investigators have suggested that manual anal dilatation may result in further scarring and progressive stenosis or incontinence and should thus be avoided in patients with Crohn's.[3,11] Currently, there is no particularly good rule of thumb for which patients may actually deteriorate with mechanical dilatation, but a trial of dilatation is a good starting point.

### Operative Management

Surgical management is generally reserved for patients with moderate-to-severe stenosis who failed attempts at conservative management. In determining proper treatment, the surgeon should try to determine the differential involvement of the anoderm as compared with the underlying sphincter mechanism. A procedure to bring in healthy perianal skin is unlikely to help the patient with a stenotic muscle unless the patient has a concomitant sphincterotomy. A simple stricture release may provide temporary symptom relief but should be avoided because subsequent scarring frequently results in stricture recurrence.[1]

In the situation of a stenosis of the anoderm, the authors' operative management consists of a flap that uses the transfer of either rectal mucosa or perianal skin to the anal canal, restoring elasticity and replacing lost or diseased nonpliable anoderm with elastic and compliant neoanoderm.[1,8] Vascular supply for these flaps is obtained from perforating vessels in the submucosal or subdermal vascular plexus or in subcutaneous tissues. These flaps are classified as advancement, rotational, or adjacent tissue transfer flaps.[1] The authors' general practice has been to treat fibrotic muscular stenosis of the anus in the setting of healthy-appearing anoderm with either unilateral or bilateral internal sphincterotomy. Relieving the circumferential fibrotic scar of the internal sphincter in these patients is a useful and effective method to reduce symptoms. In those patients with anoderm stenosis and sphincter muscle scarring, a flap procedure can be added to internal sphincterotomy.

### Mucosal advancement flaps

Several options are available to slide healthy compliant tissue into the scarred area through advancement flaps. Mucosal advancements slide healthy proximal rectal mucosa down to the area of the anal stenosis and are best suited for treating midlevel and upper anal stenosis.[1] The advancement is performed after scar tissue is excised or incised, and unilateral or bilateral internal sphincterotomy is performed if the sphincter mechanism is also scarred and stenotic. Mucosal advancement flaps have fairly minimal pain postoperatively but pose a small risk of mucosal ectropion if the flap is advanced beyond the dentate line.

A transverse incision is then made lateral and perpendicular to the dentate line extending into the anal verge.[3] The proximal rectal and anal mucosa is undermined in a cephalad direction for 2 to 5 cm. Including the underlying muscle is critical to bringing in healthy tissue that is unlikely to become ischemic and slough, leading to further scarring. The flap is advanced maintaining its vascular supply through the submucosal plexuses and sutured to the distal edge of the internal sphincter as close to the dentate line as possible and with the aim to advance the flap beyond the scarred area. Advancing the flap too distally and suturing it to the anal verge may result in an ectropion, leading to difficulty with discharge, moisture, and incontinence. In one series, 82% of 53 patients treated with mucosal advancement flaps (44 bilateral and 9 unilateral) reported good results.[3] Others have similarly reported success in 90% and 97% of patients treated with mucosal advancement flaps.[12,13]

### Anoplasty

Mucosal advancement flaps are optimal for mid-to-upper stenoses, but for more distal stenoses, flaps of healthy anal skin are more suited to be transposed into the anal canal. This method of transposition is fairly simple, with good exposure and minimal risks except for flap ischemia or necrosis. Perianal wounds can be painful for some patients but adequate analgesics should be made available and outcomes are reportedly excellent.

One very good option for anoplasty is the Y-V advancement flap. It is performed by making a Y-shaped incision with the base limb of the Y into the area of stenosis and the wide base of the Y oriented distally in the perianal skin. This wide base is shaped in a V configuration and while carefully maintaining its subdermal vascular plexus, is extensively mobilized and sutured into the vertical limb of the Y incision in the anal canal creating the final V configuration. Again, it is critical that a full-thickness flap is mobilized, generally down to the underlying fascia depending on flap location. Inadequate mobilization, tension on the flap, or loss of vascular supply leads to ischemic necrosis at the proximal tip of the flap. Other complications include suture dehiscence, ischemic contracture, and hematoma. If the proximal portion of the flap is too narrow, the patient may have insignificant widening of the stenosis. Therefore the Y-V flap is generally reserved for stenoses below the dentate line.[1] Proper technique leads to excellent or complete satisfaction in 64% to 100% of cases in which this technique is used.[7,14-16]

The V-Y advancement flap anoplasty was initially developed for the treatment of anal ectropion but is another option for the treatment of anal stenosis.[17] The V-shaped incision is made with the wide base oriented toward the dentate line. Viability of the flap depends on a vascular pedicle contained in the subcutaneous fat, making it necessary to preserve as much subcutaneous tissue as possible. The donor site is closed primarily, creating the vertical limb of the Y configuration away from the stenotic area. The flap is then transferred proximally to replace the anoderm that has been lost. The V-Y flap is best suited for widening the anal canal in patients with severe low anal stenosis.

The diamond flap first described by Caplin and Kodner[18] involves incising scar tissue and leaving a diamond-shaped defect. A diamond-shaped flap is then created distally by incising to the subcutaneous fat, with attention to maintaining the integrity of the subcutaneous vascular pedicle. The apex and borders of the flap are sutured to the mucosa and surrounding anoderm of the intra-anal portion of the defect. Advantages of this type of flap include ease of construction, maintenance of blood supply to flap, minimal tension on suture lines, and primary closure of the donor site. The donor site is then closed with primary intention. Satisfactory results with this technique have been reported in almost all patients in whom it has been attempted.[7,16,18,19]

The U-shaped flap, first described by Pearl and colleagues,[20] involves incising the scar tissue at the site of stenosis without damaging the underlying sphincter mechanism, making a broad U-shaped incision in the perianal skin adjacent to the defect, and advancing this island flap into the anal canal to cover the defect. Of 25 patients treated with U-shaped flaps (20 for anal stenosis and 5 for mucosal ectropion), 16 patients judged their results as excellent and 7, as good.[20] There were 2 failures. One patient had a long stenosis after an ileal pouch anal anastomosis and it was technically not feasible to advance the flap to the mucosa of the pouch. The second patient had persistent ulceration between the margin of the flap and the surrounding anoderm.[20] This flap is thus a good option for bringing in a wide base of healthy tissue without as much risk of ischemia to the tip as with Y-V advancements.

The "house" flap anoplasty described by Christensen and colleagues[21] is a modification of the V-Y flap for proximal stenoses or those that extend from the dentate line to the perianal skin. In these situations, a V-Y flap may not provide enough tissue to relieve the stenosis but the house flap can be very effective (**Fig. 1**). An incision is made longitudinally in the right or left lateral position, extending from the dentate line to the distal end of the stenosis. Transverse incisions are made distally and proximally perpendicular to and centered on the longitudinal incision to open the stenosis. A flap is then created in the shape of a house, with the rectangular base oriented

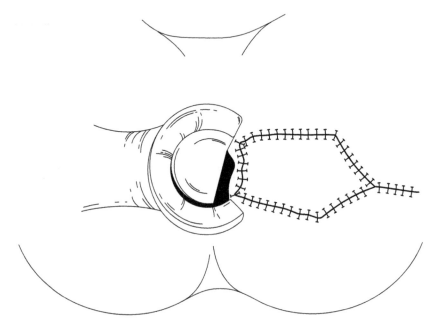

**Fig. 1.** House flap anoplasty. The longitudinal incision extends to the dentate line. The length and width of the flap should be similar in dimension. A full-thickness flap is then advanced into the anal canal toward the dentate line.

proximally and the triangular roof of the house design oriented away from the stenosis. The length of the sides of the flap (walls of the house) is equal to the longitudinal incision made in the anal canal, and the width of the base matches the width of the mucosal defect to be replaced. The width of a single flap should not exceed 25% of the circumference of the anus and thus a second flap may need to be created on the opposite side if one flap is found to insufficiently relieve the stenosis. The flap is then advanced into the anal canal, covering its entire length, and sutured into place. The donor site is closed primarily. By creating a wide base, the potential ischemic complications of having a narrow apex as seen with a Y-V flap are avoided.

This technique can be performed bilaterally for severe stenosis with good results. With a mean follow-up of 28 months, 26 of 29 (89%) consecutive patients undergoing a house advancement flap had relief of symptoms and were able to discontinue stool softeners, laxatives, and enemas.[22] There were no reports of flap necrosis, recurrent stenosis, or recurrent ectropion with this technique, although 44% of patients experienced wound separation.[22] In another review of house advancement, twenty-seven of 28 patients were satisfied with their results at mean follow-up of 26.4 months without evidence of flap necrosis or recurrent stenosis.[23]

Rotational S-plasty flaps are full-thickness flaps in which S-shaped perianal skin is rotated around the central anal canal (**Fig. 2**).[8] After all areas of scarring in the anal canal are excised, the flap is mobilized and rotated so that the apex is sutured to the anterior cut edge of the mucosa, and the side of the flap is sutured to the lateral wall. This flap is well suited for coverage of large areas.[24]

### Surgical Algorithm

If a decision is made to bring in healthy tissue via a flap procedure, no procedure is ideal for all situations. A prospective comparison between procedures is unavailable;

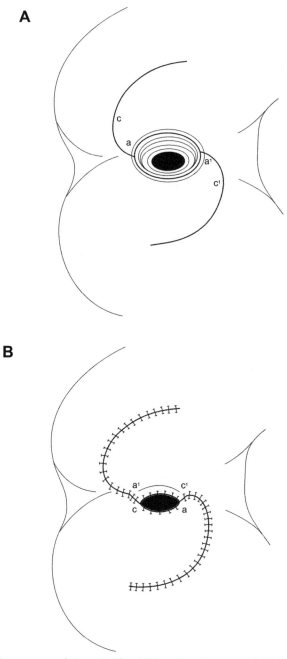

**Fig. 2.** S-plasty for severe anal stenosis. The strictured anoderm is incised and full-thickness flaps are rotated into the anal canal.

thus, choice of one procedure over another depends on surgeon comfort level and anatomic findings. Before a decision is made, the surgeon should have a thorough understanding of the contribution of the underlying sphincter mechanism and overlying anoderm to the stenosis. As discussed earlier, internal sphincterotomy to reduce the fibrosis of the underlying muscle is likely to fail if the patient had overlying anodermal scarring as is the case that bringing in healthy anodermal tissue will fail if the muscle has severe stenosis. When the stenosis is below the dentate line, a Y-V advancement flap or a house flap anoplasty is a good option, whereas the V-Y flap is best suited for middle anal canal stenoses. Y-V advancement flaps are generally ineffective for the treatment of anal stenosis of the upper anal canal. Longer stenoses are best treated with house or diamond flaps, whereas very large defects may require an S-plasty. Other complex rotational flaps based on named vascular pedicles can also be performed if a very wide area of coverage is needed or if several other procedures have already been performed. Obviously, it is up to treating surgeons to determine the flap with which they are most comfortable and the treatment that has demonstrated good success in their hands.

Following surgical treatment, it is the authors' practice to keep the wounds as dry as possible and keep the patient comfortable with appropriate analgesia. In the immediate postoperative period, all patients require some form of bowel regimen to reduce the likelihood of constipation and impaction. Following immediate surgical recovery, patients are started on a high-fiber diet and may shower as per usual routine. Few complications have been reported with most of these techniques; yet, infection, restenosis, flap necrosis, and occasional incontinence have been described. Constipation and impaction are also possible complications.

## SUMMARY

As detailed in the previous sections, anal stenosis poses a difficult problem for patients and is most commonly noted following surgical complications. The surgeon should use meticulous technique in preventing this complication by preserving anodermal skin islands and reducing electrocautery at the surgical site. Although medical options can reduce symptoms, surgical treatment is almost unavoidable when the stenosis becomes more severe and in the situation of difficult, debilitating symptoms. Good outcomes can be obtained with any one of the surgical procedures that transfers healthy tissue into the anal canal.

## REFERENCES

1. Liberman H, Thorson AG. How I do it. Anal stenosis. Am J Surg 2000;179(4): 325–9.
2. Milsom JW, MAzier WP. Classification and management of postsurgical anal stenosis. Surg Gynecol Obstet 1986;163(1):60–4.
3. Khubchandani IT. Anal stenosis. Surg Clin North Am 1994;74(6):1353–60.
4. Eu KW, Teoh TA, Seow-Choen F, et al. Anal stricture following haemorrhoidectomy: early diagnosis and treatment. Aust N Z J Surg 1995;65(2):101–3.
5. Brisinda G, Vanella S, Cadeddu F, et al. Surgical treatment of anal stenosis. World J Gastroenterol 2009;15(16):1921–8.
6. Michelassi F, Melis M, Rubin M, et al. Surgical treatment of anorectal complications in Crohn's disease. Surgery 2000;128(4):597–603.
7. Angelchik PD, Harms BA, Starling JR. Repair of anal stricture and mucosal ectropion with Y-V or pedicle flap anoplasty. Am J Surg 1993;166(1):55–9.

8. Lagares-Garcia JA, Nogueras JJ. Anal stenosis and mucosal ectropion. Surg Clin North Am 2002;82(6):1225–31.

9. Crapp AR, Alexander-Williams J. Fissure-in-ano and anal stenosis. Part I: conservative management. Clin Gastroenterol 1975;4(3):619–28.

10. Linares L, Moreira LF, Andrews H, et al. Natural history and treatment of anorectal strictures complicating Crohn's disease. Br J Surg 1988;75(7):653–5.

11. MacDonald A, Smith A, McNeill AD, et al. Manual dilatation of the anus. Br J Surg 1992;79(12):1381–2.

12. Ramajunan PS. Y-V anoplasty for severe anal stenosis. Contemp Surg 1988;33: 62–8.

13. Carditello A, Milone A, Stilo F, et al. Surgical treatment of anal stenosis following hemorrhoid surgery. Results of 150 combined mucosal advancement and internal sphincterotomy. Chir Ital 2002;54:841–4.

14. Gingold BS, Arvanitis M. Y-V anoplasty for treatment of anal stricture. Surg Gynecol Obstet 1986;162(3):241–2.

15. Rakhmanine M, Rosen L, Khubchandani I, et al. Lateral mucosal advancement anoplasty for anal stricture. Br J Surg 2002;89(11):1423–4.

16. Maria G, Brisinda G, Civello IM. Anoplasty for the treatment of anal stenosis. Am J Surg 1998;175(2):158–60.

17. Rosen L. V-Y advancement for anal ectropion. Dis Colon Rectum 1986;29(9): 596–8.

18. Caplin DA, Kodner IJ. Repair of anal stricture and mucosal ectropion by simple flap procedures. Dis Colon Rectum 1986;29(2):92–4.

19. Pidala MJ, Slezak FA, Porter JA. Island flap anoplasty for anal canal stenosis and mucosal ectropion. Am Surg 1994;60(3):194–6.

20. Pearl RK, Hooks VH 3rd, Abcarian H, et al. Island flap anoplasty for the treatment of anal stricture and mucosal ectropion. Dis Colon Rectum 1990;33(7):581–3.

21. Christensen MA, Pitsch RM Jr, Cali RL, et al. "House" advancement pedicle flap for anal stenosis. Dis Colon Rectum 1992;35(2):201–3.

22. Sentovich SM, Falk PM, Christensen MA, et al. Operative results of house advancement anoplasty. Br J Surg 1993;83(9):1242–4.

23. Alver O, Ersoy YE, Aydemir I, et al. Use of "house" advancement flap in anorectal diseases. World J Surg 2008;32(10):2281–6.

24. Ferguson J. Repair of the "Whitehead deformity" of the the anus. Surg Gynecol Obstet 1959;108(1):115–6.

# Anal Neoplasms

Kelly Garrett, MD[a], Matthew F. Kalady, MD, FASCRS[a,b,*]

## KEYWORDS

- Anal cancer • Squamous cell carcinoma • Epidermoid cancer
- Carcinoma in-situ • Anal canal • Anal margin

Anal cancer is a rare malignancy that accounts for 2% of all colorectal malignancy. Approximately 5200 cases are diagnosed annually in the United States, resulting in more than 700 deaths.[1] Diagnosis and treatment of anal cancer depends on the tumor histology and the anatomic location.

The anatomy of the anal canal and perianal region has been described and defined in a variety of ways. However, because therapy for anal and perianal tumors is determined in large part by anatomic location, understanding the anatomic landmarks in this region is critical. A key distinction is drawn between tumors located in the anal canal compared with the anal margin. The anatomic anal canal extends from the anal verge to the dentate line and is normally about 2 cm in length. In distinction, the surgical anal canal initiates at the dentate line and extends proximally to the anorectal ring. The distal rectal mucosa leads into the top of the anal canal, which is lined by transitional epithelium. The distal anal canal is lined by stratified squamous epithelium leading to the anal margin. The anal margin is essentially the perianal skin, and is defined as the area extending from the anal verge to 5 cm outward on the perineum. True skin histologically has epidermal appendages that are absent in the transitional epithelium. The anatomic distinction is clinically relevant, as it relates to lymphatic drainage. The portion of the anal canal proximal to the dentate line drains into the lymphatics of the internal iliac nodes, whereas the anal canal distal to the dentate line usually drains into the inguinal nodes.

Welton and colleagues[2] have proposed an alternative definition that divides the anal canal into intra-anal, perianal, skin, and transformation zones. Intra-anal lesions cannot be visualized in their entirety while gentle traction is applied to the buttocks. Perianal lesions can be visualized with gentle traction on the buttocks and lie within 5 cm of the anus, whereas skin lesions lie outside a 5-cm radius from the anus. Lesions that involve the transformation zone are situated in a region of variable height above the dentate line, where squamous metaplasia may be found overlying normal columnar mucosa.

[a] Department of Colorectal Surgery, Digestive Disease Institute, 9500 Euclid Avenue, A30 Cleveland Clinic, Cleveland, OH 44195, USA
[b] Department of Cancer Biology, 9500 Euclid Avenue, A30 Cleveland Clinic, Cleveland, OH 44195, USA
* Corresponding author. Department of Cancer Biology, 9500 Euclid Avenue, A30 Cleveland Clinic, Cleveland, OH 44195, USA.
E-mail address: kaladym@ccf.org (M.F. Kalady).

Surg Clin N Am 90 (2010) 147–161
doi:10.1016/j.suc.2009.09.008
0039-6109/09/$ – see front matter

A variety of lesions comprise tumors of the anal canal, with carcinoma in situ and epidermoid cancers being the most common. Less common anal neoplasms include adenocarcinoma, melanoma, gastrointestinal stromal cell tumors (GIST), neuroendocrine tumors, and Buschke-Lowenstein tumors. Treatment strategies are based on anatomic location and histopathology. In this article the different tumors and their management are discussed in turn.

## ANAL INTRAEPITHELIAL NEOPLASIA OR SQUAMOUS INTRAEPITHELIAL LESION

Many different terminologies have been used to describe anal intraepithelial neoplasia (AIN). AIN was initially adopted for nomenclature because of its similarity to cervical intraepithelial neoplasia (CIN). Like CIN, AIN is a precursor to squamous cell carcinoma (SCC), and is classified in 3 grades, AIN I, AIN II, and AIN III, which indicate low-, moderate-, and high-grade dysplasia.[3] Bowen disease is synonymous with carcinoma in situ (CIS). More recently, the term squamous intraepithelial lesion (SIL), which is subdivided into high grade (HSIL) and low grade (LSIL), has been more commonly adopted. It has been proposed that the term LSIL replace AIN I and that HSIL replace AIN II, AIN III, CIS, and Bowen disease.[4]

Infection with the human papilloma virus (HPV) is the most common risk factor for the development of AIN. HPV leads to cellular proliferation by interfering with cell cycle control mechanisms via viral genes E6 and E7. E7 binds to the retinoblastoma (Rb) tumor suppressor protein, allowing for immortalization of the cells, and E6 binds to p53, interfering with DNA repair and allowing accumulation of genetic errors.[5-7] HPV is a DNA papillomavirus with several genotypes. Types 6 and 11 have been shown to have low oncogenic potential whereas types 16, 18, 31, 33, and 35 have high oncogenic potential.

Other risk factors for developing SIL include human immunodeficiency virus (HIV) seropositivity, low CD4 counts, cigarette smoking, anal receptive intercourse, and immunosuppression. Unlike cervical neoplasia, multiple sexual partners is not an independent significant risk factor.[7-16]

AIN or SIL is often found incidentally during surgery for other unrelated problems such as hemorrhoids. However, screening programs for high-risk populations have been suggested. The specific populations that have been targeted for screening include men who have sex with men (MSM) and HIV-negative women with a history of anal intercourse or other HPV-related anogenital malignancies.[17] Screening procedures consist of anal cytology and high-resolution anoscopy (HRA), which is similar to colposcopy for CIN. Anal cytology is performed by inserting an unlubricated moistened Dacron swab in the anus to approximately 3 to 4 cm and then slowly removing it in a circular motion to sample the cells from all areas of the anal canal. Samples should be preserved quickly on slides or in a liquid medium to prevent drying. HRA uses the application of 3% acetic acid to the anal canal using a large cotton-tip applicator via an anoscope. Lugol's iodine solution can also be applied to identify normal mucosa. The anoscope should be slowly withdrawn so that all areas of the anal canal may be meticulously examined. Acetic acid is continually applied during the examination to manipulate folds, hemorrhoids, or prolapsing mucosa. Biopsies should be done on any areas that appear abnormal.[17,18]

Despite recommendations to screen for AIN in high-risk populations, the optimal screening methods have not been established. HRA is an excellent and easily performed means of detecting HSIL, but resources for HRA are limited. Anal cytology and HPV testing have been analyzed as ways to better identify those patients who might benefit from HRA.[19] Anal cytology followed by HRA for those with positive results seems to be a reasonable and feasible approach to screen large populations. Unfortunately, anal cytology has had variable reported sensitivities, with the probability of AIN in patients with negative cytology 23% for HIV-negative MSM and 45% for HIV-positive MSM.[20] In addition, the optimal use of HPV testing has yet to be defined secondarily to the different performance characteristics in HIV-positive and HIV-negative MSM.[19] The natural history of untreated SIL is not well known for the HIV-negative population. For HIV-positive patients, the disease appears to be more aggressive, with approximately 50% of LSIL lesions progressing to HSIL within 2 years for HIV-positive homosexual males.[21] Risk of progression to invasive cancer may be as high as 50% for lesions in HIV-positive patients.[22–24]

Treatment of intraepithelial lesions still remains somewhat debated. LSIL is believed to have a low malignant potential and may be followed by surveillance examination at 6-month intervals. If desired, internal lesions may be treated with a variety of chemical applications such as bichloroacetic acid or trichloroacetic acid (TCA). External lesions can be treated with imiquimod, podophyllotoxin, or cryotherapy. Cryotherapy and TCA often require more than one application.[17]

HSIL carries a more significant risk of malignant transformation and treatment is often pursued, although observation with close surveillance is an acceptable strategy. In the HIV population, dysplasia returns at high rates despite even the most thorough attempts at eradication.[18] Because there is no satisfactory treatment with low morbidity that eradicates these premalignant lesions with low recurrence, it has been suggested that patients can be followed expectantly. In a study of 40 HIV-positive men who were followed expectantly, only 3 patients developed invasive carcinoma and these were completely excised or cured with chemoradiation. Therefore, physical examination and surveillance alone may be acceptable for following patients with HIV and squamous dysplasia.[22]

Topical therapy may be effective for HSIL. 5-Fluorouracil (5-FU) cream has been used for periods of 9 to 12 weeks, with good response. However, recurrence may occur with poorly defined areas of involvement, follicular involvement, poor immune response, dense scar tissue, and recurrent or persistent HPV infection.[25] Topical 5% imiquimod cream has also demonstrated good response rates. In a study of 49 patients, an 86% complete clinical response rate was demonstrated at a mean follow-up of 19 months.[26] In 1988, the use of cryotherapy for skin cancer was suggested by Holt,[27] with 0.8% recurrence rate for Bowen disease; however, this study did not include any patients with perianal disease. Photodynamic therapy has also been suggested; however, studies are limited.[28,29]

Targeted destruction and follow-up is a more aggressive approach to identifiable lesions. Wide local excision (WLE) has been employed for discrete lesions, with the extent of resection based on preoperative mapping as first described by Strauss and Fazio[30] in 1979, although this in not routinely necessary. Mapping is done by biopsy of the anal canal at the dentate line, anal verge, and perianal skin at the 4 major points of the compass. Definitive surgical excision can be performed based on preoperative mapping or by WLE based on microscopic clearance by frozen section. Closure can be done by secondary intention, split-thickness skin graft, or advancement rotation flaps, depending on the size of the remaining defect.[30,31] HRA-directed cautery ablation has been shown to be safe and well tolerated by patients without the morbidity of a WLE. However, recurrence rates are nearly 80%, with a mean recurrence time of 12 months in HIV-positive patients.[18] The Infrared Coagulator (IRC 2100; Redfield Corporation, Rochelle Park, NJ) is an alternative surgical modality that can be used in the outpatient clinical setting with local anesthesia. This method was described by Goldstone and colleagues[32] in a 2005 study examining 68

HIV-positive MSM. Following initial treatment, 65% of patients had persistent HSIL or developed metachronous HSIL within a median of 203 days, requiring return for multiple follow-up treatments. However, in looking at individual lesions, the probability of destroying an individual HSIL lesion with its first IRC treatment was 72%.

Surveillance for patients with a history of AIN or SIL is recommended at 6-month intervals while dysplasia is still present. Follow-up examinations should include anoscopy with or without acetic acid application. The importance of close follow-up should be particularly emphasized in HIV-positive patients.[33]

## EPIDERMOID CANCERS

Epidermoid cancers are divided into 2 categories: SCC and basal cell carcinoma (BCC). Treatment of these types of cancer differs based on anatomic location. Risk factors for SCC are similar to those for AIN, which is a precursor lesion.[33]

### Squamous Cell Carcinoma of Anal Margin

SCC of the anal margin is essentially skin cancer arising from the perianal skin, and is defined as located between the distal end of the anal canal to within a 5-cm margin surrounding the anal verge. Presenting symptoms commonly are complaints of a painful lump, bleeding, pruritus, tenesmus, discharge, or fecal incontinence. Patients are often misdiagnosed, leading to a delay in treatment.[34,35] Lesions generally resemble those occurring in skin elsewhere in the body. The lesions typically have rolled, everted edges with central ulcerations, and they can vary in size from 1 cm to near obstructing lesions at the anal orifice (**Fig. 1**).[36] Staging of anal margin SCC is based on the size of the tumor and lymph node involvement. Therefore, evaluation should consist of complete digital and perianal examination as well as palpation of the femoral and inguinal lymph node basins.[3] The incidence of lymph node metastasis is directly related to tumor size, with the incidence being 0% in tumors less than 2 cm, 23% for tumors between 2 and 5 cm, and 67% in tumors larger than 5 cm.[37] Although these are slow-growing tumors, chest radiograph and computed tomography (CT) of the abdomen and pelvis should be done to assess for distant metastasis.[3]

Treatment of anal margin SCC varies depending on size and depth of invasion. In addition, the optimal treatment is difficult to discern from the literature, as anal canal and anal margin lesions have often been grouped together. In general, small,

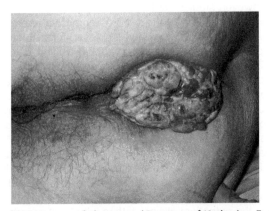

**Fig. 1.** Squamous cell carcinoma of the anus. (*Courtesy of* Katharine E. Markell, MD, San Antonio, TX.)

superficial, well-differentiated lesions are adequately treated with WLE with a 1-cm margin. However, this may be difficult to accomplish in cancers close to the anal canal.[36,38] In a study of 42 patients with epidermoid cancer of the anal margin, 74% had definitive treatment by local excision, with an 88% 5-year survival rate.[39] Salvage therapy for treatment failure after local excision can include repeat local excision, abdominoperineal resection (APR), or radiation therapy with or without chemotherapy. APR may be required for larger and deeper, less favorable lesions (T2–4 or N1), those involving the sphincter muscles, or for patients with multiple recurrences after local excision.[38,39] Primary radiation is also an option, albeit less effective than appropriate excision. Papillon and Chassard[37] describe 8 patients treated with interstitial brachytherapy and 36 patients treated with external beam irradiation (40 Gy in 10 fractions) combined with concomitant chemotherapy according to the Nigro protocol in 11 cases. Isolated local failures occurred in 7 cases and inguinal node recurrence occurred in 9 patients. Eight of the 36 patients (22%) treated with external beam radiation died of their primary disease.

### Squamous Cell Carcinoma of Anal Canal

SCC of the anal canal has several histologic variants, including squamous cell, cloacogenic or basaloid, epidermoid, or mucoepidermoid carcinomas. All lesions arise from the transitional zone of the anal canal and are nonkeratinizing. Because of their similar response to treatment and outcome, they are grouped together in terms of treatment algorithms.[36] The most common presenting symptoms include anal bleeding, pain, or the sensation of a mass. The presentation of anal canal tumors is often nonspecific and 70% to 80% are initially diagnosed as a benign anorectal condition.[40] However, up to 20% of patients may be asymptomatic.[41] Similar to that for anal margin SCC, physical examination should focus on digital examination and evaluation of the inguinal and femoral nodes. Anoscopy or proctoscopy is essential to define the location within the anal canal and to perform biopsy to confirm diagnosis. Appreciation of inguinal lymphadenopathy guides fine-needle aspiration (FNA) or core biopsy of suspicious lymph nodes to confirm malignant involvement and to guide radiation fields. Colonoscopy is required to rule out synchronous colorectal neoplasms.[33] Chest radiograph, and abdominal and pelvic CT should be done to evaluate lymphadenopathy and to exclude lung and liver metastases.[36] Endorectal ultrasound (ERUS) is useful in determining T stage and evaluating perirectal lymph node involvement, with some advantage over physical examination alone.[42] Positron emission tomography (PET) scanning may identify distant metastases that are not detected by other imaging modalities in as many as 25% of cases.[43]

Staging for SCC of the anal canal is as follows. Stage 1 is tumor less than 2 cm in greatest dimension (T1) with no regional lymph node or distant metastasis. Stage 2 is T2 (tumor >2 cm but <5 cm) or T3 (tumor >5 cm), with no regional lymph node or distant metastasis. Stage 3 is subdivided into 3A and 3B. Stage 3A is T1 to T3 with metastasis to perirectal lymph nodes (N1), or T4 tumor (tumor of any size that invades adjacent organ(s), eg, vagina, urethra, or bladder). Stage 3B is T4, N1, or any T stage with metastasis in unilateral internal iliac and/or inguinal lymph nodes (N2), or metastasis in perirectal and inguinal lymph nodes and/or bilateral internal iliac and/or inguinal lymph nodes (N3). Stage 4 is any T and any N combined with distant metastasis.[3]

Anal canal cancer historically was treated by APR. However, treatment was revolutionized in the 1970s by Nigro and colleagues,[44] who demonstrated that chemoradiation therapy not only achieved survival and recurrence rates equivalent to those achieved with surgery, but also preserved sphincter function. The Nigro protocol traditionally consisted of 5-FU (1000 mg/m$^2$/d) given as a continuous infusion for 4 days, mitomycin C (15 mg/m$^2$) as a single intravenous bolus injection, and 3000 cGy (200 cGy/d) of external beam radiation to the pelvis. 5-FU was repeated on days 20 to 31 and mitomycin C on day 29. This dosage was originally intended as neo-adjuvant therapy before APR; however, a significant number of patients were noted to have a complete pathologic response at the completion of therapy.[45] Following the introduction of this novel treatment, the Nigro protocol has become the treatment of choice for SCC of the anal canal.[38] Since then, modifications have been made to determine the optimal combined-modality treatment regimen. A phase 3, multicenter, randomized controlled trial (RTOG 98-11) was completed comparing treatment with 5-FU, mitomycin, and radiation versus 5-FU, cisplatin, and radiation. Six hundred and eighty-two patients were randomly assigned to 1 of 2 treatment groups. The 5-year disease-free survival and 5-year overall survival was 60% and 75%, respectively, for the mitomycin group compared with 70% and 70%, respectively, for the cisplatin group. The 5-year local-regional recurrence and distant metastasis rates were 25% and 15%, respectively, for mitomycin-based treatment and 33% and 19%, respectively, for cisplatin-based treatment. These findings did not support the use of cisplatin in place of mitomycin in the treatment of anal canal cancer.[46] At present, radiation combined with 5-FU and mitomycin is still considered the standard of care. European trials are further evaluating the role of cisplatin as well as radiation dose escalation. Other studies are evaluating the use of capecitabine, oxaliplatin, and cetuximab with radiation.[47]

Unfortunately, approximately 30% of patients have persistent or recurrent disease after chemoradiation for anal SCC. APR is recommended for persistent or recurrent disease, with achievable 5-year survival rates between 24% and 58%.[48]

### Basal Cell Carcinoma

BCCs of the anal margin are extremely rare and comprise 0.2% of all anorectal neoplasms.[49] Lesions are usually 1 to 2 cm in diameter, and have central ulceration with a raised pearly border. Similar to other lesions, they are often misdiagnosed as hemorrhoids or anal fissures. BCCs rarely invade or metastasize.[35,36] Histologic confirmation is important in distinguishing true BCC from the basaloid variant of SCC, which requires a more aggressive treatment.[38]

The treatment of choice is WLE, which can also be performed in patients with local recurrence. APR is reserved for advanced cases where the lesion extends into the anal canal and deep into the surrounding tissues.[36] In a 20-year review of BCC from the Mayo Clinic, 19 patients who were treated and had adequate follow-up data were identified. All patients were treated with local excision and no patients had a documented recurrence, with mean follow-up time of 72 months.[50] Another group reported recurrence rates of 24%. These patients were treated by repeat local excision, APR, or radiation, with a 5-year survival of 73%.[49]

### ANAL MELANOMA

Malignant melanoma of the anorectum was first reported by Moore in 1857.[51] Anal melanoma accounts for 0.3% to 1.6% of all melanomas and 2% to 4% of all malignant neoplasms of the anorectum.[52–54] Symptoms are generally indistinguishable from other conditions in this region.[36] The correct diagnosis is usually established at a late stage, and the symptoms have often been present for several months before diagnosis. Melanoma may be suspected when a pigmented lesion is seen in the anal canal; however; 10% to 29% may be amelanotic. Anorectal melanoma is diagnosed histologically by melanin pigment; however, immunohistochemical staining of melanoma antigen HMB-45 and S-100 protein are adjunctive for final diagnosis.[55] In poorly differentiated lesions a definitive diagnosis can be made using a Fontana stain, which stains melanin granules black.[36]

Optimal surgical management for localized anorectal melanoma remains debated. Local excision with sphincter preservation and decreased morbidity is advocated over APR because survival rates are similar with either approach. In a study from Memorial Sloan-Kettering, 46 patients treated for anorectal melanoma over a 19-year period were studied. It was noted that those undergoing local excision had similar local recurrence (26%) and 5-year disease-free survival (35%) to those patients undergoing APR (21% and 34%, respectively).[56] However, in a more recent study of 79 patients in Japan, 44% with submucosal invasion were noted to have regional lymph node metastasis. The investigators recommended local excision for patients with Stage 0 melanoma, and APR with lymph node dissection for those with Stage 1 cancers or T1 tumors.[55] In the same study, the 3- and 5-year survival rates were shown to be 34.8% and 28.8%, respectively, and the median survival time was 22 months. The authors of this article recommend WLE for localized anorectal melanoma, realizing that APR may be necessary to treat bulky tumors invading the sphincter mechanism.

## RARE ANAL NEOPLASMS
### Adenocarcinoma

Paget disease represents intraepithelial adenocarcinoma. Paget disease is extremely rare, with few cases reported in the literature. Perianal Paget disease may be in situ or with an invasive component with no separate underlying malignancy, or it may present as a downward pagetoid extension from an established adenocarcinoma. Perianal Paget disease is associated with synchronous visceral carcinomas in approximately 50% of cases, so full colonoscopic investigation for other cancers is necessary.[57–59] Typical presenting symptoms are nonspecific and comprise pruritus, irritation, and rash. Examination usually reveals red or whitish gray, elevated, crusty, scaly lesions that resemble eczema.[60] The condition resembles other benign and malignant lesions in the perianal area and therefore biopsy is diagnostic. On histological analysis distinctive Paget cells are observed, which are large, round cells with pale, vacuolated cytoplasm and reticular nucleus. These cells stain positive for periodic acid Schiff and mucicarmine.[58]

The treatment of Paget disease in the absence of invasive cancer is WLE. Adequate clear margins are important to avoid recurrence. For this reason, 4-quadrant mapping with frozen section encompassing the lesion and including the dentate line, anal verge, and perineum is recommended, similar to techniques used with Bowen disease.[57] This technique may involve circumferential excision of the perianal skin, which is not only associated with significant morbidity but also a high recurrence rate, estimated between 31% and 61%.[60] Therefore, other treatments have been suggested including radiotherapy with or without chemotherapy, photodynamic therapy, intralesional interferon-α, and topical imiquimod.[61–66] APR is recommended for localized disease that is associated with underlying carcinoma. If regional nodes are involved, then APR along with inguinal node dissection is warranted.[67] Long-term follow-up for these patients is important because recurrence of disease is common, with the overall disease-free survival rate 64% at 5 years.[68]

Adenocarcinoma can also arise in the anal canal. According to the World Health Organization, there are 3 types of anal adenocarcinoma based on presumed origin—rectal, anal gland, and duct—and those arising in chronic anal fissures.[69]

Tumors arising in the distal colorectal mucosa behave as rectal cancers and should be treated as such. Tumors arising from the anal gland or ducts and those arising in the background of a chronic fissure can mimic benign conditions of the anus, with presenting symptoms such as a lump, pruritus, or bleeding. Therefore, similar to other tumors in this location, there is often a delay in diagnosis. In a report of 21 patients with anal adenocarcinoma, 62% presented with metastatic disease and underwent palliative procedures such as diversion or radiation. The only long-term survivor had an early-stage tumor diagnosed after excision of a hemorrhoid, and was treated with WLE only. On account of poor long-term outlook with 5-year survival of 4.8%, the investigators suggest prolonged and close follow-up of patients.[70] Based on a survey of members of the American Society of Colon and Rectal Surgeons, 77% of patients analyzed had undergone APR, which at that time seemed to be the procedure of choice for locally advanced disease.[38,71] However, more recent studies have examined the addition of combined-modality therapy and have considered this a more effective approach, with better overall and disease-free survival rates.[72–75]

### Buschke-lowenstein or Verrucous Carcinoma

Verrucous carcinoma of the anus is also commonly referred to as "giant condyloma acuminatum" or "Buschke-Lowenstein tumor." This lesion usually presents as a large, exophytic, cauliflower-like mass. The size of the lesion may vary from 1 to 30 cm and may arise in the perianal skin, anal canal, or distal rectum; it was historically thought to represent a benign lesion histologically, but was considered invasive in terms of local progression and invasion into surrounding tissues and even the pelvic cavity.[36] However, large tumors may harbor an invasive component of SCC, and for this reason verrucous carcinoma is currently thought to represent the midpoint of a spectrum of disease leading from condyloma acuminate to invasive SCC.[38]

Presenting symptoms most commonly consist of a perianal mass, pain, fistula, abscess, or persistent drainage. Physical examination is diagnostic, but pelvic CT helps determine the extent of involvement.[36,76] The scope of surgical resection depends on the depth of histologic invasion. WLE is recommended for superficially invasive lesions, whereas invasion of the sphincter muscles may necessitate an APR.[77] Other treatments that have been suggested include topical podophyllin, immunotherapy with autologous vaccine preparation, intralesional, systemic, or topical interferon, and radiotherapy. However, due to the lack of adequate series of patients, optimal treatment remains controversial.[76,78]

### Gastrointestinal Stromal Tumor

Although GISTs are the most common mesenchymal neoplasms of the digestive tract, they are rarely found in the rectum and anus, with approximately 10 cases being described in the literature. With limited data available, there is no established approach to treatment. Initial local excision to define aggressiveness of the tumor as well as involvement of resection margins has been suggested. Margin positivity or high-risk tumors may further be considered for APR. The role of adjuvant therapy such as Gleevec (imatinib mesylate) is still uncertain.[79]

### Kaposi Sarcoma

Kaposi sarcoma is an uncommon malignancy, and is most often seen in patients with AIDS. Kaposi sarcoma generally presents as small brown-red to blue-red smooth nodules that may enlarge. The neoplasm is radioresponsive, and chemotherapy is generally reserved for the treatment of systemic disease.[36]

### Neuroendocrine Tumor

Colorectal neuroendocrine tumors are classified as low-grade carcinoid tumors or high-grade neuroendocrine tumors. Carcinoid tumors tend to be indolent and slow-growing, whereas high-grade neuroendocrine tumors are aggressive with poor differentiation and high mitotic rates. Pathologic recognition is important because patients may benefit from treatment with alternative chemotherapeutic agents. It is estimated that 65% to 80% of patients have distant metastases at the time of diagnosis, and prognosis is poor.[80,81] Surgical treatment consists of excision with or without chemotherapy and radiation. For Stage III and IV tumors, treatment with cisplatin and etoposide is recommended.[81]

### Sarcomas

Sarcomas represent less than 1% of malignancies in the anorectal region. Histologic diagnoses include leiomyosarcoma, fibrosarcoma, and anaplastic sarcoma. Because these tumors are resistant to radiation, the treatment of choice is APR. In a review of 9 patients undergoing radical resection for this diagnosis, there were no survivors beyond 10 years.[36,82]

## LOCAL EXCISION OF RECTAL CANCER

At the editor's request, the authors include here a section on local excision. The utility and effectiveness of local excision of rectal cancer has been debated for years, and trends in its use have waxed and waned. The goals of any rectal cancer resection are complete removal of malignancy while minimizing morbidity and preserving function. Local excision may achieve these goals in the appropriate clinical setting, but suffers from the risk of increased local recurrence. This section addresses the oncologic outcomes of local excision of rectal cancer.

### Indications for Local Excision

Many factors contribute to the decision-making process for treatment of rectal cancer including the location and stage of the tumor, patient comorbidities, availability of specialized equipment, and familiarity with surgical techniques. In general, the ideal tumor characteristics for local excision include a freely mobile T1 tumor less than 4 cm in greatest diameter, less than 40% of the bowel circumference of the bowel, and within 8 to 10 cm of the anal verge.[3] These factors favor the technical ability to achieve an adequate local excision. However, even in the best circumstances, local excision is associated with a higher rate of local recurrence, and selection of technique is based on a risk-benefit balance for each individual case.

### Techniques

Local excision may be performed using transanal excision (TAE) or transanal endoscopic microsurgery (TEM). Regardless of technique, local excision obtains a full-thickness rectal wall resection of the tumor with at least 1 cm circumferential margins. TAE is limited by the distance of the lesion from the anal verge, and is usually not recommended for tumors located more than 10 cm from the anal verge. Tumor size also influences technical ability and greater-sized lesions tend to have to higher failure rates.[83–86] In contrast, TEM is purported to allow better visualization of the tumor and is not restricted by distance from the anal verge, accessing lesions that are up to 18 cm from the anal verge.[87–89]

### Lymph Node Positivity and Local Recurrence

Local excision fails by the inability to perform an adequate lymph node harvest. Because the risk of lymph node positivity is directly related to T stage, both surgeon and patient must make an informed decision when using local excision. The risk for lymph node metastases in T1 and T2 cancers is approximately 10% and 20%, respectively.[90–93]

The local recurrence rates after local excision accordingly are reported at about 10% for T1 tumors and 25% for T2 tumors.[90,94–97] Significant predictors of lymph node metastasis are lymphovascular invasion and extension into the lower third of the submucosa, and lesions with these features should undergo radical resection.[98,99] A recent study of 35,179 patients with stage I rectal cancer demonstrated that the use of local excision had increased significantly between 1989 and 2003. However, 5-year local recurrence for local excision and radical resection was 12.5% versus 6.9% for T1 tumors and 22.1% versus 15.1% for T2 tumors.[100] Of note, clinical results from high-volume colorectal surgery units report local recurrence rates as high as 30% for T1 tumors and 47% for T2 tumors, which raises caution regarding this approach.[92,101]

Studies evaluating local recurrence after TEM have been limited by small sample size, with the larger series reporting rates of 3% to 20%, leading to the recommendation of limiting TEM use to in situ tumors and T1 lesions in healthy patients.[102–104]

### Salvage Surgery for Recurrence After Local Excision

Recurrence after initial local excision has a worse prognosis than the prognosis of the initial lesion. In a study of 52 patients with T1 low rectal cancers undergoing local excision, the 5-year recurrence rate was 29% and cancer-specific survival rate was 89%.[101] Furthermore, a study from the Memorial Sloan-Kettering Cancer Center observed that pelvic recurrences after initial local excision are often locally advanced and require extended resections, resulting in decreased survival compared with stage-matched patients.[105]

### SUMMARY ON USE OF LOCAL EXCISION OF RECTAL TUMORS

Local excision is an option for select early-stage patients with favorable tumor characteristics, but is associated with a higher rate of local recurrence. This option may be the only one open for medically compromised patients who cannot tolerate radical resection. In either case, surgeons and patients should be informed of the various limitations, benefits, and risks associated with this technique.

### REFERENCES

1. U.S. National Institutes of Health. Available at: http://www.cancer.gov/cancer topics/types/anal. Accessed July 13, 2009.
2. Welton ML, Sharkey FE, Kahlenberg MS. The etiology and epidemiology of anal cancer. Surg Oncol Clin N Am 2004;13:263–75.
3. Welton ML, Varma MG. Anal cancer. In: Wolff BG, Fleshman JW, Beck DE, et al, editors. The ASCRS textbook of colon and rectal surgery. New York: Springer Science+Business Media, LLC; 2007. p. 482–500.
4. Bullard Dunn K, Rothenberger D. Colon, rectum and anus. In: Brunicardi C, editor. Schwartz's principles of surgery. New York: McGraw Hill; 2008.
5. Werness BA, Levine AJ, Howley PM. Association of human papillomavirus types 16 and 18 E6 proteins with p53. Science 1990;248:76–9.

6. zur Hausen H. Immortalization of human cells and their malignant conversion by high risk human papillomavirus genotypes. Semin Cancer Biol 1999;9:405–11.

7. Martin F, Bower M. Anal intraepithelial neoplasia in HIV positive people. Sex Transm Infect 2001;77:327–31.

8. Critchlow CW, Surawicz CM, Holmes KK, et al. Prospective study of high grade anal squamous intraepithelial neoplasia in a cohort of homosexual men: influence of HIV infection, immunosuppression and human papillomavirus infection. AIDS 1995;9:1255–62.

9. Palefsky JM, Holly EA, Ralston ML, et al. Anal squamous intraepithelial lesions in HIV-positive and HIV-negative homosexual and bisexual men: prevalence and risk factors. J Acquir Immune Defic Syndr Hum Retrovirol 1998;17:320–6.

10. Palefsky JM, Holly EA, Ralston ML, et al. High incidence of anal high-grade squamous intra-epithelial lesions among HIV-positive and HIV-negative homosexual and bisexual men. AIDS 1998;12:495–503.

11. Palefsky JM, Shiboski S, Moss A. Risk factors for anal human papillomavirus infection and anal cytologic abnormalities in HIV-positive and HIV-negative homosexual men. J Acquir Immune Defic Syndr 1994;7:599–606.

12. Holmes F, Borek D, Owen-Kummer M, et al. Anal cancer in women. Gastroenterology 1988;95:107–11.

13. Caussy D, Goedert JJ, Palefsky J, et al. Interaction of human immunodeficiency and papilloma viruses: association with anal epithelial abnormality in homosexual men. Int J Cancer 1990;46:214–9.

14. Friedman HB, Saah AJ, Sherman ME, et al. Human papillomavirus, anal squamous intraepithelial lesions, and human immunodeficiency virus in a cohort of gay men. J Infect Dis 1998;178:45–52.

15. Ogunbiyi OA, Scholefield JH, Raftery AT, et al. Prevalence of anal human papillomavirus infection and intraepithelial neoplasia in renal allograft recipients. Br J Surg 1994;81:365–7.

16. Daling JR, Sherman KJ, Hislop TG, et al. Cigarette smoking and the risk of anogenital cancer. Am J Epidemiol 1992;135:180–9.

17. Palefsky JM, Rubin M. The epidemiology of anal human papillomavirus and related neoplasia. Obstet Gynecol Clin North Am 2009;36:187–200.

18. Chang GJ, Berry JM, Jay N, et al. Surgical treatment of high-grade anal squamous intraepithelial lesions: a prospective study. Dis Colon Rectum 2002;45:453–8.

19. Berry JM, Palefsky JM, Jay N, et al. Performance characteristics of anal cytology and human papillomavirus testing in patients with high-resolution anoscopy-guided biopsy of high-grade anal intraepithelial neoplasia. Dis Colon Rectum 2009;52:239–47.

20. Chin-Hong PV, Berry JM, Cheng SC, et al. Comparison of patient- and clinician-collected anal cytology samples to screen for human papillomavirus-associated anal intraepithelial neoplasia in men who have sex with men. Ann Intern Med 2008;149:300–6.

21. Palefsky JM, Holly EA, Hogeboom CJ, et al. Virologic, immunologic, and clinical parameters in the incidence and progression of anal squamous intraepithelial lesions in HIV-positive and HIV-negative homosexual men. J Acquir Immune Defic Syndr Hum Retrovirol 1998;17:314–9.

22. Devaraj B, Cosman BC. Expectant management of anal squamous dysplasia in patients with HIV. Dis Colon Rectum 2006;49:36–40.

23. Watson AJ, Smith BB, Whitehead MR, et al. Malignant progression of anal intra-epithelial neoplasia. ANZ J Surg 2006;76:715–7.

24. Scholefield JH, Castle MT, Watson NF. Malignant transformation of high-grade anal intraepithelial neoplasia. Br J Surg 2005;92:1133–6.

25. Graham BD, Jetmore AB, Foote JE, et al. Topical 5-fluorouracil in the management of extensive anal Bowen's disease: a preferred approach. Dis Colon Rectum 2005;48:444–50.

26. Rosen T, Harting M, Gibson M. Treatment of Bowen's disease with topical 5% imiquimod cream: retrospective study. Dermatol Surg 2007;33:427–31 [discussion: 431–2].

27. Holt PJ. Cryotherapy for skin cancer: results over a 5-year period using liquid nitrogen spray cryosurgery. Br J Dermatol 1988;119:231–40.

28. Runfola MA, Weber TK, Rodriguez-Bigas MA, et al. Photodynamic therapy for residual neoplasms of the perianal skin. Dis Colon Rectum 2000;43:499–502.

29. Petrelli NJ, Cebollero JA, Rodriguez-Bigas M, et al. Photodynamic therapy in the management of neoplasms of the perianal skin. Arch Surg 1992;127:1436–8.

30. Strauss RJ, Fazio VW. Bowen's disease of the anal and perianal area. A report and analysis of twelve cases. Am J Surg 1979;137:231–4.

31. Margenthaler JA, Dietz DW, Mutch MG, et al. Outcomes, risk of other malignancies, and need for formal mapping procedures in patients with perianal Bowen's disease. Dis Colon Rectum 2004;47:1655–60 [discussion: 1660–1].

32. Goldstone SE, Kawalek AZ, Huyett JW. Infrared coagulator: a useful tool for treating anal squamous intraepithelial lesions. Dis Colon Rectum 2005;48:1042–54.

33. Fleshner PR, Chalasani S, Chang GJ, et al. Practice parameters for anal squamous neoplasms. Dis Colon Rectum 2008;51:2–9.

34. Jensen SL, Hagen K, Harling H, et al. Long-term prognosis after radical treatment for squamous-cell carcinoma of the anal canal and anal margin. Dis Colon Rectum 1988;31:273–8.

35. Skibber J, Rodriguez-Bigas MA, Gordon PH. Surgical considerations in anal cancer. Surg Oncol Clin N Am 2004;13:321–38.

36. Gordon PH. Current status—perianal and anal canal neoplasms. Dis Colon Rectum 1990;33:799–808.

37. Papillon J, Chassard JL. Respective roles of radiotherapy and surgery in the management of epidermoid carcinoma of the anal margin. Series of 57 patients. Dis Colon Rectum 1992;35:422–9.

38. Moore HG, Guillem JG. Anal neoplasms. Surg Clin North Am 2002;82:1233–51.

39. Greenall MJ, Quan SH, Stearns MW, et al. Epidermoid cancer of the anal margin. Pathologic features, treatment, and clinical results. Am J Surg 1985;149:95–101.

40. Klas JV, Rothenberger DA, Wong WD, et al. Malignant tumors of the anal canal: the spectrum of disease, treatment, and outcomes. Cancer 1999;85:1686–93.

41. Ryan DP, Compton CC, Mayer RJ. Carcinoma of the anal canal. N Engl J Med 2000;342:792–800.

42. Giovannini M, Bardou VJ, Barclay R, et al. Anal carcinoma: prognostic value of endorectal ultrasound (ERUS). Results of a prospective multicenter study. Endoscopy 2001;33:231–6.

43. Trautmann TG, Zuger JH. Positron emission tomography for pretreatment staging and posttreatment evaluation in cancer of the anal canal. Mol Imaging Biol 2005;7:309–13.

44. Buroker TR, Nigro N, Bradley G, et al. Combined therapy for cancer of the anal canal: a follow-up report. Dis Colon Rectum 1977;20:677–8.

45. Nigro ND, Vaitkevicius VK, Buroker T, et al. Combined therapy for cancer of the anal canal. Dis Colon Rectum 1981;24:73–5.

46. Ajani JA, Winter KA, Gunderson LL, et al. Fluorouracil, mitomycin, and radiotherapy vs fluorouracil, cisplatin, and radiotherapy for carcinoma of the anal canal: a randomized controlled trial. JAMA 2008;299:1914–21.
47. Czito BG, Willett CG. Current management of anal canal cancer. Curr Oncol Rep 2009;11:186–92.
48. Papaconstantinou HT, Bullard KM, Rothenberger DA, et al. Salvage abdominoperineal resection after failed Nigro protocol: modest success, major morbidity. Colorectal Dis 2006;8:124–9.
49. Nielsen OV, Jensen SL. Basal cell carcinoma of the anus-a clinical study of 34 cases. Br J Surg 1981;68:856–7.
50. Paterson CA, Young-Fadok TM, Dozois RR. Basal cell carcinoma of the perianal region: 20-year experience. Dis Colon Rectum 1999;42:1200–2.
51. Moore WD. Recurrent melanosis of the rectum after previous removal from the verge of the anus in a man aged 65. Lancet 1857;1:290–4.
52. Longo WE, Vernava AM 3rd, Wade TP, et al. Rare anal canal cancers in the U.S. veteran: patterns of disease and results of treatment. Am Surg 1995;61: 495–500.
53. Iversen K, Robins RE. Mucosal malignant melanomas. Am J Surg 1980;139: 660–4.
54. Wanebo HJ, Woodruff JM, Farr GH, et al. Anorectal melanoma. Cancer 1981;47: 1891–900.
55. Ishizone S, Koide N, Karasawa F, et al. Surgical treatment for anorectal malignant melanoma: report of five cases and review of 79 Japanese cases. Int J Colorectal Dis 2008;23:1257–62.
56. Yeh JJ, Shia J, Hwu WJ, et al. The role of abdominoperineal resection as surgical therapy for anorectal melanoma. Ann Surg 2006;244:1012–7.
57. Beck DE, Fazio VW. Perianal Paget's disease. Dis Colon Rectum 1987;30:263–6.
58. Armitage NC, Jass JR, Richman PI, et al. Paget's disease of the anus: a clinicopathological study. Br J Surg 1989;76:60–3.
59. Sarmiento JM, Wolff BG, Burgart LJ, et al. Paget's disease of the perianal region—an aggressive disease? Dis Colon Rectum 1997;40:1187–94.
60. Tulchinsky H, Zmora O, Brazowski E, et al. Extramammary Paget's disease of the perianal region. Colorectal Dis 2004;6:206–9.
61. Burrows NP, Jones DH, Hudson PM, et al. Treatment of extramammary Paget's disease by radiotherapy. Br J Dermatol 1995;132:970–2.
62. Shieh S, Dee AS, Cheney RT, et al. Photodynamic therapy for the treatment of extramammary Paget's disease. Br J Dermatol 2002;146:1000–5.
63. Moreno-Arias GA, Conill C, Castells-Mas A, et al. Radiotherapy for genital extramammary Paget's disease in situ. Dermatol Surg 2001;27:587–90.
64. Brierley JD, Stockdale AD. Radiotherapy: an effective treatment for extramammary Paget's disease. Clin Oncol (R Coll Radiol) 1991;3:3–5.
65. Zampogna JC, Flowers FP, Roth WI, et al. Treatment of primary limited cutaneous extramammary Paget's disease with topical imiquimod monotherapy: two case reports. J Am Acad Dermatol 2002;47:S229–35.
66. Panasiti V, Bottoni U, Devirgiliis V, et al. Intralesional interferon alfa-2b as neoadjuvant treatment for perianal extramammary Paget's disease. J Eur Acad Dermatol Venereol 2008;22:522–3.
67. Shutze WP, Gleysteen JJ. Perianal Paget's disease. Classification and review of management: report of two cases. Dis Colon Rectum 1990;33:502–7.
68. McCarter MD, Quan SH, Busam K, et al. Long-term outcome of perianal Paget's disease. Dis Colon Rectum 2003;46:612–6.

69. Collaboration. Histologic typing of intestinal tumors. In: Jass JR, Sobin LH, editors. World Health Organization international histological classification of tumors. New York: Springer-Verlag; 1989. p. 42.

70. Jensen SL, Shokouh-Amiri MH, Hagen K, et al. Adenocarcinoma of the anal ducts. A series of 21 cases. Dis Colon Rectum 1988;31:268–72.

71. Abel ME, Chiu YS, Russell TR, et al. Adenocarcinoma of the anal glands. Results of a survey. Dis Colon Rectum 1993;36:383–7.

72. Lee J, Corman M. Recurrence of anal adenocarcinoma after local excision and adjuvant chemoradiation therapy: report of a case and review of the literature. J Gastrointest Surg 2009;13:150–4.

73. Li LR, Wan DS, Pan ZZ, et al. Clinical features and treatment of 49 patients with anal canal adenocarcinoma. Zhonghua Wei Chang Wai Ke Za Zhi 2006;9: 402–4.

74. Papagikos M, Crane CH, Skibber J, et al. Chemoradiation for adenocarcinoma of the anus. Int J Radiat Oncol Biol Phys 2003;55:669–78.

75. Beal KP, Wong D, Guillem JG, et al. Primary adenocarcinoma of the anus treated with combined modality therapy. Dis Colon Rectum 2003;46:1320–4.

76. Trombetta LJ, Place RJ. Giant condyloma acuminatum of the anorectum: trends in epidemiology and management: report of a case and review of the literature. Dis Colon Rectum 2001;44:1878–86.

77. Gingrass PJ, Bubrick MP, Hitchcock CR, et al. Anorectal verrucose squamous carcinoma: report of two cases. Dis Colon Rectum 1978;21:120–2.

78. De Toma G, Cavallaro G, Bitonti A, et al. Surgical management of perianal giant condyloma acuminatum (Buschke-Lowenstein tumor). Report of three cases. Eur Surg Res 2006;38:418–22.

79. Nigri GR, Dente M, Valabrega S, et al. Gastrointestinal stromal tumor of the anal canal: an unusual presentation. World J Surg Oncol 2007;5:20.

80. Khansur TK, Routh A, Mihas TA, et al. Syndrome of inappropriate ADH secretion and diplopia: oat cell (small cell) rectal carcinoma metastatic to the central nervous system. Am J Gastroenterol 1995;90:1173–4.

81. Bernick PE, Klimstra DS, Shia J, et al. Neuroendocrine carcinomas of the colon and rectum. Dis Colon Rectum 2004;47:163–9.

82. Molnar L, Bezsnyak I, Daubner K, et al. Anorectal sarcomas. Acta Chir Hung 1985;26:85–91.

83. Bailey HR, Huval WV, Max E, et al. Local excision of carcinoma of the rectum for cure. Surgery 1992;111:555–61.

84. Frost DB, Wong R, Rao A. A retrospective comparison of transanal surgery and endocavitary radiation for the treatment of 'early' rectal adenocarcinoma. Arch Surg 1993;128:1028–32.

85. Willett CG, Compton CC, Shellito PC, et al. Selection factors for local excision or abdominoperineal resection of early stage rectal cancer. Cancer 1994;73: 2716–20.

86. Bleday R, Breen E, Jessup JM, et al. Prospective evaluation of local excision for small rectal cancers. Dis Colon Rectum 1997;40:388–92.

87. Dias AR, Nahas CS, Marques CF, et al. Transanal endoscopic microsurgery: indications, results and controversies. Tech Coloproctol 2009;13:105–11.

88. Demartines N, von Flue MO, Harder FH. Transanal endoscopic microsurgical excision of rectal tumors: indications and results. World J Surg 2001;25: 870–5.

89. Palma P, Freudenberg S, Samel S, et al. Transanal endoscopic microsurgery: indications and results after 100 cases. Colorectal Dis 2004;6:350–5.

90. Blumberg D, Paty PB, Guillem JG, et al. All patients with small intramural rectal cancers are at risk for lymph node metastasis. Dis Colon Rectum 1999;42: 881–5.

91. Brodsky JT, Richard GK, Cohen AM, et al. Variables correlated with the risk of lymph node metastasis in early rectal cancer. Cancer 1992;69:322–6.

92. Mellgren A, Sirivongs P, Rothenberger DA, et al. Is local excision adequate therapy for early rectal cancer? Dis Colon Rectum 2000;43:1064–71 [discussion: 1071–4].

93. Garcia-Aguilar J, Mellgren A, Sirivongs P, et al. Local excision of rectal cancer without adjuvant therapy: a word of caution. Ann Surg 2000;231:345–51.

94. Taylor RH, Hay JH, Larsson SN. Transanal local excision of selected low rectal cancers. Am J Surg 1998;175:360–3.

95. Varma MG, Rogers SJ, Schrock TR, et al. Local excision of rectal carcinoma. Arch Surg 1999;134:863–7 [discussion: 867–8].

96. Sengupta S, Tjandra JJ. Local excision of rectal cancer: what is the evidence? Dis Colon Rectum 2001;44:1345–61.

97. Chorost MI, Petrelli NJ, McKenna M, et al. Local excision of rectal carcinoma. Am Surg 2001;67:774–9.

98. Nascimbeni R, Burgart LJ, Nivatvongs S, et al. Risk of lymph node metastasis in T1 carcinoma of the colon and rectum. Dis Colon Rectum 2002;45:200–6.

99. Rothenberger DA, Garcia-Aguilar J. Role of local excision in the treatment of rectal cancer. Semin Surg Oncol 2000;19:367–75.

100. You YN, Baxter NN, Stewart A, et al. Is the increasing rate of local excision for stage I rectal cancer in the United States justified?: a nationwide cohort study from the National Cancer Database. Ann Surg 2007;245:726–33.

101. Madbouly KM, Remzi FH, Erkek BA, et al. Recurrence after transanal excision of T1 rectal cancer: should we be concerned? Dis Colon Rectum 2005;48:711–9 [discussion: 719–21].

102. Stipa F, Burza A, Lucandri G, et al. Outcomes for early rectal cancer managed with transanal endoscopic microsurgery: a 5-year follow-up study. Surg Endosc 2006;20:541–5.

103. Maslekar S, Pillinger SH, Monson JR. Transanal endoscopic microsurgery for carcinoma of the rectum. Surg Endosc 2007;21:97–102.

104. Borschitz T, Heintz A, Junginger T. Transanal endoscopic microsurgical excision of pT2 rectal cancer: results and possible indications. Dis Colon Rectum 2007; 50:292–301.

105. Weiser MR, Landmann RG, Wong WD, et al. Surgical salvage of recurrent rectal cancer after transanal excision. Dis Colon Rectum 2005;48:1169–75.

# Retrorectal Tumors

Kelli Bullard Dunn, MD*

**KEYWORDS**

• Retrorectal • Presacral tumor • Congenital cyst • Chordoma

Tumors occurring in the retrorectal (presacral) space are rare. The true incidence of these tumors is unknown, but several retrospective series suggest that between 1 and 6 patients are diagnosed annually in major referral centers.[1–5] One study found that retrorectal tumors represented about 1 in 40,000 hospital admissions.[6] The retrorectal space contains multiple embryologic remnants derived from various tissues, and tumors that develop in this space are both grossly and histologically heterogeneous. Most lesions are benign, but malignant neoplasms are not uncommon. Malignancy is more common in the pediatric population than in adults, and solid lesions are more likely to be malignant than are cystic lesions.

Retrorectal tumors often go undetected because of nonspecific symptoms. Most benign lesions are asymptomatic. Pain or obstruction occur occasionally. Other symptoms, such as postural headache (associated with anterior meningocele), are considerably rarer.[6] Most of these lesions are palpable on digital rectal examination. Once detected, radiologic evaluation (especially pelvic magnetic resonance imaging [MRI]) is invaluable in surgical planning. Most retrorectal tumors ultimately require surgical resection (without preoperative biopsy), although biopsy can be considered for unresectable lesions or in patients who will not tolerate surgery.

## ANATOMY

The retrorectal or presacral space lies between the upper two-thirds of the rectum and the sacrum, above the rectosacral fascia. It is bound by the rectum anteriorly, the presacral fascia posteriorly, and the endopelvic fascia laterally (lateral ligaments). The superior border of the space is the posterior peritoneal reflection of the rectum and the inferior border is Waldeyer fascia (**Fig. 1**). This region contains structures derived from embryonic neuroectoderm, notochord, and hindgut, and many tumors arise from embryonic remnants. As a result, retrorectal tumors are clinically diverse.[1,7] In addition, the complexity of pelvic anatomy can make surgical management challenging.

Department of Surgical Oncology, Roswell Park Cancer Institute and the University at Buffalo, State University of New York, Elm and Carlton Streets, Buffalo, NY 14263, USA
* Corresponding author.
*E-mail address:* kelli.bullarddunn@roswellpark.org

Surg Clin N Am 90 (2010) 163–171
doi:10.1016/j.suc.2009.09.009
0039-6109/09/$ – see front matter © 2010 Elsevier Inc. All rights reserved.

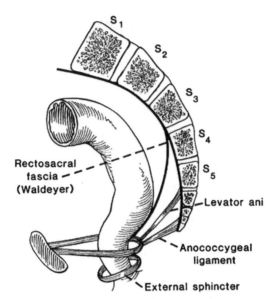

**Fig. 1.** The boundaries of the retrorectal (presacral) space are the rectum anteriorly, the presacral fascia posteriorly, the endopelvic fascia laterally (lateral ligaments), the posterior peritoneal reflection superiorly, and Waldeyer fascia inferiorly. (*From* Nicholls J, Dozios RR, editors. Surgery of the colon and rectum. Edinburgh: Churchill Livingstone, 1997; with permission.)

## CONGENITAL LESIONS

Congenital lesions are most common, comprising approximately two-thirds of retrorectal tumors. These lesions are thought to arise from the remnants of embryonic tissues and include cystic (developmental cysts, duplication cysts, and anterior meningoceles) and solid lesions (chordomas, teratomas, and adrenal rest tumors).[2,6,8]

## DEVELOPMENTAL CYSTS

Developmental cysts constitute most congenital lesions and may arise from all 3 germ cell layers. These lesions have been reported to be more common in women than in men.[6,8] Developmental cysts are further classified as dermoid and epidermoid cysts. Tailgut cysts are often classified as developmental cysts, but are probably more closely related to enterogenous duplication cysts.

## DERMOID AND EPIDERMOID CYSTS

Dermoid and epidermoid cysts are benign lesions that arise from the ectoderm. These cysts are lined with squamous epithelium (epidermoid) or a combination of squamous epithelium and various cutaneous appendages (dermoid), and they may communicate with the skin creating a postanal dimple (**Fig. 2**). These lesions have a high rate of infection (up to 30%),[9] and infected cysts can be easily mistaken for perirectal abscess, pilonidal disease, or fistulae in ano. Recurrence after surgical therapy suggests that there may be an underlying congenital cyst.[10]

## DUPLICATION CYSTS

Enterogenous cysts arise from the primitive gut. Sequestration of the hindgut during embryogenesis results in thin-walled, multilocular cysts lined by columnar epithelium.

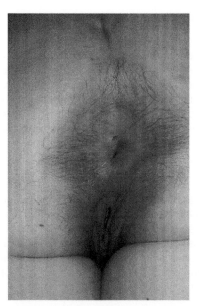

**Fig. 2.** Dermoid and epidermoid cysts may communicate with the skin forming a postanal dimple. Infected cysts, especially those that communicate with the skin, are often confused with pilonidal disease or fistulae in ano. (*Courtesy of* W Douglas Wong, MD, Memorial Sloan Kettering Cancer Institute, New York, NY.)

Tailgut cysts (retrorectal cystic hamartomas) are similar in origin, arising from a portion of the embryonic tail that fails to regress (**Fig. 3**).[11] Rectal duplication cysts also occur and possess all components of the intestinal wall. Most of these lesions are benign, although rare malignant degeneration has been reported.[12–15]

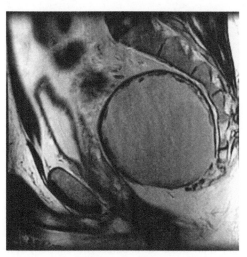

**Fig. 3.** Sagittal MRI image of a large tailgut cyst. (*Courtesy of* W Douglas Wong, MD, Memorial Sloan Kettering Cancer Institute, New York, NY.)

## ANTERIOR MENINGOCELE

Anterior meningocele and myelomeningocele arise from herniation of the dural sac through a defect in the anterior sacrum. This unilateral sacral defect results in the pathognomonic "scimitar sign" (sacrum with a rounded concave border without any bony destruction) on plain radiographs (**Fig. 4**). In addition to nonspecific symptoms, patients with anterior meningocele may present with headache; these headaches are often positional or related to changes in intra-abdominal pressure or defecation.[1,6,16] Aspiration of an anterior meningocele should be strictly avoided because of the risk of causing meningitis.[1,7,10]

## CHORDOMA

Chordomas arise from the notochord and are the most common malignant tumor of the retrorectal space.[4] Chordomas frequently present with pain and are thought to be more common in men. Chordomas can occur anywhere in the spine, but the most common single site is the sacrococcygeal region (30%–50%).[17] These tumors are slow-growing, invasive cancers that show characteristic bony destruction (**Fig. 5**). Radical resection offers the best hope for cure, but local recurrence rates are high, and 10-year survival is only 9% to 35%.[6,18–20]

## TERATOMA

Teratomas are true neoplasms and contain tissue from each germ cell layer. They can be cystic or solid and often contain both components. Like developmental cysts,

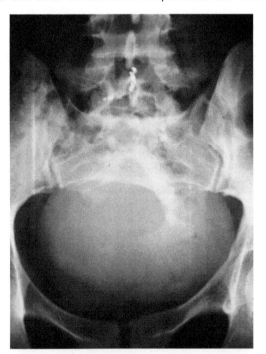

**Fig. 4.** The "scimitar sign," a unilateral sacral defect without bony destruction, is pathogno-monic for anterior meningocele (*Reprinted from* Bou-Assaly W. AJR teaching file: child with chronic constipation. Am J Roentgenol 2007;189; with permission.)

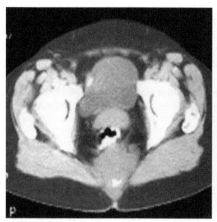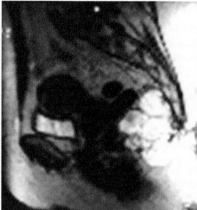

**Fig. 5.** Computed tomographic and MRI images of a chordoma demonstrating characteristic multilobular appearance and bony destruction. (*Courtesy of* W Douglas Wong, MD, Memorial Sloan Kettering Cancer Institute, New York, NY.)

teratomas are more common in female than in male patients. Many teratomas possess germ-cell elements that are capable of malignant degeneration, and up to 10% of retrorectal teratomas progress to cancer if left untreated.[1] Teratomas are more common in children than in adults, but when found in adults, they are more likely to be malignant.[7,19] Teratomas classically possess various tissue types, including respiratory, nervous system, and gastrointestinal structures. These lesions are usually tightly attached to the coccyx and resection requires en bloc coccygectomy.[1]

### ADRENAL REST TUMOR

Adrenal rest tumors are extremely rare, and, although congenital in nature, are often classified as "miscellaneous." They are treated as ectopic adrenal tumors (including pheochromocytoma).[1]

### NEUROGENIC LESIONS

Neurogenic lesions typically arise from peripheral nerves and represent about 10% of retrorectal tumors. These tumors include neurofibromas and sarcomas, neurilemmomas, ependymomas, schwannomas, and ganglioneuromas. Ependymomas are most common. Pain and neurologic dysfunction are often presenting symptoms and are related to the route of the involved nerve. Radical resection (often resulting in significant disability) is usually required, but overall survival seems to be good.[1,6,8]

### OSSEOUS LESIONS

Osseous lesions also make up about 10% of retrorectal lesions and include osteomas, bone cysts, and neoplasms, such as osteogenic sarcoma, Ewing tumor, chondromyxosarcoma, and giant cell tumors. Although benign lesions in this region are often amenable to radical resection, local recurrence can be problematic. Malignant lesions in this location are typically advanced and have poor prognosis.[1,5,6,21]

## INFLAMMATORY LESIONS

Inflammatory lesions may be solid or cystic (abscess) and usually represent extensions of infection either in the perirectal space or in the abdomen (infected congenital cysts are not considered primarily inflammatory). Foreign body granulomas may result from barium or suture material. Pelvic or perineal sepsis can track into this space. Crohn disease and diverticulitis may also manifest with retrorectal inflammation. Finally, more uncommon inflammatory conditions (tuberculosis and granulomatous disease) have been reported in this area.[1,5]

## MISCELLANEOUS

Miscellaneous lesions in the retrorectal space include a wide variety of benign and malignant masses (**Box 1**). Treatment and prognosis are usually related to the natural history of the underlying disease.[21]

### Clinical Presentation and Evaluation

Symptoms of retrorectal tumors are often nonspecific and are related to the location and size of the lesion. Most benign cystic lesions are asymptomatic and are discovered on routine rectal examination.[6] Some authors have suggested that the observed higher incidence of these lesions in women may be related to selection bias resulting from annual pelvic and rectal examinations.[1] Infection or bony invasion may produce pain (lower back, rectal/pelvic, or lower extremity). Postural headache or headache associated with changes in intra-abdominal pressure, as occurs with defecation, are suggestive of anterior meningocele. Large masses (cystic or solid) may cause obstruction, leading to constipation, straining, or overflow incontinence. Rarely, large neoplasms can cause obstructed labor and lead to life-threatening dystocia.[22]

Evaluation begins with a careful rectal examination. Almost all retrorectal masses can be palpated and the location, size, and proximal extent of the tumor are critical for surgical planning. Flexible sigmoidoscopy or colonoscopy are useful for detecting full-thickness rectal involvement. Plain radiographs are often obtained and are occasionally useful; for example, the "scimitar sign" is pathognomonic for anterior meningocele. Computed tomographic scans have been used extensively, but with recent advances in technology, pelvic MRI is emerging as the most sensitive and specific imaging study. A myelogram is occasionally necessary if there is central nervous system involvement.[7]

The role of biopsy is a critical, and often misunderstood, aspect of evaluating retrorectal lesions. In general, biopsy is almost never indicated. For resectable lesions, surgical resection is the best diagnostic and therapeutic option.[1] For cystic lesions, needle biopsy or aspiration may result in infection; in meningocele, this can cause meningitis. Biopsy of malignant lesions (especially chordoma) can result in tumor spread and seeding of the needle track.[4,6] If a patient has undergone needle biopsy of a chordoma, it is important to excise the biopsy track at the time of resection.[1] Unresectable tumors are the main indication for biopsy to direct nonoperative therapy. Biopsy can also be helpful in patients with significant medical comorbidity that precludes pelvic surgery. Occasionally, to exclude metastatic disease, biopsy may be appropriate for a patient with a history of another malignancy.

### Treatment

For patients who are medically fit for an operation and in whom the lesion seems resectable, treatment of retrorectal lesions is almost always surgical resection. The approach depends on the nature and location of the lesion. Lesions that do not extend

**Box 1**
**Classification of retrorectal masses**

Congenital
    Developmental cyst
        Epidermoid cyst
        Dermoid cyst
    Teratoma
    Chordoma
    Anterior meningocele
    Rectal duplication
    Adrenal rest tumors
Neurogenic
    Neurofibroma
    Neurolemmoma
    Ependymoma
    Ganglioneuroma
    Neurofibrosarcoma
Osseous
    Osteoma
    Osteogenic sarcoma
    Sacral bone cyst
    Ewing tumor
    Giant cell tumor
    Chondromyxosarcoma
Inflammatory
    Granuloma
    Perineal abscess
    Pelvirectal abscess
    Fistula
    Chorionic granulomas
Miscellaneous
    Metastatic disease
    Lymphangioma
    Desmoid tumor
    Leiomyoma
    Fibrosarcoma
    Endothelioma

below S4 (high lesions) can be resected transabdominally (anterior approach). Lower lesions can be resected transsacrally (posterior approach). If the upper extent of the lesion can be palpated on rectal examination, it is likely to be resectable transsacrally. Larger lesions or those in an intermediate position may require a combined abdominal and sacral operation. Invasion of the rectum requires rectal resection. Sacrococcygeal invasion requires coccygectomy or sacrectomy. In these complicated cases, a multidisciplinary team, including a colon and rectal surgeon, neurosurgeon or orthopedic surgeon, and plastic surgeon is critical.[1,9,23] Although experience with minimally invasive approaches to resection of these tumors is limited, laparoscopic resection and transanal endoscopic microsurgery have been reported.[24–27] The reader is directed to a surgical textbook or atlas for a more detailed description of these operations.

Medical or radiation therapy are fairly ineffective in treating primary retrorectal lesions. Malignancies in this location are frequently resistant to chemotherapy and radiation. Radiation is occasionally useful for palliation. In contrast, metastases to this area (especially from colorectal carcinoma) often respond to combination chemoradiation therapy.

Long-term outcome after resection of a retrorectal lesion depends on the type of tumor and on adequate resection at the initial operation. For benign lesions, survival is excellent, but local recurrence is common. Recurrent lesions can often be resected for cure. Teratomas often involve the coccyx, and in this setting, coccygectomy can reduce the risk of local recurrence. Prognosis after resection of malignant lesions is variable and reflects the biology of the underlying tumor. For chordoma, local recurrence is common, and reports of long-term survival are highly variable, ranging from 43% to 75% 5-year survival and 9% to 35% 10-year survival.[6,17–20] Other malignancies tend to have poorer prognosis.

## SUMMARY

Retrorectal tumors are rare and heterogeneous. Signs and symptoms are often vague and nonspecific, although almost all lesions are palpable on digital rectal examination. In most cases, surgical resection will be required, and radiologic imaging (especially MRI) can be critical for surgical planning. Biopsy should be avoided unless the lesion seems unresectable. Finally, resection of retrorectal tumors can be complicated and the use of a multidisciplinary team is invaluable.

## REFERENCES

1. Hobson KG, Ghaemmaghami V, Roe JP, et al. Tumors of the retrorectal space. Dis Colon Rectum 2005;48(10):1964–74.
2. Uhlig BE, Johnson RL. Presacral tumors and cysts in adults. Dis Colon Rectum 1975;18(7):581–9.
3. Johnson WR. Postrectal neoplasms and cysts. Aust N Z J Surg 1980;50(2):163–6.
4. Cody HS 3rd, Marcove RC, Quan SH. Malignant retrorectal tumors: 28 years' experience at Memorial Sloan-Kettering Cancer Center. Dis Colon Rectum 1981;24(7):501–6.
5. Freier DT, Stanley JC, Thompson NW. Retrorectal tumors in adults. Surg Gynecol Obstet 1971;132(4):681–6.
6. Jao SW, Beart RW Jr, Spencer RJ, et al. Retrorectal tumors. Mayo Clinic experience, 1960–1979. Dis Colon Rectum 1985;28(9):644–52.
7. Bullard Dunn K, Rothenberger D. Colon, rectum, and anus. In: Brunicardi C, editor. Schwartz's principles of surgery. 9th edition. New York: McGraw Hill, in press.

8. Stewart RJ, Humphreys WG, Parks TG. The presentation and management of presacral tumours. Br J Surg 1986;73(2):153–5.

9. Abel ME, Nelson R, Prasad ML, et al. Parasacrococcygeal approach for the resection of retrorectal developmental cysts. Dis Colon Rectum 1985;28(11): 855–8.

10. Singer MA, Cintron JR, Martz JE, et al. Retrorectal cyst: a rare tumor frequently misdiagnosed. J Am Coll Surg 2003;196(6):880–6.

11. Hjermstad BM, Helwig EB. Tailgut cysts. Report of 53 cases. Am J Clin Pathol 1988;89(2):139–47.

12. Springall RG, Griffiths JD. Malignant change in rectal duplication. J R Soc Med 1990;83(3):185–7.

13. Krivokapic Z, Dimitrijevic I, Barisic G, et al. Adenosquamous carcinoma arising within a retrorectal tailgut cyst: report of a case. World J Gastroenterol 2005; 11(39):6225–7.

14. Tampi C, Lotwala V, Lakdawala M, et al. Retrorectal cyst hamartoma (tailgut cyst) with malignant transformation. Gynecol Oncol 2007;105(1):266–8.

15. Shivnani AT, Small W Jr, Benson A 3rd, et al. Adenocarcinoma arising in rectal duplication cyst: case report and review of the literature. Am Surg 2004;70(11): 1007–9.

16. Williams B. Cerebrospinal fluid pressure changes in response to coughing. Brain 1976;99(2):331–46.

17. McMaster ML, Goldstein AM, Bromley CM, et al. Chordoma: incidence and survival patterns in the United States, 1973–1995. Cancer Causes Control 2001;12(1):1–11.

18. Bergh P, Kindblom LG, Gunterberg B, et al. Prognostic factors in chordoma of the sacrum and mobile spine: a study of 39 patients. Cancer 2000;88(9):2122–34.

19. Finne CO. Presacral tumors and cysts. In: Cameron J, editor. Current surgical therapy. 3rd edition. Toronto: BC Decker; 1989. p. 736–43.

20. Miyahara M, Saito T, Nakashima K, et al. Sacral chordoma developing two years after low anterior resection for rectal cancer. Surg Today 1993;23(2):144–8.

21. Gordon P. Retrorectal tumors. In: Gordon P, Nivatvongs S, editors. Principles and practice of surgery for the colon, rectum, and anus. St Louis (MO): Quality Medical Publishing, Inc; 1999. p. 427–45.

22. Sobrado CW, Mester M, Simonsen OS, et al. Retrorectal tumors complicating pregnancy. Report of two cases. Dis Colon Rectum 1996;39(10):1176–9.

23. Bohm B, Milsom JW, Fazio VW, et al. Our approach to the management of congenital presacral tumors in adults. Int J Colorectal Dis 1993;8(3):134–8.

24. Gunkova P, Martinek L, Dostalik J, et al. Laparoscopic approach to retrorectal cyst. World J Gastroenterol 2008;14(42):6581–3.

25. Chen Y, Xu H, Li Y, et al. Laparoscopic resection of presacral teratomas. J Minim Invasive Gynecol 2008;15(5):649–51.

26. Palanivelu C, Rangarajan M, Senthilkumar R, et al. Laparoscopic and perineal excision of an infected "dumb-bell" shaped retrorectal epidermoid cyst. J Laparoendosc Adv Surg Tech A 2008;18(1):88–92.

27. Zoller S, Joos A, Dinter D, et al. Retrorectal tumors: excision by transanal endoscopic microsurgery. Rev Esp Enferm Dig 2007;99(9):547–50.

# Rectal Foreign Bodies

Joel E. Goldberg, MD, FACS[a],*, Scott R. Steele, MD, FACS, FASCRS[b]

**KEYWORDS**

- Rectal foreign bodies • Perforation
- Transanal approach • Endoscopy

Rectal foreign bodies often pose a challenging diagnostic and management dilemma that begins with the initial evaluation in the emergency department and continues through the postextraction period. Numerous objects ranging from billy clubs, varied fruits and vegetables, nails, light bulbs, and a turkey baster to a propane tank have been described as retained rectal foreign bodies. Because of the wide variety of objects and the variable trauma that can be caused to the local tissues of the rectum and distal colon, a systematic approach to the diagnosis and management of the retained rectal foreign body is essential. One of the most common problems encountered in the management of rectal foreign bodies is the delay in presentation, as many patients may be embarrassed and reluctant to seek medical care. Moreover, in the emergency room, patients may often be less than truthful regarding the reason for their visit, leading to extensive workups and further delays. Even after extraction, rectal foreign bodies can lead to delayed perforation or significant bleeding from the rectum. Hence, a stepwise approach to the diagnosis, removal, and postextraction evaluation is essential.

## EPIDEMIOLOGY

Although retained rectal foreign bodies have been reported in patients of all ages, genders, and ethnicities, more than two-thirds of patients with rectal bodies are men in their 30s and 40s, and patients as old as 90 years were also reported.[1–3] The literature is replete with single-center case studies because this is generally a rare problem that does not lend itself to a systematic or prospective analysis (**Table 1**). A report from one major teaching hospital spanning a 10-year period reported approximately 1 rectal foreign body per month.[4] The incidence is even lower in smaller community-based hospitals.

[a] Division of General and Gastrointestinal Surgery, Section of Colon and Rectal Surgery, Brigham and Women's Hospital, Harvard Medical School, 75 Francis Street, Boston, MA 02115, USA
[b] Department of General Surgery, Colon and Rectal Surgery, Madigan Army Medical Center, Fort Lewis, WA 98431, USA
* Corresponding author.
*E-mail address:* jgoldberg1@partners.org (J.E. Goldberg).

Surg Clin N Am 90 (2010) 173–184
doi:10.1016/j.suc.2009.10.004
0039-6109/09/$ – see front matter © 2010 Published by Elsevier Inc.

**Table 1**
Rectal foreign body series

| Author (Year) | Number of Patients | Male/ Female | Age (Mean or Median in y) | Insertion (Anal/ Ingestion) | Extraction (Transanal/ Abdominal) | Stoma (Number) | Morbidity/Mortality (Percentage) |
|---|---|---|---|---|---|---|---|
| Rodriguez (2007)[2] | 30 | 20/10 | 42.5 | 16/14 | 23/7 | 6 | 14/0 |
| Clarke (2005)[3] | 13 | 13/0 | 45 | 13/0 | 8/5 | 2 | NA |
| Lake (2004)[4] | 87 | 85/5 | 40 | 87/0 | 79/8 | 2 | 1/0 |
| Ruiz (2001)[10] | 17 | 14/3 | 46.3 | 17/0 | 10/7 | 5 | 0/0 |
| Biriukov (2000)[11] | 112 | 111/1 | 16–80 | 112/0 | 107/6 | NA | NA |
| Ooi (1998)[1] | 30 | 25/5 | 46 | 30/0 | 27/3 | 1 | 7/0 |
| Cohen (1996)[12] | 48 | 45/3 | 33.6 | 48/0 | 42/6 | 5 | 0/0 |
| Yaman (1993)[13] | 29 | 28/1 | 42.5 | 22/7 | 27/2 | 2 | 17/0 |
| Marti (1986)[14] | 8 | NA | 38 | 8 | NA | NA | 0/0 |
| Nehme Kingsley (1985)[15] | 51 | 51/0 | 19–94 | 51/0 | 50/1 | 0 | 0/0 |
| Barone (1983)[16] | 101 | 101/0 | 16–48 | 101/0 | 89/12 | 11 | NA/1 |
| Crass (1981)[17] | 29 | 26/3 | 10–84 | 29/0 | 15/14 | 10 | 14/3 |
| Sohn (1977)[18] | 11 | 11/0 | 35 | 11/0 | 7/4 | 4 | 10/0 |
| Barone (1976)[19] | 28 | 26/2 | 16–56 | 28/0 | 23/5 | 5 | 14 |

*Abbreviation:* NA, not available.

*Data from* Steele SR, Goldberg JE. Rectal foreign bodies. In: Basow DS, editor. UpToDate. Waltham (MA): UpToDate, Inc; 2009. For more information visit http://www.uptodate.com.

*Data from* Refs.[1–4,10–19]

**Table 2**
**AAST rectal organ injury scale**

| Grade I | Hematoma: contusion or hematoma without devascularization and/or partial-thickness laceration |
|---|---|
| Grade II | Laceration ≤50% circumference |
| Grade III | Laceration>50% circumference |
| Grade IV | Full-thickness laceration with extension into the perineum |
| Grade V | Devascularized segment |

*Data from* Moore EE, Cogbill TH, Malangoni MA, et al. Organ injury scaling, II: Pancreas, duodenum, small bowel, colon, and rectum. J Trauma 1990;30:1427.

## CLASSIFICATION

Although the American Association for the Surgery of Trauma (AAST) rectal organ injury scale is generally used for blunt and penetrating trauma, its use for injury secondary to rectal foreign bodies is appropriate (**Table 2**). The treatment of all rectal injuries depends on the degree of injury, which is classified according to presence of hematoma, the percent circumference laceration, and whether or not there is devascularization of the rectum and perforation/extension into the perineum.[5] Another useful classification of rectal foreign bodies has been to categorize them as voluntary versus involuntary and sexual versus nonsexual (**Table 3**). By far the most common category of rectal foreign bodies is objects that are inserted voluntarily and for sexual stimulation. Numerous objects have been described in the literature, and a partial listing from the literature and the authors' experience includes vibrators, dildos, a turkey baster, a Billie club, cucumbers, apples, light bulbs, Christmas ornaments, a camping stove, knives, trailer hitch, nails, bottles, utensils, and a pill bottle. Involuntary sexual foreign bodies are almost exclusively in the domain of rape and sexual assault. The most infamous case is that of Haitian immigrant Abner Louima who was assaulted by 4 New York City Police Department officers after a scuffle at a nightclub in Brooklyn, New York, in 1997. He was repeatedly sodomized with a broomstick handle, resulting in rectal and bladder injuries that required several operations and more than 2 months stay in the hospital.[6] The second most common type of rectal foreign body is best known as body packing and is commonly used by drug traffickers. A person known as a mule swallows several packages of drugs (usually heroin or cocaine) wrapped in plastic bags and/or condoms. The potential complications from body packing include impaction, obstruction, perforation, and even rupture of

**Table 3**
**Classification of rectal foreign bodies**

| | Voluntary | | Involuntary |
|---|---|---|---|
| Sexual | Vibrators, dildos, varied other objects | | Rape or assault (ie, the Abner Louima case where New York City Police Department assaulted/sodomized him with a broom stick in 1997). |
| Nonsexual | Body packing of illicit drugs | | The mentally ill or children: retained thermometers; enema tips; oral ingestion, such as bones, toothpicks, plastic objects |

the packages resulting in systemic absorption of the drugs, which can result in overdose and even death of the mule.[7] Involuntary nonsexual foreign bodies are generally found in the elderly, children, or the mentally ill. The objects are usually retained thermometers and enema tips; aluminum foil wrapping from pill containers; and orally ingested objects, such as tooth picks, chicken bones, plastic objects such as erasers or pill bottle caps, and even coins or small plastic toys. Any of these mechanisms or objects can cause severe injury. Therefore, all retained rectal foreign bodies should be treated as potentially hazardous. Despite the potential for severe injury, most rectal injuries from foreign bodies result in grade I or grade II injuries.

## EVALUATION AND MANAGEMENT
### History and Physical Examination

Patients with rectal foreign bodies are embarrassed and often reluctant to state the true nature of their emergency room visit. As a result, they may present with a chief complaint of rectal pain or abdominal pain, bright red blood per rectum, inability to have a bowel movement, and rectal mucous leakage. In most cases, patients present several hours to days after the placement of the rectal foreign body, and on occasion, the foreign body has even been successfully removed but the patient has delayed symptoms of bleeding, perforation, or even incontinence.[1,4] When suspected, physicians need to bring up the possibility of a retained or removed rectal foreign body in a nonconfrontational way. This may be difficult, especially in the case of nonvoluntary placement, and physicians should also be prepared to provide emotional support. Yet, valuable information may be gained from a description of the object(s), timing of event, and history of repetitive trauma from either placement or attempted removal.

Physical examination of the patient with a rectal foreign body can present with a wide spectrum of findings. If the object is distal and no significant trauma is present, then the examination can be quite benign. But if there is perforation above the peritoneal reflection, the patient can present with frank peritonitis. Often, the rectal foreign body can be palpated in either the left or right lower quadrant of the abdomen. The rectal examination has similar variability to the abdominal examination. The foreign body may be palpable in the distal rectum or, if higher up, the surgeon may not be able to feel it on digital examination. Bright red blood per rectum is often seen but is not always present, and should not be interpreted as minimal injury potential when absent. Careful attention should also be paid to the status of the sphincter, especially in patients without a prior history of foreign body placement and in those nonvoluntary cases. In patients without sphincter injury, the rectal sphincter may have increased tone secondary to muscular spasm as a result of the foreign object. In other cases, the sphincter may have obvious damage with visible injury to both the internal and external sphincter. In either case, a careful examination and documentation of resting and squeeze tone and sensation is important.

### Laboratory and Radiologic Evaluation

In general, laboratory evaluation is not very helpful in the patient with a rectal foreign body. If the patient has a suspected perforation, the white blood cell (WBC) count may be elevated and/or acidosis may be present on chemistry. However, these laboratory tests are not very helpful, as the physical examination will be more revealing as to the extent of injury. In select cases, elevated WBC count or acidosis may be suggestive of occult injuries, such as mucosal ischemia from pressure necrosis, or an extraperitoneal rectal perforation, both of which may not be immediately obvious on examination. Laboratory tests should be limited to those that are necessary in case an operation is

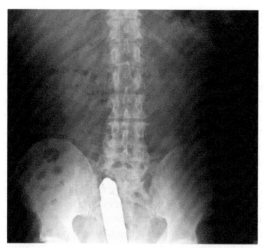

**Fig. 1.** Rectal dildo on abdominal plain film. (*Courtesy of* Joel Goldberg, MD, Boston, MA.)

needed. Hence, a clot in the blood bank and general chemistries that may be useful to the anesthesia provider should be ordered. Radiologic evaluation is far more important than any laboratory test. A flat and upright series of the abdomen will show the location of the object and the presence or absence of pneumoperitoneum (**Figs. 1** and **2**).

## Management

The first step in the evaluation and management of a patient with a rectal foreign body is to determine whether or not a perforation occurred. When a perforation is suspected, it should be determined as soon as possible whether the patient is stable or unstable. The history and physical examination helps to determine if the patient has peritonitis, whereas the plain radiographs may help localize the object and rule out free air. These steps in conjunction with each other allow one to decide if the situation is a surgical

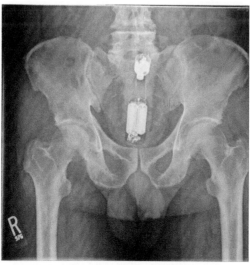

**Fig. 2.** Rectal vibrator on abdominal plain film. (*Courtesy of* Joel Goldberg, MD, Boston, MA.)

emergency or if a more measured approach can be taken. Hypotension, tachycardia, severe abdominopelvic pain, and fevers are indicative of a perforation. If there is free air or obvious peritonitis indicating a perforation, then the patient needs immediate resuscitation with intravenous fluids and broad-spectrum antibiotics. A Foley catheter and nasogastric tube should be placed, and appropriate blood samples should be sent to the laboratory for evaluation, including a complete blood count, chemistries, and a type and crossmatch. If the patient appears stable and has normal vital signs but a perforation is suspected, a computed tomographic (CT) scan often helps determine if there has been a rectal perforation (**Fig. 3**). This is often the case for perforations below the level of the peritoneal reflection. Rectal wall thickening, mesorectal air, fluid collections, and fat stranding are all indications of a full-thickness injury and should be considered as indicative until proved otherwise. When a foreign body is removed or absent in the rectal vault, rigid proctoscopy or endoscopic evaluation may reveal the rectal injury or the foreign body located higher in the rectosigmoid.

In clinically stable patients without evidence of perforation or peritonitis, the rectal foreign body should be removed either in the emergency department or in the operating room, if general anesthesia is needed. If the object is proximally located and the patient is stable, then a trial of nonoperative management and observation to see if the object passes more distally should be attempted. Although the use of stimulants and enemas has been described, their routine use has not been endorsed by most practitioners because there is the theoretical risk of causing more extensive rectal wall injury, perforation, or even possibly propelling the object more proximally in the colon. Many rectal foreign bodies fail to pass on their own and need to be extracted in either the emergency room or the operating room. Most objects can be removed transanally, and if not, then a transabdominal approach is used.[4] The authors recommend direct visualization with rigid proctoscopy or flexible sigmoidoscopy for all patients after the object has been removed to evaluate the status of the rectum and rule out ischemia or wall perforation.

## EXTRACTION TECHNIQUES
### Transanal Approach

When attempting to remove a rectal foreign body transanally, the most important factor in successful extraction is patient relaxation. This can be achieved with a perianal nerve block, a spinal anesthetic, or either of these in combination with intravenous conscious sedation. All of these techniques allow the patient to relax, decrease anal

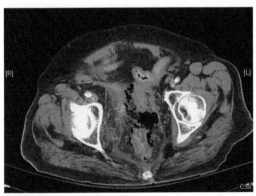

**Fig. 3.** Rectal perforation with extraperitoneal air seen on CT scan. (*Courtesy of* Joel Goldberg, MD, Boston, MA.)

sphincter spasm, and improve visualization and exposure. In general, a perianal nerve block similar to that used for anorectal surgery works quite well. The authors favor using lidocaine (Xylocaine) 1% with epinephrine and bupivacaine 0.5% with epinephrine in a 50:50 mix. A superficial block and then an intersphincteric block circumferentially around the anal verge are performed. Finally, a pudendal nerve block is performed. The branches of the pudendal nerve that innervate the anal sphincter complex approach the sphincter complex from a posterolateral location. A pudendal nerve block is done by infiltrating the tissues deeply in a fanlike technique approximately 1 cm medial to the ischial tuberosities in the posterolateral location bilaterally. Approximately 2 to 5 mL of the local anesthetic mix is used on each side.

Only after the patient has been appropriately sedated and anesthetized should attempts be made to remove the object. The high lithotomy position in candy cane stirrups facilitates removal of most objects and has the added benefit of allowing for downward abdominal pressure to aid in extraction of the foreign body. Although the size and location of the object may be determined by the preprocedure films, a digital rectal examination is the critical first step in evaluating the patient with a rectal foreign body, allowing the surgeon to see if the object is within reach of the anal verge. The anal canal should then be gently dilated to 3 fingers' breadth. If the foreign body can be easily palpated, it is amenable to transanal extraction using one of many clamps and instruments. If not easily grasped with a hand, the authors prefer to use a Kocher clamp or a ring forceps to take hold of the object and to bring it down to the anal verge where it can be grasped with the surgeon's hand and then be removed easily. After successful removal of a rectal foreign body, the mucosa of the colon and rectum needs to be examined. A rigid sigmoidoscopy is recommended, although some advocate a flexible sigmoidoscopy. The goal is to completely evaluate the mucosa of the distal colon and rectum to make sure that there is no active bleeding, additional foreign bodies, or full-thickness injury to the bowel mucosa. A repeat plain film of the abdomen is often warranted to ensure that no perforation took place during the extraction process. Because the surgeon will encounter various differing objects, there are many methods to be aware of that may aid in the removal of the foreign body, depending on its size and shape.

### Blunt and Sharp Objects

The best method for the removal of a blunt object is to grasp the object using one of the clamps mentioned earlier or, better yet, using the surgeon's hand, depending on the laxity of the anal canal and the success of the anal block. If the patient has a lax anal sphincter, there is a good block, and the patient is adequately sedated, then the object is often easily removed. Frequently, the patient can be asked to perform the Valsalva maneuver to see if that maneuver helps propel the object closer to the anal canal. Smooth objects, such as bottles, fruits and vegetables, dildos, and vibrators, cannot always be grasped, and caution should be taken to ensure that they are not broken inside the patient. In the cases of fruits and vegetables, however, either grasping or breaking apart the object is a well-described technique that aids in the removal of the foreign body. Some smooth foreign bodies create a seal with the rectal mucosa. When downward traction is placed on the object, a vacuum force is created that prevents the removal of the object. In this case, it has been shown that placing a Foley catheter alongside the object and inflating the balloon above it helps in extraction in 2 ways. First, once the balloon is inflated above the object, air can be insufflated and the suction vacuum seal is broken. The balloon is then left inflated and is used to pull the object down toward the rectum. In the case of a jar, a larger ballooned implement (Sengstaken-Blakemore or Minnesota tube) can be inserted into the jar and the balloon can be inflated inside the jar and thereby can be used to extract the jar. Obstetric vacuum extractors have even been described to grasp the object, widen the canal, and release the rectal seal.[1–4,8–19] Removal of sharp objects can prove even more difficult, as they pose an additional risk for both the patient and the surgeon. These objects should be removed with the utmost care under direct visualization through a rigid or flexible endoscope. Once again, the rectal mucosa must be closely examined for tears, bleeding, and perforation.

### Body Packers

The ingestion of illicit drugs in small packets poses a particularly challenging dilemma as the surgeon has to balance extracting the foreign object with using too much force that could result in the rupture of the packets. Most body packers use condoms that are filled with drugs and then swallowed (**Fig. 4**). Clamps are not recommended when attempting to remove these, as the packets are easily ruptured. If the packets are not within reach of the surgeon's hand and there is no systemic toxicity, the patient should be admitted and observed and the packets will eventually pass to a point where the surgeon can remove them manually. Should signs or symptoms of perforation or drug ingestion/toxicity be observed, then exploratory laparotomy for removal of the remaining packets and aggressive medical treatment for the overdose is warranted.

### Endoscopy

Flexible endoscopy is reserved for objects that are located more proximally in the rectum or the distal sigmoid colon. Endoscopy also provides excellent visualization of the mucosa to evaluate for subtle and gross changes in the rectal mucosa. Lake and colleagues[4] reported on the location of the foreign body and need for surgery.

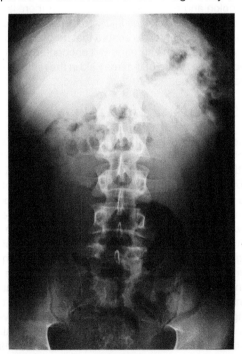

**Fig. 4.** Body packing with sigmoid colon condoms seen on plain films. (*Courtesy of* Koenraad Mortele, MD, Boston, MA.)

When the object was present in the sigmoid colon, 55% of cases required surgery, whereas only 24% required surgery when the object was present in the rectum. Endoscopy can serve as a middle ground in many cases to avoid surgical exploration by enabling evaluation and therapeutic removal of objects that may have been nonamenable to transanal extraction. Once the object is identified with the flexible endoscope, it can be grasped with a polypectomy snare, much like using a lasso (**Fig. 5**). The scope can also be used to place air in the vault, breaking the seal much like the Foley catheter. Once successful extraction has been accomplished, the endoscope should be passed again to evaluate the bowel mucosa for any inadvertent injuries.

### Surgery

If the local perianal block and sedation are unsuccessful in the emergency department, the patient needs to be brought to the operating room for a general or spinal anesthetic to aid in the removal of the object. In many cases, even deeper conscious sedation is successful to provide the relaxation needed to aid in removal. Once again, downward pressure on the object in the left iliac fossa greatly aids in moving the object toward the rectum and stabilizing it when attempting to grab it from below. After anesthesia has been applied and the patient is adequately relaxed, if the foreign body cannot be removed from below then a laparotomy is indicated. Surgery is also indicated in all patients who present with perforation (free air), sepsis, or peritonitis. Some surgeons have also described laparoscopy as an aid to push the object more distally into the rectum for a transanal removal.[20,21] In the absence of a perforation,

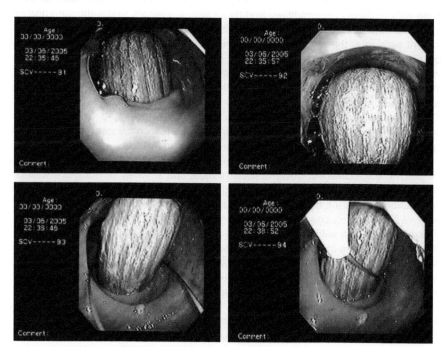

**Fig. 5.** Rectal billy club and endoscopic extraction with colonoscopy snare. (*Courtesy of* Justin Maykel, MD, Worcester, MA. *Reproduced from* Steele SR, Goldberg JE. Rectal foreign bodies. In: Basow DS, editor. UpToDate. Waltham (MA): UpToDate, Inc; 2009; with permission. For more information visit http://www.uptodate.com.)

once inside the abdomen, the first step is to attempt to milk the object distally into the rectum. If this fails, then a colotomy and removal of the foreign object is needed. This colotomy can be primarily repaired and often no diversion is needed. Diversion is reserved for patients with frank peritonitis and instability, perforation with extensive fecal contamination, and proper surgical judgment. After removal of the object, the entire length of the bowel needs to be inspected to make sure there are no inadvertent injuries.

## POSTREMOVAL MANAGEMENT AND COMPLICATIONS

The most dangerous complication of a rectal foreign body is perforation. When patients present with a rectal perforation, they should at first be stabilized like any trauma patient. After stabilization, management depends on 3 factors: first, whether the patient is clinically stable or unstable, second, whether the perforation is in an intraperitoneal or extraperitoneal location, and last, whether there is significant fecal soilage or not. A good rule of thumb is to manage a rectal perforation from a foreign body in the same way as a colorectal bullet or stab wound. The historical principles of treating a rectal injury are diversion, debridement, distal washout, and drainage (4 "D's"). Each of these procedures depends on the degree of contamination, the amount of time since the perforation, and the extent and location of the injury. Clearly, the surgeon needs to individualize the care of these patients. The trauma literature has shown that primary repair with and without diversion for intraperitoneal injuries is acceptable and depends on the principles outlined earlier.[22,23] Unstable patients, those with multiple comorbidities, and those with significant tissue damage and delayed presentation more often require a diversion. On the other hand, patients who present early after the insult, those with minimal tissue damage, and those with little to no contamination can be managed with primary repair and washout. Small extraperitoneal injuries can also be managed with observation, avoidance of oral feeding, and antibiotics. After several days, a gentle diatrizoate (Gastrografin) enema should be performed to see if the perforation has healed.[24] Like the trauma literature, the 4 "D's" of rectal trauma management are highly controversial as to which, if any, are required. The authors recommend consideration for each component, with individualization as per surgeon experience, judgment, and comfort level.

Postremoval observation depends on several factors, such as the clinical status of the patient, comorbidities, delay in presentation, and whether or not there was any resultant trauma to the rectum or surrounding tissue. Postextraction endoscopy and plain radiographs are a must before discharging any patient who had a foreign body removal. Even with routine transanal extraction, the authors recommend several hours of close observation with serial abdominal examinations and plain films as indicated. Major complications from rectal foreign bodies are rare, but can be life threatening if missed. Bleeding from lacerations in the rectal mucosa are generally self-limited but can on occasion require repeat examination under anesthesia and suture ligation. Perforation can result in a laparotomy and even a colostomy, which then requires a repeat operation for colostomy reversal. Death from sepsis and multisystem organ failure has been reported.[25] If a major laparotomy is performed, the patient is also at risk for cardiovascular morbidity and wound complications (ie, infection and hernia). In addition, traumatic disruption of the anal sphincter can result in mild to severe fecal incontinence, depending on the degree of the injury.[26] Attempts for surgical correction of any sphincter injury should be delayed until adequate time has passed to evaluate any resultant defect and clinical symptoms.

After a foreign body incident, and especially with sexual assault, patients will often experience a wide range of emotions from shock, disbelief, denial, embarrassment, and guilt to flashbacks, fear, anger, and stress. Long-term consequences may occur, such as substance abuse or psychological problems. As such, the authors recommend offering all patients counseling by an experienced mental heath care provider.

## SUMMARY

Rectal foreign bodies present a difficult diagnostic and management dilemma. This is often because of the delayed presentation, wide variety of objects that cause the damage, and the wide spectrum of injury patterns that range from minimal extraperitoneal mucosal injury to free intraperitoneal perforation, sepsis, and even death. The evaluation of the patient with a rectal foreign body needs to progress in an orderly fashion, with appropriate examination, laboratory and radiographic evaluation, and resuscitation with intravenous fluids and antibiotics. In the nonperforated stable patient, the object should be removed in the emergency department with a local block and/or conscious sedation via the transanal approach. If this fails, then the patient should go to the operating room for a deeper anesthetic and attempt at transanal extraction. Surgery with a laparotomy should be reserved for patients with perforation or ischemic bowel or cases of failed transanal attempts. Colostomy is not mandatory in all patients, with care being based on their overall condition, length of time since perforation, comorbidities, concomitant injuries, and surgical judgment. After removal of the foreign body, the authors suggest a period of observation, a rigid or flexible endoscopy to evaluate for rectal injury, and repeat plain films to examine for evidence of injury and perforation that may have occurred during the extraction process.

## REFERENCES

1. Ooi BS, Ho YH, Eu KW, et al. Management of anorectal foreign bodies: a cause of obscure anal pain. Aust N Z J Surg 1998;68:852.
2. Rodriguez-Hermosa JI, Codina-Cazador A, Ruiz B, et al. Management of foreign bodies in the rectum. Colorectal Dis 2007;9:543.
3. Clarke DL, Buccimazza I, Anderson FA, et al. Colorectal foreign bodies. Colorectal Dis 2005;7:98.
4. Lake JP, Essani R, Petrone P, et al. Management of retained colorectal foreign bodies: predictors of operative intervention. Dis Colon Rectum 2004;47:1694.
5. Moore EE, Cogbill TH, Malangoni MA, et al. Organ injury scaling, II: pancreas, duodenum, small bowel, colon, and rectum. J Trauma 1990;30:1427.
6. Brenner Marie. Incident in the 70th precinct. Vanity Fair; December 1997.
7. Traub SJ, Hoffman RS, Nelson LS. Body packing—the internal concealment of illicit drugs. N Engl J Med 2003;349:2519.
8. Johnson SO, Hartranft TH. Nonsurgical removal of a rectal foreign body using a vacuum extractor. Report of a case. Dis Colon Rectum 1996;39:935.
9. Feigelson S, Maun D, Silverberg D, et al. Removal of a large spherical foreign object from the rectum using an obstetric vacuum device: a case report. Am Surg 2007;73:304.
10. Ruiz de Castillo J, Selles Dechent R, Millan Scheiding M, et al. Colorectal trauma caused by foreign bodies introduced during sexual activity: diagnosis and management. Rev Esp Enferm Dig 2001;93:631.
11. Biriukov IuV, Volkov OV, An VK, et al. [Treatment of patients with foreign bodies in rectum]. Khirurgiia (Mosk) 2000;7:41 [in Russian].

12. Cohen JS, Sackier JM. Management of colorectal foreign bodies. J R Coll Surg Edinb 1996;41:312.

13. Yaman M, Deitel M, Burul CJ, et al. Foreign bodies in the rectum. Can J Surg 1993;36:173.

14. Marti MC, Morel P, Rohner A. Traumatic lesions of the rectum. Int J Colorectal Dis 1986;1:152.

15. Nehme Kingsley A, Abcarian H. Colorectal foreign bodies. Management update. Dis Colon Rectum 1985;28:941.

16. Barone JE, Yee J, Nealon TF Jr. Management of foreign bodies and trauma of the rectum. Surg Gynecol Obstet 1983;156:453.

17. Crass RA, Tranbaugh RF, Kudsk KA, et al. Colorectal foreign bodies and perforation. Am J Surg 1981;142:85.

18. Sohn N, Weinstein MA, Gonchar J. Social injuries of the rectum. Am J Surg 1977;134:611.

19. Barone JE, Sohn N, Nealon TF Jr. Perforations and foreign bodies of the rectum: report of 28 cases. Ann Surg 1976;184:601.

20. Berghoff KR, Franklin ME Jr. Laparoscopic-assisted rectal foreign body removal: report of a case. Dis Colon Rectum 2005;48:1975.

21. Rispoli G, Esposito C, Monachese TD, et al. Removal of a foreign body from the distal colon using a combined laparoscopic and endoanal approach: report of a case. Dis Colon Rectum 2000;43:1632.

22. Demetriades D, Murray JA, Chan L, et al. Penetrating colon injuries requiring resection: diversion or primary anastomosis? An AAST prospective multicenter trial. J Trauma 2001;50:765.

23. Herr MW, Gagliano RA. Historical perspective and current management of colonic and intraperitoneal rectal trauma. Curr Surg 2005;62:187.

24. Fry RD, Shemesh EI, Kodner IJ, et al. Perforation of the rectum and sigmoid colon during barium-enema examination. Management and prevention. Dis Colon Rectum 1989;32:759.

25. Waraich NG, Hudson JS, Iftikhar SY. Vibrator-induced fatal rectal perforation. N Z Med J 2007;120:U2685.

26. Madiba TE, Moodley MM. Anal sphincter reconstruction for incontinence due to non-obstetric sphincter damage. East Afr Med J 2003;80:585.

# Fecal Incontinence

Anders Mellgren, MD, PhD, FACS, FASCRS

**KEYWORDS**

- Fecal incontinence • Sphincteroplasty
- Sacral nerve stimulation • Injectable biomaterials • Evaluation

Fecal incontinence is defined as the loss of voluntary control of feces (liquid or solid) from the bowel. The condition is socially embarrassing and the prevalence varies between 1% and 21% in different studies.[1–4] This prevalence increases with age: 0.5% to 1% in people younger than 65 years and 3% to 8% in people older than 65 years.[1,5,6] Multiple factors may contribute to the development of fecal incontinence, including obstetric, traumatic, or neurologic damage, spinal injuries, mental disorders, or problems with loose stool consistency. Consistently, obstetric injury is the most common cause, although fecal incontinence may not manifest until years later.

Following evaluation, therapy usually begins with dietary and lifestyle modifications and medical therapy. The addition of exogenous fiber supplements or medications that thicken and harden stool, such as loperamide, may be of significant benefit for patients with loose stools and fecal incontinence. By simply adding bulking agents, many patients experience such noticeable improvements that an extensive evaluation becomes unnecessary. Another nonsurgical therapy is biofeedback, which entails "retraining" the pelvic floor in proper defecation. This therapy is painless, risk-free, and can be successful in patients with mild or moderate symptoms.

Patients not responding to nonsurgical treatments should usually be evaluated with specialized testing modalities and assessed with standardized questionnaires. Endoanal ultrasonography can delineate possible anal sphincter injuries, anorectal manometry can assess anal sphincter function, and measurement of pudendal nerve motor latencies can assess the function in the pudendal nerves. In some patients, defecography or dynamic magnetic resonance imaging (MRI) can be of value when assessing overall pelvic floor function and identifying concomitant pelvic floor defects that may be contributing to symptoms.

Overlapping sphincteroplasty is the most common surgical therapy for fecal incontinence. This surgery works for an isolated sphincter injury, which is repaired with an overlapping technique while preserving the scar tissue to provide extra bulk and strength. This technique is not useful in patients without sphincter injuries or in patients with multiple sphincter lesions in different locations. Recent studies have demonstrated that outcome after sphincteroplasty may deteriorate over time,[7] although it

Division of Colon and Rectal Surgery, University of Minnesota, Pelvic Floor Center, 2800 Chicago Avenue South, # 300, Minneapolis, MN 55407, USA
*E-mail address:* amellgren@crsal.org

Surg Clin N Am 90 (2010) 185–194
doi:10.1016/j.suc.2009.10.006
0039-6109/09/$ – see front matter © 2010 Published by Elsevier Inc.

may provide significant symptomatic improvement for many patients, especially in the short term.

Previously, the only surgical alternative to overlapping sphincteroplasty has been a diverting colostomy. However, novel surgical techniques have been developed and are increasingly used in the treatment of fecal incontinence. More extensive procedures, such as the stimulated graciloplasty and the artificial anal sphincter, were originally developed to treat patients with severe fecal incontinence. Although these continue to be practiced and provide excellent outcomes to many patients, they require more in-depth operations and follow-up. More recently, less invasive techniques, such as sacral nerve stimulation and injectable biomaterials, have been used in the treatment of fecal incontinence. This article briefly covers each of these aspects, to highlight the complex nature of the distal 5 to 10 cm of the distal alimentary tract and to provide further insight into managing patients with fecal incontinence.

## EVALUATION

Normal continence is an intricate process that involves the coordinated interaction between multiple different neuronal pathways and the pelvic and perineal muscula-ture. Many other factors, including systemic disease, emotional effect, bowel motility, stool consistency, evacuation efficiency, pelvic floor stability, and sphincter integrity, play a role in normal regulation. Failure at any level may result in an impaired ability to control gas or stool. Invaluable information can be gathered from physical examina-tion. At this assessment, it is imperative for the physician to be able to differentiate normal findings from abnormal ones, a skill that can only be acquired from a complete perineal examination of the many different types of patients seen by surgeons, not just those with fecal incontinence. However, even a well-performed physical examination has limitations. Anal inspection and digital rectal examination are poor for detecting sphincter defects, especially those less than 90°. Furthermore, specific questions relating to the overall health and bowel function of the patient need to be ascertained. Even with the most in-depth history taking and physical examination, fecal inconti-nence often demands further workup with ancillary studies.

This highlights the value of an integrated approach. The patient presenting with fecal incontinence may have a plethora of concomitant pelvic floor defects that will affect their current function and may affect results of future therapy. As such, physicians need to have an organized approach to evaluation for optimal management of these patients and to avoid pitfalls that may ultimately lead to failed outcomes. Studies, such as endoanal ultrasound, MRI, and defecography, are useful in identifying sphincter defects and in demonstrating concomitant pathology in up to 43% of patients undergoing workup for fecal incontinence. Anorectal manometry and anorec-tal electrophysiology testing also provide anal canal pressures and information regarding nerve function, respectively. Although each of these procedures provides valuable additional information, they do have some drawbacks. Manometry lacks specific correlation with any specific anatomic defect, and it has associated wide vari-ations in normal pressures that differ with age and gender. Manometry similarly has variable efficacy in correlating with postoperative symptomatic improvement. Anal electromyography has shown inconsistent effects on predicting success following repair, thus limiting its overall use. Pudendal neuropathy, when present, is highly vari-able for predicting improvements in continence following repair. Unilateral neuropathy has conflicting correlation with manometric or fecal incontinence severity scores. Bilateral neuropathy, in general, correlates with worse scores and decreased mean resting but not squeeze pressures. Unfortunately, the presence of neuropathy may not predict outcome of repair, and normal pudendal nerve terminal motor latencies do not exclude problems with pelvic dysfunction. Although individual tests may not be prognostic, when treated as part of the entire incontinence evaluation, they may provide valuable information when considering surgery and counseling patients as to potential postoperative outcomes.

Test availability may be a determining factor for the studies that can be performed. If access is limited, endoanal ultrasonography, with the goal of identifying a sphincter injury, is the most likely examination to affect the treatment recommendation. However, limiting evaluation to one test has the risk of missing other significant factors that could influence treatment outcome. Although the understanding of incontinence and appropriate evaluation has improved, the most effective and efficient algorithm remains to be identified.

## BIOFEEDBACK

Pelvic floor exercises with biofeedback are often beneficial when combined with the addition of dietary modifications. Biofeedback educates patients regarding pelvic floor coordination, recognition of sensory thresholds, and conditioning of the pelvic musculature, and it helps develop improved pelvic floor habits.[8–10] Biofeedback may be performed in various ways, but most often, it involves placement of a pressure-sensitive probe transanally to monitor the strength and coordination of the sphincter and levator ani muscles. By transmitting data from the probe to a monitor, patients are able to see a representation of the pelvic floor activity during defecation. Through a series of exercises and visual feedback, improvements can be made in muscle control and overall defecation. It is thought that biofeedback may also improve rectal sensation. A study from St Mark's Hospital has demonstrated that biofeedback is beneficial in treating urge incontinence and passive fecal incontinence.[11] A randomized controlled trial at the same institution has shown that biofeedback did not offer any additional benefit to patients when compared with those offered standard care (advise on diet, fluids, evacuation techniques, bowel training, and antidiarrheal medications).[12] Although similar studies with somewhat contradictory results may create doubt as to biofeedback's effectiveness, this may be more or a reflection of patient selection, motivation, and compliance with the therapy. At a minimum, biofeedback is risk-free and safe and may provide drastic improvements for those suffering from fecal incontinence, especially those experiencing concomitant minor obstructed defecation symptoms.

## ANAL SPHINCTEROPLASTY

Surgery may be indicated for patients with significant symptoms who have failed medical management. Most importantly, surgical repair of the anal sphincter is indicated only for patients with a defined sphincter injury. Those with patulous but intact sphincters receive no benefit from sphincteroplasty or attempts to "tighten things up." Several patients undergoing anal sphincteroplasty have persisting mild symptoms postoperatively. Thus, patients with significant preoperative symptoms are better candidates for this treatment option than patients with mild incontinence symptoms. Several different validated scoring systems, such as the Fecal Incontinence Severity Index, Fecal Incontinence Quality of Life, and Cleveland Clinic Incontinence (Wexner) score help in gauging pre- and postoperative dysfunction. In patients with significant symptoms, this operation is fairly simple, with an associated short hospital stay and satisfactory short-term results. Several studies have demonstrated good or excellent short-term results in two-thirds of patients (**Table 1**). However, results tend to

**Table 1**
**Results of anal sphincteroplasty**

|  | Year | Good or Excellent Outcome (%) |
|---|---|---|
| Oliveira et al[13] | 1996 | 71 |
| Malouf et al[7] | 2000 | 49 |
| Halverson and Hull[14] | 2002 | 25 |
| Bravo Gutierrez et al[15] | 2004 | 6 |
| Trowbridge et al[16] | 2006 | 11 |

worsen over time and are satisfactory in less than half the patients after longer follow-up.[7,8] Although this should not be a reason to avoid surgical repair in appropriate candidates, patients must be made aware of expected outcomes.

Anal sphincteroplasty is usually performed in the prone jack-knife position. Full bowel preparation is usually preferred, and studies have indicated better results with use of perioperative antibiotic prophylaxis. An overlapping technique is usually preferred and the internal and external anal sphincters can be repaired en bloc or separately (**Figs. 1** and **2**). Dissection anteriorly above the level of scar tissue with proper mobilization of the sphincters laterally provides excellent apposition of scar and muscle for ideal results. To avoid damage to the pudendal nerves innervating the region, care should be taken to avoid too aggressive a dissection posterior-laterally.

Early suboptimal outcomes have been associated with persisting sphincter defects at postoperative workup. Deterioration of continence function over time after surgical repair is unfortunately fairly common. Several studies have demonstrated suboptimal late outcomes.[7,14,15] Yet, many patients experience at least some degree of improvement. In combination with an adequate bulking regimen, properly selected patients may experience significantly improved quality of life.

## STIMULATED GRACILOPLASTY

Muscle transposition of the gracilis muscle was tried initially in the 1950s, but its outcome was limited by the inability to consciously maintain tonic contraction of the

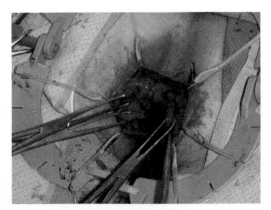

**Fig. 1.** Sphincter muscles dissected free in preparation for overlapping repair. (*Courtesy of* Justin A. Maykel, MD, Worcester, MA.)

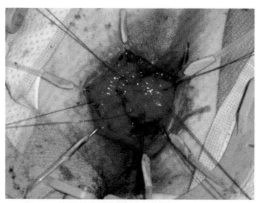

**Fig. 2.** Overlapping sphincter repair with horizontal mattress sutures in place. (*Courtesy of Justin A. Maykel, MD, Worcester, MA.*)

neosphincter over long periods of time. This has since been overcome by electrical stimulation of the transposed muscle. This technique involves mobilization of the gracilis muscle from the medial leg by detaching it distally at the knee, with a superior-based neurovascular pedicle. This muscle is then tunneled around the existing sphincter complex. An electronic pulse generator applies continuous low-grade current to aid tonic contraction of the muscle. It is thought that this continuous stimulation converts the skeletal muscle fibers of the gracilis to smooth muscle, allowing sustained contraction to aid in continence.

Success rates after stimulated gracioplasty have been satisfactory in several studies, but complication rates have been substantial. In one of the first reports, Baeten and coworkers[17] reported successful outcomes in 70% of 52 patients. In another multi-center study from 12 centers, Madoff and coworkers[18] reported similar success rates in 139 patients. Complication rates were however high; reported complications included pain, stimulator problems, wound complications, and so forth. At present, only a few select centers perform this procedure, and it is not approved in the United States.

## ARTIFICIAL ANAL SPHINCTER

Artificial sphincters were initially developed for the treatment of urinary incontinence.[19] This device has subsequently been modified and adapted for treatment of fecal incontinence. After perineal dissection, the device is placed around the existing sphincter complex. A tunnel is then constructed to hold a connecting reservoir and pump that controls filling (contraction) and emptying (relaxation) of the sphincter. Reports have demonstrated excellent results with good functional improvement and a significant increase in patient quality of life.[20,21] The largest series has been reported by Wong and coworkers[22] with 78 of 112 patients (70%) retaining a functioning device (after 7 successful reimplantations). Similar to the stimulated gracioplasty, complication rate was high at 87%, including patients who needed surgery (46%) or device explantation (37%). With a longer follow-up period, Altomare and colleagues[23] have reported more disappointing long-term results. Patients undergo a trial period of learning to control the sphincter, and most require minor adjustments to the apparatus.

The artificial sphincter is an approved treatment in the United States. This treatment option is used for end-stage fecal incontinence in selected patients who do not have other treatment alternatives, except for colostomy. The artificial anal sphincter is primarily used at specialist centers or those with dedicated interest and experience, because complication rates are substantial, especially in inexperienced hands.

## SACRAL NERVE STIMULATION

Like the artificial sphincter, sacral nerve stimulation (SNS) was initially developed to be used in urinary dysfunction.[24] The first stimulators were implanted in 1981 for urinary urge incontinence and nonobstructive urinary retention.[25,26] Since that time, several additional clinical benefits have been discovered, including re-establishment of pelvic floor muscle awareness, resolution of pelvic floor muscle tension and pain, decreased vestibulitis and vulvodynia, decreased bladder pain (for interstitial cystitis), and normalization of bowel function.[27]

In 1995, Matzel and coworkers[28] were the first to report the benefits of SNS in fecal incontinence. SNS treatment for fecal incontinence has traditionally been restricted to patients with an intact external sphincter and symptoms of fecal incontinence. However, recent evidence has challenged the limitations of these indications. Case reports and small studies indicate that SNS may also be beneficial in patients with disrupted sphincters.

The exact mechanism behind the success of SNS is unclear. SNS applies a low-amplitude electrical current to a sacral nerve through an electrode that is placed through a corresponding sacral foramen. The stimulation of the sacral nerves leads to recruitment of the pelvic floor musculature and pelvic organs, leading to improvement in pelvic floor function.[25,29] The third sacral foramen is the level at which an optimal response is most commonly elicited.[25] The third sacral nerve root contains afferent sensory and efferent autonomic motor nerves and voluntary somatic fibers, which may, alone or in harmony, create the beneficial effect elicited by SNS.[25] Additionally, there is a local spinal reflex arc effect, leading to increased rectal blood flow, reduced rectal sensory threshold, and improved balloon expulsion time.[30–33]

SNS is a 2-stage procedure. The first stage of the procedure may be completed under local or general anesthesia. With the patient in prone position, several of the S2 to S4 foramina are cannulated and tested for optimal response, and an electrode is left in one or several foramina.[33,34] Fluoroscopy may be used to confirm the position of the electrodes. The best response is frequently found in the S3 foramen and a typical S3 response is characterized clinically by plantar flexion of the patient's ipsilateral first toe and the "bellows response" of the pelvic floor.[33,34] A portable stimulator is then used to stimulate the implanted electrodes.[33] This tined lead is introduced with percutaneous technique and it has self-retaining flanges that minimize lead migration.[34,35] The second stage is completed in the operating room under local or general anesthesia. The procedure is completed with the patient in the prone position. A tined lead with self-retaining flanges is introduced with percutaneous technique and it is connected to a permanent stimulator surgically placed in a deep subcutaneous position in the gluteal region.[25] If the tined lead was used already during the testing phase, the external extension is removed and the lead already in place is connected to the permanent stimulator. The pulse generator can be activated and controlled by using an external programmer or via a hand-held device.[33]

Several studies have investigated the efficacy of SNS in fecal incontinence. Most of the studies are case series from specialized centers, whose patients had previously failed conservative management and experienced at least one episode of fecal incontinence each week.[25] An intact external sphincter was required in most studies. SNS for fecal incontinence has demonstrated encouraging results in published studies.[25] Approximately 80% of patients demonstrate success at the initial stage and qualify for permanent implant.[36–40] Most included patients (70%–88%) are women and the follow-up period ranges from 1 month to more than 8 years.[25] More than 75% of study participants reported greater than 50% improvement in continence episodes, whereas 41% to 75% of patients reported complete continence to liquid and solid stool.[36–40] Moderate increase in anal pressures and improved sensory function to rectal distension have been reported in some studies.

In a recent Cochrane review, 2 double-blind crossover studies of SNS for fecal incontinence were reviewed.[26] Leroi and coworkers[41] studied 34 patients following SNS for fecal incontinence. Patients were randomized, following implantation of the electrode, to "on" or "off" stimulation for periods of 1 month. Although patients were "blinded", they chose which period they preferred. Without unblinding the study, the preferred mode was continued by patients for 3 additional months. Participants receiving stimulation experienced a significant reduction in symptoms compared with the "off" cohort. Stimulation led to decrease in fecal incontinence episodes and symptom severity, and improved quality of life scores. Vaizey and coworkers[42] reported similar results in a study with similar design, but their study included only 2 participants.

In a recent study, Tjandra and coworkers[43] randomized patients with fecal incontinence to receive SNS or the best supportive therapy including pelvic floor exercises, bulking agents, and dietary modification. The study arms were evenly randomized and patients were followed for a period of 12 months. Patients randomized to receive SNS enjoyed a significant improvement in quality of life scores and incontinent episodes, and benefits were sustained throughout the follow-up period. Although future research is still needed to define the exact mechanisms underlying its success, SNS is one of the promising, exciting modalities for many incontinent patients who have previously been left with few other options.

## INJECTABLE BIOMATERIALS

Injection of bulk-enhancing agents into the anal canal area is being evaluated after some successful use in patients with urinary incontinence. This therapy can be performed in an outpatient setting without anesthesia. The agent is usually injected intersphincterically or submucosally. Different agents have been evaluated, including collagen, silicon beads, carbon beads, dextranomer/hyaluronic acid, and so forth. Results have demonstrated a low rate of complications and a mild-to-moderate effect on incontinence symptom improvement.[44–47] Unfortunately, this treatment option is still only available in investigational studies in the United States, whereas it is approved for clinical use in Europe. Being in its infancy, further recommendations and description of injectables' ultimate role in the care of incontinent patients remain to be described.

## SUMMARY

Fecal incontinence is a debilitating and socially embarrassing condition. Significant advances in the evaluation and treatment of this condition have been made in recent years and several new treatment modalities are in the pipeline to be made available to affected patients. Surgeons who care for these patients should have a thorough understanding of the medical, nonoperative, and operative components and the various studies available to properly select a treatment plan and optimize outcomes.

## REFERENCES

1. Nelson R, Norton N, Cautley E, et al. Community-based prevalence of anal incontinence. JAMA 1995;274:559–61.

2. Ho YH, Muller R, Veitch C, et al. Faecal incontinence: an unrecognised epidemic in rural North Queensland? Results of a hospital-based outpatient study. Aust J Rural Health 2005;13:28–34.

3. Siproudhis L, Pigot F, Godeberge P, et al. Defecation disorders: a French population survey. Dis Colon Rectum 2006;49:219–27.

4. Kalantar JS, Howell S, Talley NJ. Prevalence of faecal incontinence and associated risk factors; an underdiagnosed problem in the Australian community? Med J Aust 2002;176:54–7.

5. Enck P, Bielefeldt K, Rathmann W, et al. Epidemiology of faecal incontinence in selected patient groups. Int J Colorectal Dis 1991;6:143–6.

6. Perry S, Shaw C, McGrother C, et al. Prevalence of faecal incontinence in adults aged 40 years or more living in the community. Gut 2002;50:480–4.

7. Malouf AJ, Norton CS, Engel AF, et al. Long-term results of overlapping anterior anal-sphincter repair for obstetric trauma. Lancet 2000;355:260–5.

8. Madoff RD, Parker SC, Varma MG, et al. Faecal incontinence in adults. Lancet 2004;364:621–32.

9. Norton C, Cody JD, Hosker G. Biofeedback and/or sphincter exercises for the treatment of faecal incontinence in adults. Cochrane Database Syst Rev 2006;(3):CD002111.

10. Norton C, Hosker G, Brazzelli M. Biofeedback and/or sphincter exercises for the treatment of faecal incontinence in adults. Cochrane Database Syst Rev 2000;(4): CD002111.

11. Norton C, Kamm MA. Outcome of biofeedback for faecal incontinence. [erratum appears in Br J Surg 2000 Feb;87(2):249]. Br J Surg 1999;86:1159–63.

12. Norton C, Chelvanayagam S, Wilson-Barnett J, et al. Randomized controlled trial of biofeedback for fecal incontinence. Gastroenterology 2003;125:1320–9.

13. Oliveira L, Pfeifer J, Wexner SD. Physiological and clinical outcome of anterior sphincteroplasty. Br J Surg 1996;83:502–5.

14. Halverson AL, Hull TL. Long-term outcome of overlapping anal sphincter repair. Dis Colon Rectum 2002;45:345–8.

15. Bravo Gutierrez A, Madoff RD, Lowry AC, et al. Long-term results of anterior sphincteroplasty. Dis Colon Rectum 2004;47:727–31.

16. Trowbridge ER, Morgan D, Trowbridge MJ, et al. Sexual function, quality of life, and severity of anal incontinence after anal sphincteroplasty. Am J Obstet Gynecol 2006;195:1753–7.

17. Baeten CG, Geerdes BP, Adang EM, et al. Anal dynamic graciloplasty in the treatment of intractable fecal incontinence. N Engl J Med 1995;332:1600–5.

18. Madoff RD, Rosen HR, Baeten CG, et al. Safety and efficacy of dynamic muscle plasty for anal incontinence: lessons from a prospective, multicenter trial. Gastroenterology 1999;116:549–56.

19. Scott FB, Bradley WE, Timm GW. Treatment of urinary incontinence by an implantable prosthetic urinary sphincter. J Urol 1974;112:75–80.

20. Lehur PA, Glemain P, Bruley des Varannes S, et al. Outcome of patients with an implanted artificial anal sphincter for severe faecal incontinence. A single institution report. Int J Colorectal Dis 1998;13:88–92.

21. Parker SC, Spencer MP, Madoff RD, et al. Artificial bowel sphincter: long-term experience at a single institution. Dis Colon Rectum 2003;46:722–9.

22. Wong WD, Congliosi SM, Spencer MP, et al. The safety and efficacy of the artificial bowel sphincter for fecal incontinence: results from a multicenter cohort study. Dis Colon Rectum 2002;45:1139–53.

23. Altomare DF, Binda GA, Dodi G, et al. Disappointing long-term results of the artificial anal sphincter for faecal incontinence. Br J Surg 2004;91:1352–3.
24. Tanagho EA, Schmidt RA. Bladder pacemaker: scientific basis and clinical future. Urology 1982;20:614–9.
25. Jarrett MED, Mowatt G, Glazener CMA, et al. Systematic review of sacral nerve stimulation for faecal incontinence and constipation. Br J Surg 2004;91: 1559–69.
26. Mowatt G, Glazener C, Jarrett M. Sacral nerve stimulation for faecal incontinence and constipation in adults. Cochrane Database Syst Rev 2007;(3):CD004464.
27. Pettit PD, Thompson JR, Chen AH. Sacral neuromodulation: new applications in the treatment of female pelvic floor dysfunction. Curr Opin Obstet Gynecol 2002; 14:521–5.
28. Matzel KE, Stadelmaier U, Hohenfellner M, et al. Electrical stimulation of sacral spinal nerves for treatment of faecal incontinence. Lancet 1995;346:1124–7.
29. Tanagho EA. Concepts of neuromodulation. Neurourol Urodyn 1993;12:487–8.
30. Kenefick NJ, Emmanuel A, Nicholls RJ, et al. Effect of sacral nerve stimulation on autonomic nerve function. Br J Surg 2003;90:1256–60.
31. Kenefick NJ, Vaizey CJ, Cohen RC, et al. Medium-term results of permanent sacral nerve stimulation for faecal incontinence. Br J Surg 2002;89:896–901.
32. Ganio E, Ratto C, Masin A, et al. Neuromodulation for fecal incontinence: outcome in 16 patients with definitive implant. The initial Italian Sacral Neurostimulation Group (GINS) experience. Dis Colon Rectum 2001;44:965–70.
33. Tan JJ, Chan M, Tjandra JJ. Evolving therapy for fecal incontinence. Dis Colon Rectum 2007;50:1950–67.
34. Tjandra JJ, Lim JF, Matzel K. Sacral nerve stimulation: an emerging treatment for faecal incontinence. ANZ J Surg 2004;74:1098–106.
35. Matzel KE, Stadelmaier U, Hohenfellner M, et al. Chronic sacral spinal nerve stimulation for fecal incontinence: long-term results with foramen and cuff electrodes. Dis Colon Rectum 2001;44:59–66.
36. Leroi AM, Michot F, Grise P, et al. Effect of sacral nerve stimulation in patients with fecal and urinary incontinence. Dis Colon Rectum 2001;44:779–89.
37. Ganio E, Luc AR, Clerico G, et al. Sacral nerve stimulation for treatment of fecal incontinence: a novel approach for intractable fecal incontinence. Dis Colon Rectum 2001;44:619–29.
38. Jarrett MED, Varma JS, Duthie GS, et al. Sacral nerve stimulation for faecal incontinence in the UK. Br J Surg 2004;91:755–61.
39. Rosen HR, Urbarz C, Holzer B, et al. Sacral nerve stimulation as a treatment for fecal incontinence. Gastroenterology 2001;121:536–41.
40. Uludag O, Koch SM, van Gemert WG, et al. Sacral neuromodulation in patients with fecal incontinence: a single-center study. Dis Colon Rectum 2004;47:1350–7.
41. Leroi A-M, Parc Y, Lehur P-A, et al. Efficacy of sacral nerve stimulation for fecal incontinence: results of a multicenter double-blind crossover study. Ann Surg 2005;242:662–9.
42. Vaizey CJ, Kamm MA, Roy AJ, et al. Double-blind crossover study of sacral nerve stimulation for fecal incontinence. Dis Colon Rectum 2000;43:298–302.
43. Tjandra JJ, Chan MK, Yeh CH, et al. Sacral nerve stimulation is more effective than optimal medical therapy for severe fecal incontinence: a randomized, controlled study. Dis Colon Rectum 2008;51:494–502.
44. Stojkovic SG, Lim M, Burke D, et al. Intra-anal collagen injection for the treatment of faecal incontinence. Br J Surg 2006;93:1514–8.

45. Tjandra JJ, Lim JF, Hiscock R, et al. Injectable silicone biomaterial for fecal incontinence caused by internal anal sphincter dysfunction is effective. Dis Colon Rectum 2004;47:2138–46.

46. de la Portilla F, Fernández A, León E, et al. Evaluation of the use of PTQ implants for the treatment of incontinent patients due to internal anal sphincter dysfunction. Int J Colorectal Dis 2008;10:89–94.

47. Kenefick NJ, Vaizey CJ, Malouf AJ, et al. Injectable silicone biomaterial for faecal incontinence due to internal anal sphincter dysfunction. [retraction in Kenefick NJ, Vaizey CJ, Malouf AJ, Norton CS, Marshall M, Kamm MA. Gut. 2006 Dec;55(12):1824; PMID: 17171815]. Gut 2002;51:225–8.

# Overview of Pelvic Floor Disorders

M. Shane McNevin, MD, FASCRS[a,b,*]

KEYWORDS

• Pelvic floor disorders • Rectocele • Entercele
• Rectal prolapse

Pelvic floor disorders are an underdiagnosed source of morbidity and decreased quality of life for women,[1] while it is a much less common disorder in men. In the United States, almost 24% of women report at least one pelvic floor disorder, which, unfortunately, increases with age, parity, and obesity.[2,3] The demand for pelvic floor services is expected to grow at twice the rate of the population in the coming decades as the relative proportion of the elderly increases and physicians become more aware of these disorders.[4]

Patients with pelvic floor disorders typically present with symptoms of pelvic organ prolapse, dysfunctional bowel, or bladder evacuation. In the general population, approximately 16% of women experience urinary incontinence, 9% experience fecal incontinence, and 3% experience pelvic organ prolapse.[2] This appears to be most related to pregnancy carriage and childbirth, regardless of route.[5–8] In addition to problems with bowel continence, patients with poor posterior or central pelvic floor support may also complain of symptoms of obstructed defecation. In these cases, patients often cite excessive straining to no avail, feeling of inability to expel the stool without digitizing, or chronic pelvic pain with bowel movements. Furthermore, while constipation is reported in 32% of adult women in the general population, the relative percentage of this complaint is increased even more by the presence of advanced genital organ prolapse and posterior colpocele.[9,10] To add to the problem, each pelvic floor complaint has a high propensity to coexist with others, making multispecialty evaluation and care essential.[9–12]

Even for those patients without defined anatomic defects, functional disorders of the gastrointestinal tract or pelvic floor unrelated to prior obstetric experience are also common.[12–15] This often manifests with chronic pain or functional bowel complaints similar to obstructive defecation or slow-transit constipation.

This article focuses on disorders of the posterior and central pelvic floor compartments. Symptom complex, diagnostic testing, nonoperative and operative management of common pelvic floor disorders are reviewed.

[a] Providence Continence Center, Spokane, WA, USA
[b] Surgical Specialists of Spokane, 105 W 8th Avenue Suite 7060, Spokane, WA 99204, USA
* Surgical Specialists of Spokane, 105 W 8th Avenue Suite 7060, Spokane, WA 99204.
*E-mail address:* skmcnevin@comcast.net

Surg Clin N Am 90 (2010) 195–205
doi:10.1016/j.suc.2009.10.003
0039-6109/09/$ – see front matter

## PELVIC FLOOR DIAGNOSTICS

As with many disease processes, it is increasingly recognized that patients with pelvic floor complaints benefit from a multispecialty evaluation focusing on colorectal, gynecologic, and urologic surgical care. Often, isolated evaluation leads to identification of only one component of a multisystem process. Operative fixation of one may lead to "failure" or, more likely, unmasking an existing problem (ie, worsening urinary incontinence following repair of rectal prolapse). Thus, a thorough history and physical examination of these patients is imperative to identify all elements creating problems. Yet, physical examination, while important, is historically poor for identification of many common pelvic floor problems. Therefore, comprehensive pelvic floor testing in a stand-alone laboratory facilitates this evaluation, and is a very efficient and convenient process for the patient.[16] Tests germane to the posterior pelvis and frequently used by the colorectal surgeon are discussed below.

## SYMPTOM ASSESSMENT

Patients with disorders of the central and posterior compartments of the pelvic floor often present with complaints of pelvic organ prolapse or disordered gastrointestinal elimination—either fecal incontinence or obstructed defecation. A careful history and physical examination is key to establishing a working clinical diagnosis and directing diagnostic testing. Often, patients present with vague complaints and it is vital that a careful description of the patient's symptoms in their own words be obtained to better define the clinical scenario.

Symptoms of pelvic organ prolapse manifest as protrusion of anorectal or vaginal tissue past the anal verge or vaginal introitus. This may exist alone or in combination with symptoms of dysfunctional bowel elimination. Constipation symptoms related to pelvic floor dysfunction usually manifest as obstructed defecation. The history is quite typical in most cases. Patients describe excessive and prolonged straining at stool, pain with defecation, the need for manual perineal support (splinting), and incomplete evacuation of the rectum.

Patients with disorders of bowel continence present with the involuntary loss of bowel contents. History should differentiate true incontinence from pseudoincontinence. In the latter, patients have the ability to adequately hold in gas or stool, but complain of mucus or stool seepage (often following bowel movements) or difficulties with good perianal hygiene. For patients with true incontinence, further differentiating among overflow incontinence, incontinence with a normal pelvic floor, and incontinence with an abnormal pelvic floor is helpful to direct testing and plan appropriate interventions.

Once the primary symptoms are clear, proceeding with a careful gastrointestinal, gynecologic, obstetric, and urologic history is paramount to determine the cause of the complaints. Patients with primary gastrointestinal or gynecologic pathology or prior surgery are frequently troubled by bowel evacuation disorders and pelvic organ prolapse. Additionally, patients with pelvic floor disorders often experience sexual dysfunction that can be exacerbated by pelvic floor reconstruction. The majority of pelvic floor disorders are related to remote obstetric injuries; hence, a careful history of parity, mode of delivery, and complications of delivery is useful. Finally, patients with symptoms referable to the posterior and central compartments frequently have coexisting dysfunction of the anterior compartment that benefit from concomitant treatment. Assessments of urologic and gynecologic symptoms facilitate this evaluation.

As such, both symptom severity and impact on quality of life should be determined because they are helpful to direct therapy and assess response. Symptoms of pelvic floor dysfunction significantly impair quality of life, yet don't typically have an impending risk to health or longevity. Decisions regarding the need for treatment and the acceptable risk of that treatment should take this fact into account, especially when counseling patients and choosing proper operative candidates. Currently, objective measures of pelvic floor disorders are imperfect, although standardized, validated measures of both fecal incontinence and obstructed defecation exist.[17,18] Recognizing their limitations, these metrics still have a role in research protocols, documenting treatment efficacy, and are also useful for patients undergoing pelvic floor treatment in comprehensive nonacademic pelvic floor centers.

## ENDOANAL ULTRASOUND

Endoanal ultrasound is the primary diagnostic modality for patients undergoing evaluation for fecal incontinence. It allows for more accurate determination of defects in the internal and external anal sphincter, and length of the anal canal, than other modalities.[19] The external sphincter appears as a circumferential hyperechoic structure in the anal canal, while the internal sphincter appears as the hypoechoic inner circle. Sphincter defects are demonstrated by "graying" or incomplete rings representing scarring, which are commonly seen in the anterior midline with childbirth injuries (**Fig. 1**).

## ANORECTAL MANOMETRY

Anorectal manometry is traditionally used for evaluation of patients with fecal incontinence. It allows for a precise definition of resting and squeeze pressures of the anal canal, and length of the high-pressure zone of the anus. Additional information obtained is the presence of the rectoanal inhibitory reflex denoting appropriate anorectal innervation. This data point can also be used as a screening tool for Hirschsprung disease, with its absence suggesting aberrant innervation to be confirmed

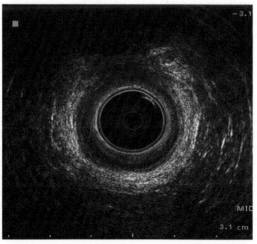

**Fig. 1.** Endoanal ultrasound demonstrating an anterior external anal sphincter defect as demonstrated by the incomplete hyperechoic ring. (*Courtesy of* Susan C. Parker, MD.)

with a rectal biopsy. Rectal sensory thresholds also provide valuable information regarding rectal volume at first sensation, urge to defecate, and maximal tolerable volume. These data points define both the frequency and urgency of defecation and are typically lower in poor compliance patients (ie, prior radiation therapy or chronic proctitis).

## PUDENDAL NERVE TERMINAL MOTOR LATENCY TESTING

Pudendal nerve testing is conducted using the St Mark's probe and is diagnostic of injury to this peripheral nerve supplying voluntary control to the anal sphincter complex. Prolongation of electrical impulse through this nerve may have impacts on fecal control and is prognostically relevant for patients undergoing anal sphincter reconstruction.[20] It is easily performed by placing the glove with the electrode attached into the anal canal on each ischial tuberosity and measuring the total time for the reflex arc following stimulation.

## ANORECTAL ELECTROMYOGRAPHY

Anorectal electromyography is primarily useful for the evaluation of patients with obstructed defecation. It senses electrical activity in the pelvic floor musculature during rest, squeeze, and push, and can be useful to identify patients with paradoxic contraction of the puborectalis.[21] In this situation, the normal relaxation of the levator ani muscles that occurs with Valsalva is paradoxically contracted, causing difficulty with defecation. Patients with abnormal electromyography should undergo confirmatory testing with dynamic defecography.

## DYNAMIC DEFECOGRAPHY

Dynamic defecography provides the most detailed functional anatomic view of the pelvis. Traditionally, this has been performed in the upright position using lateral fluoroscopic view as the patient expels a thickened barium paste from the rectum. Ingestion of oral contrast to opacify the small bowel, placement of contrast material in the vagina and bladder, and injection of intraperitoneal contrast into the peritoneum to better define anatomy have also been described. This is an invaluable test for evaluation of symptoms of obstructed defecation and pelvic organ prolapse.[21–23]

Magnetic resonance imaging defecography has been recently developed and is gaining increased support as an improved alternative to traditional techniques of defecography.[23–27]

## BIOFEEDBACK

Biofeedback is an essential component of a comprehensive pelvic floor center. It is a technique using operant conditioning that reinforces positive behavior, thereby retraining the pelvic floor to optimize function. Therapy at this point is nonstandardized with respect to techniques, frequency of encounters, and duration of therapy. In many cases, a several week cycle of multiple pelvic floor exercises combined with a transanal probe displaying visual feedback to monitor pelvic floor activity during the squeeze-relax-push cycle is used. Therapy is typically performed by nurses or physical therapists with advanced training and interest in pelvic floor disorders. Outcomes can be very dependent on the affect of the therapist and patient acceptance of this technique. Many patients with functional disorders of the bowel and bladder undergo successful nonoperative treatment with biofeedback.[28–32]

## MANAGEMENT OF SPECIFIC DISORDERS OF THE PELVIC FLOOR

Pelvic floor disorders are ubiquitous and increasing in frequency. While a cause of significant morbidity and reduction in quality of life, they rarely have any impact on overall physical health or longevity. It is therefore essential to accurately identify the specific complaints associated with the pelvic disorder and the impact of those complaints on quality of life. Diagnostic and therapeutic intervention should only be undertaken when the reduction in quality of life is to such a degree that it outweighs morbidity and functional consequences of the treatment modality. Goals of therapy should be relief of symptoms and restoration of normal pelvic floor anatomy.

### RECTOCELE

Rectoceles arise from loss of anterior rectal support from the rectovaginal septum. This can occur as a result of an age-related decline in tissue integrity or a traumatic disruption typically related to prior obstetric trauma. Somewhat clouding the situation, approximately 80% of adult women have rectoceles–the majority of which are small, asymptomatic, and require no treatment. Larger rectoceles (>2 cm) typically come to clinical attention owing to symptoms of vaginal prolapse, obstructed defecation, or a combination of the two. Patients may also complain of anorectal or vaginal pain and sexual dysfunction. In addition, many patients with symptomatic rectoceles note the need for posterior vaginal wall or perineal pressure to have a bowel movement. Careful history and physical examination to define the specific presenting symptoms, their impact on quality of life, and patient expectations of treatment are critical to determine the optimum treatment plan.

Patients with symptomatic rectoceles noted on history and physical examination should undergo confirmatory imaging with dynamic or MRI defecography before intervention. Patients with primary complaints of vaginal prolapse and a confirmed rectocele may be offered surgical reconstruction with the expectation of reliable relief of their symptoms. For patients not fit for surgery or desiring a less invasive alternative, pessary use may be considered. Reports have supported repair via the transvaginal, transrectal, and transperineal approaches with levator plication (levatoroplasty). While all approaches reliably relieve the symptoms of vaginal prolapse, it is at the cost of appreciable operative morbidity and recurrence risk, vaginal anatomic distortion, and a significant risk of dyspareunia where the procedures differ.[33–37] Attempts to alleviate these disadvantages have led to the concept of rectovaginal septal repair or discrete fascial defect repair.[38,39] A more controversial approach that is gaining increased acceptance is mesh-based reconstruction of the rectovaginal septum using either prosthetic or biologic mesh systems. These may be particularly advantageous in cases of recurrent prolapse or patients at high risk of primary failure.[40–43]

Patients with primary complaints of obstructed defecation should understand that surgical reconstruction of the rectocele has less reliable improvement in functional bowel complaints. Many of these patients may be successfully managed nonoperatively by stool bulking with fiber and biofeedback.[44] For patients failing nonoperative therapy, all of the aforementioned rectocele repair techniques have been used with varying success and durability. Another alternative for those with rectoceles, with or without internal rectal prolapse as defined by defecography, and refractory symptoms of obstructed defecation who have failed nonoperative therapy is the Stapled Transanal Rectal Resection (STARR) procedure. This approach uses a transluminal gastrointestinal stapling device to resect the redundant anterior and posterior rectal walls, thereby restoring normal rectal anatomy and reducing rectal volume. Results have been overall positive, though appreciable operative morbidity (up to 36%) and long-term functional consequences including urgency, bleeding, recurrence, rectovaginal fistula, persistent obstructive defecation, sepsis, and incontinence have all been described.[45–48]

## ENTEROCELE OR VAGINAL VAULT PROLAPSE

Enterocele and vaginal vault prolapse may exist in isolation of each other, but are coexistent in the majority of cases. Enterocele is most commonly located posteriorly between the vagina and rectum, and contains small bowel or omentum. It may be congenital or, more commonly, acquired through either a pulsion or traction phenomenon. It may also be iatrogenic in etiology, mostly related to prior vaginal surgery. Vaginal vault prolapse results from a loss of apical vaginal fixation allowing descent of the vaginal vault and may be acquired in a similar fashion. Patients typically present with complaints of vaginal wall protrusion and symptoms of obstructed defecation. Chronic pelvic and low back pain may also result, are typically worse throughout the day and while upright, and are classically relieved with recumbency. Dyspareunia is also a frequent complaint, and can be quite debilitating. As with other pelvic floor disorders, careful history and physical examination is essential to clarify symptoms and their severity and thereby determine the appropriate therapy. If an enterocele is clinically suspected, confirmation with pelvic floor testing either dynamic or MRI defecography is again helpful.

For symptomatic patients with a confirmed enterocele or vaginal vault prolapse, intervention is appropriate. For patients unfit for surgery or desiring a nonoperative approach, a pessary and lifestyle alteration is an alternative. For patients with symptoms refractory to this approach or desiring definitive management, operative intervention is required. The surgical approach can be either transabdominal or transvaginal, and is often determined by overall patient performance status. With either approach, patients without prior uterine resection are often treated with hysterectomy in conjunction with apical vaginal support and enterocele closure. For younger patients with good performance status, an abdominal approach offers a more durable and functionally better repair. The gold standard is abdominal sacral colpopexy with either prosthetic or biologic mesh support. A number of plication procedures to manage the enterocele sac may be concomitantly performed.[49] With surgeons increasingly facile with advanced laparoscopic or robotic techniques, this procedure has become less invasive in recent years.[50,51] Patients with poor performance status or patients with relative contra-indications for abdominal surgery are considered for a transvaginal approach. For patients without any desire to preserve sexual function, a vaginal obliterative procedure, colpocleisis, is an attractive approach for its relative ease and safety.[52] Traditionally, the transvaginal approach has used sacrospinous ligament fixation to support the vaginal apex concomitant with high ligation of the enterocele sac. As with the various native tissue repairs described for rectoceles, concerns regarding durability and vaginal function have plagued native tissue repairs for vaginal vault prolapse.[53,54] Similar to rectocele, transvaginal prosthetic or biologic mesh repairs are still controversial, though gaining increased acceptance. Reports documenting early results have showed improved durability and acceptable morbidity rates of these mesh-based repairs.[55]

## RECTAL PROLAPSE

Full-thickness procidentia is a disturbing syndrome of eversion of the rectum through the anal verge. It is vastly more common in females, with an increasing incidence with age. Unfortunately, the cause of the disorder remains idiopathic. The primary symptom initiating physician contact is rectal protrusion, either spontaneously or with Valsalva. This can be associated with anorectal pain or a mucoid, bloody discharge. Patients also frequently complain of symptoms of obstructed defecation or fecal incontinence. Examination is usually diagnostic with a characteristic patulous anus and protrusion of the full thickness of the rectal wall with concentric mucosal folds. If a patient is unable to demonstrate the prolapse in the examination room, a Valsalva test on the commode usually produces the prolapse. It is important to avoid examination in the prone jackknife position, as this may not demonstrate the full extent (or any) of the prolapse, even for advanced prolapse. Occasionally, radiographic imaging with dynamic or MRI defecography is required to demonstrate the procidentia. All patients should undergo endoscopic evaluation irrespective of treatment intention, as an uncommon but important association of prolapse occurs with rectal polyps, tumors, or colitis.

As with the other pelvic floor disorders, patient symptoms dictate the need for surgical intervention. A small, asymptomatic prolapse does not necessarily require surgical correction. For patients with symptomatic rectal prolapse, surgical intervention is indicated. Abdominal and perineal approaches have been well described. Like other forms of pelvic organ prolapse, the approach is largely determined by patient performance status. The perineal approach has the advantage of lower perioperative morbidity, but at the cost of higher recurrence and poorer functional results.[56,57] In general, elderly patients, those with significant medical comorbidities, or those with contraindications for abdominal surgery are chosen for the perineal approach. Usually, a perineal rectosigmoidectomy or Delorme procedure is then performed. The perineal rectosigmoidectomy involves the full-thickness resection of the prolapse with a coloanal anastomosis, whereas the Delorme procedure uses a mucosectomy of the prolapsed segment and rectal muscular wall plication. Both procedures can be performed under general or spinal anesthesia. The perineal rectosigmoidectomy has the advantage of a lower recurrence rate and improved continence, but is associated with a higher anastomotic complication rate.[56,58]

Younger, more active patients are more suited to the abdominal approach, and are largely treated with either a rectopexy alone or rectopexy with sigmoid resection. Both procedures involve rectal mobilization with preservation of the lateral rectal stalks and suture fixation of the rectum to the upper sacrum. As with many other surgical procedures, laparoscopic and robotic techniques are now common and efficacious for abdominal approaches to chronic rectal prolapse.[56] A particularly vexing problem with the abdominal rectopexy alone is the development of postoperative constipation. Patients should be questioned preoperatively for a history significant constipation, as this may alter the operative approach. Attempts to minimize this postoperatively involve the addition of the sigmoid colectomy and preservation of the lateral rectal stalks.[56] A newer technique seeking to alleviate this problem is ventral rectopexy, which appears to have similar rates of morbidity and recurrence, with less postoperative constipation.[59] This procedure may be performed with various minor technical differences; however, in general, involves an anterior nerve-sparing dissection (ie, in the rectal-vaginal septum) to the pelvic floor with mesh fixation of the ventral rectum, posterior vagina and vaginal fornix to the sacral promontory.

## FUNCTIONAL DISORDERS OF THE PELVIC FLOOR

Functional disorders of the pelvic floor result in typical symptoms of obstructed defecation unassociated with an anatomic abnormality of the pelvic floor. These are exceedingly common and often vexing problems to treat.

### Paradoxic Puborectalis

During normal defecation mechanics, relaxation of the pelvic floor occurs allowing the pelvic floor to descend and the distal rectum to shift posteriorly thereby straightening the anorectal angle. Inappropriate contraction of the puborectalis muscle decreases the anorectal angle and obstructs the rectal outlet, inhibiting rectal evacuation. This is felt to be a learned phenomenon seen typically in patients who neglect the call to defecate. Diagnosis is suggested by physical examination when the puborectalis is felt to contract inappropriately when the patient is asked to strain or push during digital rectal examination. Confirmatory testing with a combination of anorectal electromyogram and dynamic defecography is diagnostic. Biofeedback is the treatment of choice with improvement in 40% to 60% of patients that are able to complete the therapy.[60,61]

### Abnormal Perineal Descent

As opposed to inappropriate contraction of the puborectalis, excessive relaxation of the levator ani can also result in difficulties with rectal evacuation and fecal incontinence. Physical examination and dynamic defecography are diagnostic. Treatment remains conservative with dietary manipulation, cathartics, and biofeedback. Unfortunately, outcomes of these conservative measures are relatively poor with less than 30% experiencing major symptomatic improvement.[62]

### SUMMARY

Pelvic floor disorders are an underdiagnosed and undertreated cause of major morbidity and reduction in quality of life that appear to be increasing in frequency with our aging population. Specialized, multidisciplinary pelvic floor diagnostic and treatment facilities can have a pronounced impact on the care of these patients. Careful history and physical examination are important to determine appropriate diagnostic and therapeutic intervention. Many patients can be treated with simple dietary modification and pelvic floor retraining with biofeedback. While many efficacious surgical reconstructive options are available, careful selection of patients optimizes results.

### REFERENCES

1. Handa VL, Cundiff G, Chang HH, et al. Female sexual function and pelvic floor disorders. Obstet Gynecol 2008;111(5):1045–52.
2. Nygaard I, Barber MD, Burgio KL, et al. Pelvic floor disorders network. Prevalence of symptomatic pelvic floor disorders in US women. JAMA 2008;300(11): 1311–6.
3. MacLennan AH, Taylor AW, Wilson DH, et al. The prevalence of pelvic floor disorders and their relationship to gender, age, parity and mode of delivery. BJOG 2000;107(12):1460–70.
4. Walters MD. Pelvic floor disorders in women: an overview. Rev Med Univ Navarra 2004;48(4):9–12, 15–7.
5. Borello-France D, Burgio KL, Richter HE, et al. Pelvic floor disorders. Fecal and urinary incontinence in primiparous women. Obstet Gynecol 2006;108(4):863–72.
6. Lukacz ES, Lawrence JM, Contreras R, et al. Parity, mode of delivery and pelvic floor disorders. Obstet Gynecol 2006;107(6):1253–60.
7. NIH state of the science conference statement on prevention of fecal and urinary incontinence in adults. NIH Consensus State Sci Statements 2007;24(1):1–37.

8. Uustal Fornell E, Wingren G, Kjolhede P. Factors associated with pelvic floor dysfunction with emphasis on urinary and fecal incontinence and genital prolapse: an epidemiologic study. Acta Obstet Gynecol Scand 2004;83(4):383–9.
9. Soligo M, Salvatore S, Emmanuel AV, et al. Patterns of constipation in urogynecology: clinical importance and pathophysiologic insights. Am J Obstet Gynecol 2006;195(1):50–5.
10. Jelovsek JE, Barber MD, Paraiso MF, et al. Functional bowel and anorectal disorders in patients with pelvic organ prolapse. Am J Obstet Gynecol 2005;193(6):2105–11.
11. Meschia M, Buonaguidi A, Pifarotti P, et al. Prevalence of anal incontinence in women with symptoms of urinary incontinence and genital prolapse. Obstet Gynecol 2002;100(4):719–23.
12. Nichols CM, Ramakrishnan V, Gill EJ, et al. Anal incontinence in women with and those without pelvic floor disorders. Obstet Gynecol 2005;106(6):1266–71.
13. Whitehead WE, Wald A, Diamant NE, et al. Functional disorders of the anus and rectum. Gut 1999;45(Suppl 2):II55–9.
14. Whitehead WE. Functional anorectal disorders. Semin Gastrointest Dis 1996;7(4):230–6.
15. Bharucha AE, Wald A, Enck P, et al. Functional anorectal disorders. Gastroenterology 2006;130(5):1510–8.
16. Kapoor DS, Sultan AH, Thakar R, et al. Management of complex pelvic floor disorders in a multispecialty pelvic floor clinic. Colorectal Dis 2008;10(2):118–23.
17. Altomare DF, Spazzafumo L, Rinaldi M, et al. Set-up and statistical validation of a new scoring system for obstructed defecation syndrome. Colorectal Dis 2008;10(1):84–8.
18. Rockwood TH, Church JM, Fleshman JW, et al. Patient and surgeon ranking of the severity of symptoms associated with fecal incontinence: the fecal incontinence severity index. Dis Colon Rectum 1999;42(12):1525–32.
19. Sultan AH, Kamm MA, Hudson CN, et al. Endosonography of the anal sphincter: normal anatomy and comparison with manometry. Clin Radiol 1994;49:368–74.
20. Ricciardi R, Mellgren AF, Madoff RD, et al. The utility of pudendal nerve terminal motor latencies in idiopathic incontinence. Dis Colon Rectum 2006;49(6):852–7.
21. Andromanakos N, Skandalakis P, Troupis T, et al. Constipation of anorectal outlet obstruction: pathophysiology, evaluation and management. J Gastroenterol Hepatol 2006;21(4):638–46.
22. Jorge JM, Habr-Gama A, Wexner SD. Clinical applications and techniques of cinedefecography. Am J Surg 2001;182(1):93–101.
23. Ganeshan A, Anderson EM, Upponi S, et al. Imaging of obstructed defecation. Clin Radiol 2008;63(1):18–26.
24. Stoker J, Bartram CI, Halligan S. Imaging of the posterior pelvic floor. Eur Radiol 2002;12(4):779–88.
25. Seynaeve R, Billiet I, Vossaert P, et al. MR imaging of the pelvic floor. JBR-BTR 2006;89(4):182–9.
26. Fletcher JG, Busse RF, Riederer SJ, et al. Magnetic resonance imaging of anatomic and dynamic defects of the pelvic floor in defecatory disorders. Am J Gastroenterol 2003;98(2):399–411.
27. Rentsch M, Paetzel C, Lenhart M, et al. Dynamic magnetic resonance imaging defecography: a diagnostic alternative in the assessment of pelvic floor disorders in proctology. Dis Colon Rectum 2001;44(7):999–1007.
28. Ko CY, Tong J, Lehman RE, et al. Biofeedback is effective therapy for fecal incontinence and constipation. Arch Surg 1997;132(8):829–33.

29. Jorge JM, Habr-Gama A, Raivio P, et al. The role of biofeedback therapy in functional proctologic disorders. Scand J Surg 2004;93(3):184–90.

30. Kairaluoma M, Raivio P, Kupila J, et al. The role of biofeedback therapy in functional proctologic disorders. Scand J Surg 2004;93(3):184–90.

31. Heymen S, Jones KR, Ringel Y, et al. Biofeedback treatment of fecal incontinence: a critical review. Dis Colon Rectum 2001;44(5):728–36.

32. Palsson OS, Heymen S, Whitehead WE. Biofeedback treatment for functional anorectal disorders: a comprehensive efficacy review. Appl Psychophysiol Biofeedback 2004;29(3):153–74.

33. Mellgren A, Anzen B, Nilsson B-Y, et al. Results of rectocele repair. Dis Colon Rectum 1995;38:7–13.

34. Khunchandani IT, Clancy JP III, Rosen L, et al. Endorectal repair of rectocele revisited. Br J Surg 1997;84:89–91.

35. Segal JL, Karram MM. Evaluation and management of rectoceles. Curr Opin Urol 2002;12(4):345–52.

36. Komesu YM, Rogers RG, Kammerer-Doak DN, et al. Posterior repair and sexual function. Am J Obstet Gynecol 2007;197(1):101–6.

37. Cundiff GW, Fenner D. Evaluation and treatment of women with rectocele: focus on associated defecatory and sexual dysfunction. Obstet Gynecol 2004;104(6):1403–21.

38. Zbar AP, Lienemann A, Fritsch H, et al. Rectocele: pathogenesis and surgical management. Int J Colorectal Dis 2003;18(5):369–84.

39. Paraiso MF, Barber MD, Muir TW, et al. Rectocele repair: a randomized trial of three surgical techniques including graft augmentation. Am J Obstet Gynecol 2006;195(6):1762–71.

40. D'Hoore A, Vanbeckevoort D, Penninckx F. Clinical, physiological and radiological assessment of the rectovaginal septum reinforcement with mesh for complex rectocele. Br J Surg 2008;95(10):1264–72.

41. Caquant F, Collinet P, Debodinance P, et al. Safety of transvaginal mesh procedure: retrospective study of 684 patients. J Obstet Gynaecol Res 2008;34(4):449–56.

42. Gauruder-Burmester A, Koutouzidou P, Rohne J, et al. Follow up after polypropylene mesh repair of anterior and posterior compartments in patients with recurrent prolapse. Int Urogynecol J Pelvic Floor Dysfunct 2007;18(9):1059–64.

43. Fatton B, Amblard J, Debodinance P, et al. Transvaginal repair of genital prolapse: preliminary results of a new tension free vaginal mesh (Prolift technique)—a case series multicentric study. Int Urogynecol J Pelvic Floor Dysfunct 2007;18(7):743–52.

44. Hausamann R, Steffen T, Weishaupt D, et al. Rectocele and intussusception: is there any coherence in symptoms or additional pelvic floor disorders? Tech Coloproctol 2009. [Epub ahead of print].

45. Renzi A, Talento P, Giardello C, et al. Stapled transanal rectal resection (STARR) by a new dedicated device for the surgical treatment of obstructed defecation syndrome caused by rectal intussusception and rectocele: early results of a multicenter prospective study. Int J Colorectal Dis 2008;23(10):999–1005.

46. Arroyo A, Gonzalez-Argente FX, Garcia-Domingo M, et al. Prospective multicenter trial of stapled transanal rectal resection for obstructed defecation syndrome. Br J Surg 2008;95(12):1521–7.

47. Pescatori M, Gagliardi G. Postoperative complications after procedure for prolapsed hemorrhoids (PPH) and stapled transanal rectal resection (STARR) procedure. Tech Coloproctol 2008;12(1):7–19.

48. Stolfi VM, Micossi C, Sieri P, et al. Retroperitoneal sepsis and mediastinal and subcutaneous emphysema complicating stapled transanal rectal resection (STARR). Tech Coloproctol 2009;13(1):69–71.

49. Woodruff AJ, Roth CC, Winters JC. Abdominal sacral colpopexy: surgical pearls and outcomes. Curr Urol Rep 2007;8(5):399–404.

50. Claerhout F, De Ridder D, Roovers JP, et al. Medium term anatomic and functional results of laparoscopic sacral colpopexybeyond the learning curve. Eur Urol 2008. [Epub ahead of print].

51. Kramer BA, Whelan CM, Powell TM, et al. Robot-assisted laparoscopic sacral colpopexy as management of pelvic organ prolapse. J Endourol 2009;23(4): 855–8.

52. Fitzgeral MP, Richter HE, Bradley CS, et al. Pelvic floor disorders network. Pelvic support, pelvic symptoms and patient satisfaction after colpocleisis. Int Urogynecol J Pelvic Floor Dysfunct 2008 Dec;19(12):1603–9.

53. Aigmueller T, Riss P, Dungl A, et al. Long term follow-up after vaginal sacrospinous ligament fixation: patient satisfaction, anatomical results and quality of life. Int Urogynecol J Pelvic Floor Dysfunct 2008;19(7):965–9.

54. Chen HY, Chiu TH, Ho M, et al. Analysis of risk factors associated with surgical failure of sacrospinous ligament suspension for uterine or vaginal vault prolapse. Int Urogynecol J Pelvic Floor Dysfunct 2009;20(4):387–91.

55. Lucioni A, Rapp DE, Gong EM, et al. The surgical technique and early postoperative complications of the Gynecare Prolift pelvic floor repair system. Can J Urol 2008;15(2):4004–8.

56. Tou S, Brown SR, Malik AI, et al. Surgery for complete rectal prolapse in adults. Cochrane Database Syst Rev 2008;(4):CD001758.

57. Deen KI, Grant E, Billingham C, et al. Abdominal resection rectopexy with pelvic floor repair versus perineal rectosigmoidectomy with pelvic floor repair for full thickness rectal prolapse. Br J Surg 1994;81(2):302–4.

58. Agachan F, Reisman P, Pfeifer J, et al. Comparison of three perineal procedures for treatment of rectal prolapse. South Med J 1997;90(9):925–32.

59. Samaranayake CB, Luo C, Plank AW, et al. Systematic review on ventral rectopexy for rectal prolapse and intussusception. Colorectal Dis 2009. [Epub ahead of print].

60. Rao SS. Constipation: evaluation and treatment of colonic and anorectal motility disorders. Gastrointest Endosc Clin N Am 2009;19(1):117–39.

61. Rao SS. Dyssenrgic defecation and biofeedback therapy. Gastroenterol Clin North Am 2008;37(3):569–86.

62. Harewood GC, Coulie B, Camelleri M, et al. Descending perineum syndrome: audit of clinical and laboratory features and outcome of pelvic floor retraining. Am J Gastroenterol 1999;94(1):126–30.

# Index

*Note:* Page numbers of article titles are in **boldface** type.

### A

Abnormal perineal descent, 202
Abscess(es), anorectal, **45–68,** 86–89. See also *Anal abscess.*
Adenocarcinoma, 153–154
Adrenal rest tumor, 167
Advancement flap, in anal abscess and fistula-in-ano management, 56–57
AIN. See *Anal intraepithelial neoplasia (AIN).*
Anal abscess, **45–68**
    classification of, 46–48
    described, 45, 48–49
    pathophysiology of, 45–46
    treatment of, 48–63
        advancement flap in, 56–57
        fibrin glue in, 52–54
        fistula plug in, 54–56
        fistulotomy in, 60–63
        medical, 49–51
        newer methods, 63
        preoperative planning, 51–52
        setons in, 58–60
Anal canal, anatomy of, 1–3
Anal cancer, STDs related to, 105–110
Anal ectropion, after hemorrhoidal surgery, 28
Anal fissure, **33–44**
    Crohn's disease and, 40–41
    described, 33
    HIV and, 41
    pathogenesis of, 34–35
    treatment of
        botulinum toxin type A in, 36–37
        calcium channel blockers in, 36
        nitroglycerin in, 35–36
        nonoperative, 35–37
        operative, 37–40
    without anal hypertonicity, 40
Anal incontinence, physiology of, 8–9
Anal intraepithelial neoplasia (AIN), 148–150
    STDs related to, 105–110
Anal melanoma, 152–153
Anal neoplasms, **147–161**
    adenocarcinoma, 153–154

Anal neoplasms (*continued*)
    AIN, 148–150
    anal melanoma, 152–153
    Buschke-lowenstein carcinoma, 154
    described, 147–148
    epidermoid cancers, 150–152. See also *Epidermoid cancers.*
    gastrointestinal stromal tumor, 154
    Kaposi sarcoma, 154
    local excision of, 155–156
        indications for, 155
        lymph node positivity after, recurrence related to, 156
        recurrence after, salvage surgery for, 156
        techniques, 155
    neuroendocrine tumor, 155
    rare, 153–155
    sarcomas, 155
    verrucous carcinoma, 154
Anal sphincter, artificial, in fecal incontinence management, 189–190
Anal sphincteroplasty, in fecal incontinence management, 187–188
Anal stenosis, **137–145**
    causes of, 137–138
    described, 137–138
    diagnosis of, 138–139
    prevention of, 139
    treatment of, 139–144
        anoplasty in, 140–142
        mucosal advancement flaps in, 140
        nonoperative, 139
        operative, 140–142
        surgical algorithm in, 142, 144
Anal strictures, after hemorrhoidal surgery, 28
Anal ulcer, 85–86
Anoplasty, in anal stenosis management, 140–142
Anorectal Crohn's disease, **83–97**
    described, 83
    epidemiology of, 83–84
    presentations of, 84–90
    protectomy and, 89–90
    restorative proctocolectomy and, 90
    skin tags, 84–85
    types of, 84–90
Anorectal electromyography, in pelvic floor disorders evaluation, 198
Anorectal manometry, in pelvic floor disorders evaluation, 197–198
Anorectum, anatomy and physiology of, **1–15**
Anterior meningocele, retrorectal, 166
Artificial anal sphincter, in fecal incontinence management, 189–190

**B**

Basal cell carcinoma, 152
Biofeedback

in fecal incontinence management, 187
in pelvic floor disorders evaluation, 198
Biomaterial(s), injectable, in fecal incontinence management, 191
Bioprosthetics, in rectovaginal fistula management, 78
Bipolar diathermy, for hemorrhoids, 23–24
Bleeding, after hemorrhoidal surgery, 27
Body packers, removal of, 180–181
Botulinum toxin type A, for anal fissure, 36–37
Buschke-lowenstein carcinoma, 154


C

Calcium channel blockers, for anal fissure, 36
Cancer(s)
    anal, STDs related to, 105–110
    epidermoid, 150–152. See also *Epidermoid cancers.*
    in pilonidal sinus, 121–122
    rectal. See also *Anal neoplasms.*
    rectovaginal fistula due to, 70
Carcinoma. See *Cancer(s).*
Chancroid, 101–102
Chlamydia, STDs related to, 102
Chordoma, 166
Compliance, in physiologic testing of pelvic floor, rectum, and sphincters, 12–13
Condyloma, STDs related to, 104–105
Congenital lesions, retrorectal, 164
Continence, loss of, after hemorrhoidal surgery, 28
Crohn's disease
    anal fissures and, 40–41
    anorectal, **83–97.** See also *Anorectal Crohn's disease.*
    fistulizing, rectovaginal fistula due to, 70
    rectovaginal fistula and, treatment of, 72–74
Cyst(s), retrorectal
    dermoid, 164
    developmental, 164
    duplication, 164–165
    epidermoid, 164


D

Defecation, physiology of, 9
Defecography
    dynamic, in pelvic floor disorders evaluation, 198
    in physiologic testing of pelvic floor, rectum, and sphincters, 11–12
Dermoid cysts, retrorectal, 164
Developmental cysts, retrorectal, 164
Diathermy, bipolar, for hemorrhoids, 23–24
Diet, in hemorrhoid management, 20
Doppler-guided transanal hemorrhoidal ligation, in hemorrhoid management, 25–26
Duplication cysts, retrorectal, 164–165
Dynamic defecography, in pelvic floor disorders evaluation, 198

**E**

Ectropion, anal, after hemorroidal surgery, 28
Electromyography (EMG)
      anorectal, in pelvic floor disorders evaluation, 198
      in physiologic testing of pelvic floor, rectum, and sphincters, 10–11
EMG. See *Electromyography (EMG)*.
Endoanal ultrasound, in pelvic floor disorders evaluation, 197
Endoscopy, in rectal foreign body removal, 180–181
Enteritis, STDs related to, 103
Enterocele(s), management of, 200
Epidermoid cancers, 150–152
      basal cell carcinoma, 152
      squamous cell carcinoma
            of anal canal, 151–152
            of anal margin, 150–151
Epidermoid cysts, retrorectal, 164


**F**

FCD. See *Fistulizing Crohn's disease (FCD)*.
Fecal incontinence, **185–194**
      defined, 185
      described, 185–186
      evaluation of, 186–187
      management of
            anal sphincteroplasty in, 187–188
            artificial anal sphincter in, 189–190
            biofeedback in, 187
            injectable biomaterials in, 191
            sacral nerve stimulation in, 190–191
            stimulated graciloplasty in, 188–189
Fibrin glue, in anal abscess and fistula-in-ano management, 52–54
Fissure(s)
      anal, **33–44.** See also *Anal fissure*.
      anorectal, 85
Fistula(s)
      anorectal, 86–89
      rectovaginal, **69–82.** See also *Rectovaginal fistula*.
Fistula plug, in anal abscess and fistula-in-ano management, 54–56
Fistula-in-ano, **45–68**
      classification of, 46–48
      pathophysiology of, 45–46
      treatment of, 48–63
            advancement flap in, 56–57
            described, 45, 48–49
            fibrin glue in, 52–54
            fistula plug in, 54–56
            fistulotomy in, 60–63
            medical, 49–51
            newer methods, 63

preoperative planning, 51–52
    setons in, 58–60
Fistulizing Crohn's disease (FDC), rectovaginal fistula due to, 70
Fistulotomy, in anal abscess and fistula-in-ano management, 60–63
Foreign bodies, rectal, **173–184.** See also *Rectal foreign bodies.*


**G**

Gastrointestinal stromal tumor, 154
Glue(s), fibrin, in anal abscess and fistula-in-ano management, 52–54
Gonorrhea, 103
Graciloplasty, stimulated, in fecal incontinence management, 188–189
Granuloma inguinale, STDs related to, 102


**H**

Harmonic Scalpel, in hemorrhoid management, 25
Hemorrhoid(s)
    anorectal, 85
    classification of, 18–19
    clinical presentation of, 19–20
    described, 17
    differential diagnosis of, 19
    during pregnancy, 30
    external, thrombosed, clinical presentation of, 19–20
    IBD and, 29
    internal, treatment of, office-based, 21–24
    pathophysiology of, 17–18
    prevalence of, 17
    prolapsed, treatment of, 26–27
    rectal varices due to, 29
    strangulation/crisis, 29–30
    symptomatic, **17–32**
    treatment of, 20–27
        bipolar diathermy in, 23–24
        creams in, 20–21
        dietary/lifestyle changes in, 20
        IPC in, 23–24
        medical, 20–21
        phlebotonics in, 24
        rubber band ligation in, 21–23
        sclerotherapy in, 23
        surgical, 24–27
            complications following, 27–28
            Doppler-guided transanal hemorrhoidal ligation, 25–26
            Harmonic Scalpel in, 25
            LigaSure in, 25
            open/closed excision in, 24–25
Herpes simplex virus-1 (HSV-1), 100–101
HIV. See *Human immunodeficiency virus (HIV).*
HSV-1. See *Herpes simplex virus-1 (HSV-1).*

Human immunodeficiency virus (HIV)
    anal fissures and, 41
    STDs related to, 102
Human papillomavirus (HPV), STDs related to, 104–110
    AIN, 105–110
    condyloma, 104–105
    described, 99


    I

IBD. See *Irritable bowel disease (IBD)*.
Incontinence
    anal, physiology of, 8–9
    fecal, **185–194.** See also *Fecal incontinence*.
Infection(s)
    rectovaginal fistula due to, 71
    wound, after hemorrhoidal surgery, 27–28
Inflammatory lesions, retrorectal, 168
Infrared photocoagulation (IPC), for hemorrhoids, 23–24
Injectable biomaterials, in fecal incontinence management, 191
IPC. *See* Infrared photocoagulation (IPC).
Irritable bowel disease (IBD)
    hemorrhoids due to, 29
    rectovaginal fistula due to, 70


    K

Kaposi sarcoma, 154


    L

Lesion(s)
    retrorectal
        congenital, 164
        inflammatory, 168
        neurogenic, 167
        osseous, 167
    squamous intraepithelial, 148–150
LGV. See *Lymphogranuloma venereum (LGV)*.
Lifestyle changes, in hemorrhoid management, 20
LigaSure, in hemorrhoid management, 25
Lymphogranuloma venereum (LGV), 103


    M

Magnetic resonance (MR) defecography, in physiologic testing of pelvic floor, rectum, and sphincters, 11–12
Manometry
    anorectal, in pelvic floor disorders evaluation, 197–198
    in physiologic testing of pelvic floor, rectum, and sphincters, 10
Melanoma, anal, 152–153

Meningocele(s), anterior, retrorectal, 166
Mucosal advancement flaps, in anal stenosis management, 140


**N**

Neoplasm(s), anal, **147–161.** See also *Anal neoplasms.*
Nerve stimulation techniques, in physiologic testing of pelvic floor, rectum,
     and sphincters, 12
Neuroendocrine tumor, 155
Neurogenic lesions, retrorectal, 167
Nitroglycerin, for anal fissure, 35–36
Non–human papillomavirus (non-HPV), STDs related to, 100–104
     chancroid, 101–102
     chlamydia, 102
     described, 99
     enteritis, 103
     gonorrhea, 103
     granuloma inguinale, 102
     HIV, 102
     HSV-1, 100–101
     LGV, 103
     proctitis, 102–103
     proctocolitis, 103
     syphilis, 101
     ulceration, 100–102


**O**

Obstetric trauma, rectovaginal fistula due to, 69–70
Osseous lesions, retrorectal, 167


**P**

Paget disease, 153–154
Paradoxic puborectalis, 202
Pelvic floor disorders
     abnormal perineal descent, 202
     described, 195
     diagnosis of, 196–198
          anorectal EMG in, 198
          anorectal manometry in, 197–198
          biofeedback in, 198
          dynamic defecography in, 198
          endoanal ultrasound in, 197
          physiologic testing in, 9–13
          pudendal nerve terminal motor latency testing in, 198
          symptom assessment in, 196–197
     functional disorders, 201–202
     management of, 199–201
          enterocele, 200
          rectal prolapse, 200–201

Pelvic (*continued*)
    rectocele, 199–200
    vaginal vault prolapse, 200
  overview of, **195–205**
  paradoxic puborectalis, 202
Pelvic floor muscles, anatomy of, 3
Perianal spaces, anatomy of, 3–4
Perineal descent, abnormal, 202
Perirectal spaces, anatomy of, 3–4
Phlebotonics, in hemorrhoidal management, 24
Photocoagulation, infrared, in hemorrhoidal management, 23–24
Pilonidal disease, **113–124**
  causes of, 113–114
  diagnosis of, 113–114
  management of, 114–121
    nonoperative, 114–115
    surgical, 115–121
  recurrent, management of, 121
Pilonidal sinus, carcinoma in, 121–122
Pregnancy, hemorrhoids during, 30
Proctitis, STDs related to, 102–103
Proctocolectomy, restorative, anorectal Crohn's disease after, 90
Proctocolitis, STDs related to, 103
Prolapse, rectal, management of, 200–201
Protectomy, anorectal Crohn's disease after, 89–90
Pruritus ani, **125–135**
  approach to patient with, 133
  classification of, 125
  defined, 125
  incidence of, 125
  primary "idiopathic," 126–129
    management of
      injectable therapy in, 128–129
      routine, 126–127
      topical, 127–128
  secondary, 129–133
    anal, 132–133
    colorectal, 132–133
    dermatologic, 130–132
    in systemic diseases, 132
    infectious, 129–130
    local irritants, 132
Puborectalis, paradoxic, 202
Pudendal nerve terminal motor latency testing, in pelvic floor disorders evaluation, 198


  R

Radiation, rectovaginal fistula due to, 70
Radiation therapy, in rectovaginal fistula management, 77–78
Radiography, of rectovaginal fistula, 72
Rectal cancer, **147–161.** See also *Anal neoplasms.*

Rectal foreign bodies, **173–184**
    classification of, 175–176
    described, 173
    epidemiology of, 173–174
    evaluation of, 176–177
    management of, 177–182
        extraction techniques, 178–182
            body packers, 180
            endoscopy in, 180–181
            for blunt and sharp objects, 179–180
            surgical, 181–182
            transanal approach, 178–179
        postremoval, 182–183
Rectal prolapse, management of, 200–201
Rectocele(s), management of, 199–200
Rectovaginal fistula, **69–82**
    anatomic classification of, 71
    causes of, 69–71
    Crohn's, treatment of, 72–74, 76–77
    described, 69
    evaluation of, 71–72
    postoperative, 70–71
    radiography of, 72
    treatment of
        bioprosthetics in, 78
        radiation therapy in, 77–78
        surgical, 74–78
            perineal repair, 75
            transanal repair, 74–75
            transvaginal repair, 75–76
Rectum
    anatomy of, 1
    arterial supply to, 4
    innervation of, 6–8
    lymphatic drainage from, 6
    physiologic testing of, 9–13
    varices of, hemorrhoids and, 29
    venous drainage from, 4
Restorative proctocolectomy, anorectal Crohn's disease after, 90
Retrorectal tumors, **163–171**
    adrenal rest tumor, 167
    anatomy of, 163
    anterior meningocele, 166
    chordoma, 166
    congenital lesions, 164
    dermoid cysts, 164
    described, 163
    developmental cysts, 164
    duplication cysts, 164–165
    epidermoid cysts, 164
    inflammatory lesions, 168

Retrorectal tumors (*continued*)
   miscellaneous lesions, 168–170
   neurogenic lesions, 167
   osseous lesions, 167
   teratoma, 166–167
Rubber band ligation, for hemorrhoids, 21–23

   **S**

Sacral nerve stimulation, in fecal incontinence management, 190–191
Sarcoma(s), 155
   Kaposi, 154
Sclerotherapy, for hemorrhoids, 23
Seton(s), in anal abscess and fistula-in-ano management, 58–60
Sexually transmitted diseases (STDs)
   HPV–related, 104–110
   non–HPV–related, 100–104
Sinus(es), pilonidal, carcinoma in, 121–122
Skin tags, anorectal, 84–85
Sphincter(s)
   anal, artificial, in fetal incontinence management, 189–190
   physiologic testing of, 9–13
Sphincteroplasty, anal, in fecal incontinence management, 187–188
Squamous cell carcinoma
   of anal canal, 151–152
   of anal margin, 150–151
Squamous intraepithelial lesion, 148–150
STDs. See *Sexually transmitted diseases (STDs)*.
Stenosis(es), anal, **137–145.** See also *Anal stenosis*.
Stimulated graciloplasty, in fecal incontinence management, 188–189
Stricture(s), anorectal, 86
Syphilis, 101

   **T**

Teratoma(s), 166–167
Trauma
   obstetric, rectovaginal fistula due to, 69–70
   vaginal, rectovaginal fistula due to, 69–70
Tumor(s). See also specific tumors.
   adrenal rest, 167
   gastrointestinal stromal, 154
   neuroendocrine, 155
   retrorectal, **163–171**

   **U**

Ulcer(s)
   anal, 85–86
   non–HPV–related STDs and, 100–102
Ultrasound
   endoanal, in pelvic floor disorders evaluation, 197
   in physiologic testing of pelvic floor, rectum, and sphincters, 12
Urinary retention, after hemorrhoidal surgery, 27

## V

Vaginal trauma, rectovaginal fistula due to, 69–70
Vaginal vault prolapse, management of, 200
Varice(s), rectal, hemorrhoids and, 29
Verrucous carcinoma, 154

## W

Wound infections, after hemorrhoidal surgery, 27–28

# Moving?

## Make sure your subscription moves with you!

To notify us of your new address, find your **Clinics Account Number** (located on your mailing label above your name), and contact customer service at:

**Email: journalscustomerservice-usa@elsevier.com**

**800-654-2452** (subscribers in the U.S. & Canada)
**314-447-8871** (subscribers outside of the U.S. & Canada)

**Fax number: 314-447-8029**

**Elsevier Health Sciences Division**
**Subscription Customer Service**
**3251 Riverport Lane**
**Maryland Heights, MO 63043**

*To ensure uninterrupted delivery of your subscription, please notify us at least 4 weeks in advance of move.